Cytokines and B Lymphocytes

Cytokines and B Lymphocytes

edited by

R. E. CALLARD
Institute of Child Health,
London, WC1N 1EH

ACADEMIC PRESS
Harcourt Brace Jovanovich, Publishers
London   San Diego   New York   Boston
Sydney   Tokyo   Toronto

ACADEMIC PRESS LIMITED
24–28 Oval Road
London NW1 7DX

United States Edition published by
ACADEMIC PRESS INC.
San Diego, CA 92101

ISBN 0–12–155145–8

Typeset by Paston Press, Loddon, Norfolk
and printed in Great Britain by Galliard (Printers) Ltd, Great Yarmouth, Norfolk

Contents

List of Contributors   vii

1   Introduction   1
     Robin E. Callard

2   The physico-chemical properties of B cell
     growth and differentiation factors and their
     receptors   11
     Robin E. Callard, Andrew J. H. Gearing and
     Richard J. Armitage

3   Receptor signalling in B lymphocytes   . . .   39
     Kevin Rigley and Margaret Harnett

4   Role of cytokines in the ontogeny, activation
     and proliferation of B lymphocytes   65
     Thierry DeFrance and Jacques Banchereau

5   Cytokine regulation of B-cell differentiation   .   115
     Richard J. Armitage, Kenneth H. Grabstein and
     Mark R. Alderson

6   Collaboration between T and B cells   143
     Virginia M. Sanders and Ellen S. Vitetta

7   Immunoglobulin isotype regulation 173
     Judy M. Teale and D. Mark Estes

8   Autocrine aspects of the B lymphocyte
     regulation 195
     John Gordon

9   Cytokine action on B cells in disease 215
     Sergio Romagnani

10   B cell assays for growth and differentiation
     factors 253
     John G. Shields and Jean-Yves Bonnefoy

     Index   267

List of contributors

Mark R. Alderson   Immunex Corporation, 51 University Street, Seattle, Washington 98101, USA.

Richard J. Armitage   Immunex Corporation, 51 University Street, Seattle, Washington 98101, USA.

Jacques Bancherau   Schering-Plough (UNICET), Laboratory for Immunological Research, 27 Chemin des Peupliers, 69570 Dardilly, France.

Jean-Yves Bonnefoy   Glaxo Institute for Molecular Biology, 46 Route des Acacias, 1211 Geneva 24, Switzerland.

Robin E. Callard   Department of Immunology, Institute of Child Health, 30 Guildford Street, London WC1N 1EH, UK.

Thierry DeFrance   Schering-Plough (UNICET), Laboratory for Immunological Research, 27 Chemin des Peupliers, 69570 Dardilly, France.

D. Mark Estes   Department of Microbiology, The University of Texas, Health Science Center at San Antonio, 7703 Floyd Curl Drive, San Antonio, Texas 78284–7758, USA.

Andrew J. H. Gearing   British Biotechnology, Watlington Road, Cowley Road, Oxford, OX4 5LY, UK.

John Gordon   Department of Immunology, The Medical School, Vincent Drive, Birmingham, B15 2TJ, UK.

Kenneth H. Grabstein   Immunex Corporation, 51 University Street, Seattle, Washington 98101, USA.

Margaret Harnett   Division of Immunology, National Institute for Medical Research, The Ridgeway, Mill Hill, London, NW7 1AA, UK.

Kevin Rigley   Department of Immunology, Institute of Child Health, 30 Guildford Street, London, WC1N 1EH, UK.

Sergio Romagnani   Department of Clinical Immunology and Allergology, University of Florence, Instituto di Clinica, Medica 3, Policclinico di Careggi, 50134 Firenze, Italy.

Virginia M. Sanders   NIEHS, mail-drop C1–04, PO Box 12233, Research Triangle Park, North Carolina 27709, USA.

John G. Shields   Glaxo Institute for Molecular Biology, 46 Route des Acacias, 1211 Geneva 24, Switzerland.

Judy M. Teale   Department of Microbiology, The University of Texas, Health Science Center at San Antonio, 7703 Floyd Curl Drive, San Antonio, Texas 78284-7758, USA.

Ellen S. Vitetta   Department of Microbiology, University of Texas, Southwestern Medical Center, Dallas, Texas 75235, USA.

1
Introduction

ROBIN E. CALLARD

Aims of this book

It is common in books about cytokines to describe in detail the physico-chemical and biological properties of each one in turn, rather than discuss the way in which they interact with a particular physiological system or tissue. This is not the approach taken here. Instead, the emphasis throughout is on how cytokines, in combination with other activation signals, regulate B cell growth and subsequent differentiation into antibody-forming cells. One chapter is devoted to the physico-chemical properties of the different cytokines and their receptors, as this information is not available from any other single reference source. The rest of the chapters deal individually with B cell activation, proliferation, differentiation, T–B cell collaboration, isotype selection, autocrine stimulation, the role of cytokines in disease, and B cell assays for cytokines. In each case, responses of both human and murine B cells are considered so that both their similarities and their differences are made clear.

For the most part, only cytokines which have been cloned and fully characterized are included in this book. This is mainly to avoid the uncertainties and ambiguities associated with the less well characterized factors, but also because now is an appropriate time to summarize the many discoveries made with recombinant cytokines over the past few years.

A brief historical perspective

The regulation of antibody responses has been a major subject of investigation for about a hundred years. During this time, there have been a number of significant milestones that have led to our current understanding and point to the direction for future research. Before the discovery of T cells and B cells in the late 1960s, investigations into the regulation of antibody

CYTOKINES AND B LYMPHOCYTES
ISBN 0–12–155145–8

responses were mostly concerned with the roles of antigen, antibody, and antigen–antibody complexes. At this time, the animal was treated largely as a "black box", with little understanding of the cellular mechanisms under-lying immunoregulation. It was not until the small lymphocyte was un-equivocally shown to be the precursor to antibody-secreting cells (Gowans and McGregor, 1965; Gowans and Uhr, 1966), and the discovery that T cell collaboration was required for optimal antibody responses by B cells (Claman *et al.*, 1966; Miller and Mitchell, 1968; Mitchell and Miller, 1968), that cellular models of immunoregulation came into fashion. These import-ant findings triggered an explosion of cellular regulation studies during the 1970s, culminating in the extremely complex and sometimes bizarre network models of interacting T cells to account for help and suppression of antibody responses.

The main achievement of this period was to recognize that immuno-regulation depended on complex cellular interactions. However, the way in which the participating cells communicated was not known, and in the end the various models failed because they did not address immunoregulation at a molecular level. With the realization that T cells can exert their influence on B cells by defined molecular entities (cytokines and cell surface inter-action molecules), immunoregulation entered the molecular era. In the space of 10 years, more than a dozen cytokines that regulate B cell growth and differentiation have been identified. Although, in some ways, the complexities of cytokine biology have even exceeded the byzantine nature of the cellular network theories, the application of cDNA and gene cloning techniques has allowed precise definition of both the molecules concerned and their cell-surface receptors. These advances have opened the way to investigations of the transmembrane signalling events, intracellular bio-chemistry and specific gene regulation, which ultimately determine how any one B cell will respond to the combination of molecular signals received at the cell surface.

Cytokine models of B cell growth and differentiation

In the past, it has been common to think of B cell differentiation as a linear transition from a homogeneous population of resting B cells to antibody-secreting cells (Figure 1). According to this model, ligand (antigen or anti-Ig) binding to surface Ig primes the B cell for subsequent and discrete phases of proliferation and maturation in response to specific growth and differen-tiation signals. This simple model has been useful, but is now clearly inadequate to account for the complexity and diversity of B cell responses. It is now known that many different signals in various synergistic and/or

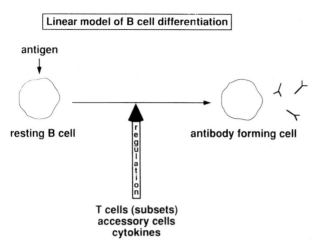

Figure 1 In early models, B cell differentiation was represented by a linear transition from a homogeneous population of B cells stimulated by antigen into antibody-forming cells, with each discrete step of proliferation and differentiation regulated by T cells, accessory cells and cytokines.

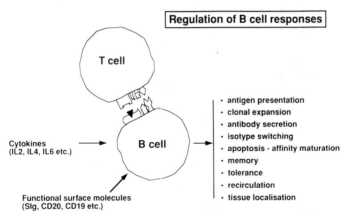

Figure 2 It is now known that B cells can respond in a number of different ways as illustrated. Each response is regulated by signals received at the cell surface from regulatory T cells, cytokines, and other ligands binding to functional cell-surface molecules. Cognate T cell interactions are known to involve T cell-receptor recognition of antigen, in association with MHC class II antigens, CD4 binding to non-polymorphic determinants on MHC class II, LFA-1 binding to ICAM-1/ICAM-2, and CD2 binding to LFA-3. In each case binding seems able to deliver a specific signal to the B cell. The other functional cell surface antigens (CD19, CD20, etc.) are known to be signal transducing molecules, but their natural ligands are so far unknown.

inhibitory combinations are received at the B cell surface from interactions with T cells, cytokines and other ligands (Figure 2). It is also important to appreciate that B cell responses are far more diverse and complex than had previously been recognized. In addition to proliferation and differentiation into antibody-secreting cells, many other functions—such as antigen presentation by B cells, antibody affinity maturation, generation of memory, tolerance, re-circulation, and microenvironmental localization—must also be subject to regulation (Figure 2). When this complexity is taken into account, it is clear why earlier efforts to understand B cell regulation in terms of interacting T cell subsets were not very successful.

Cytokines play only a part in these diverse B cell responses and must not be considered in isolation. Interactions with other signals delivered by ligand binding to functional cell-surface antigens are also important for determining B cell responses (Valentine et al., 1988; Brown et al., 1989). Moreover, any one cytokine may have different (enhancing and inhibiting) effects depending on what other signal the cell has received. For example, interferon γ (IFN-γ) can induce proliferation by B cells stimulated with anti-IgM (Romagnani et al., 1986; Defrance et al., 1986), or inhibit B cell responses to interleukin 4 (Rabin et al., 1986a). Similarly, interleukin 4 (IL-4) activates B cells and promotes B cell proliferation (Paul and Ohara, 1987), but inhibits B cell responses to IL-2 (Defrance et al., 1988; Llorente et al., 1989).

Most in vitro techniques for investigating cytokine action on B cell growth and differentiation require co-stimulation of B cells with, for example, anti-Ig, to polyclonally mimic the action of antigen. The rationale behind this approach is the idea that activation through surface Ig in combination with T cell-derived cytokines is a model for T cell help to antigen-stimulated B cells. To my mind there are two major problems with this model.

First, it seems unlikely that the conditions employed to stimulate B cells with polyclonal crosslinking ligands (anti-Ig, dextran sulphate, lipopolysaccharide, Staphylococcus aureus Cowan I, etc.) in any way reflects the nature or local concentrations of most T cell-dependent antigens presented to B cells in vivo. In fact, concentrations of rabbit anti-Ig up to 1,000-fold less than required in co-stimulation assays with B cell growth factors (10 ng ml^{-1} compared with 10 μg ml^{-1}) have been used successfully with rabbit Ig-specific T cell lines to stimulate B cell immunoglobulin production (Tony and Parker, 1985). Interestingly, very low doses of anti-Ig (100 pg ml^{-1}), when coupled to dextran, are also able to stimulate B cell responses (Brunswick et al., 1988), but without activation of the phosphoinositide signalling pathway (Brunswick et al., 1989).

Secondly, it is now known that antigen binding to B cell surface Ig is internalized, processed and then re-expressed on the surface in association with major histocompatibility complex (MHC) class II for presentation to T cells (Gosselin *et al.*, 1988; Lanzavecchia, 1988). Proliferation and differentiation occur after this step in response to signals delivered by T cells and T cell-derived cytokines (Figure 3). This model is supported by a recent study, in which co-stimulation of quiescent B cells with anti-Ig and IL-4 was shown to prime B cells to proliferate in response to subsequent stimulation with immobilized antibodies to MHC class II plus additional cytokines (IL-4, IL-5 and mixed lymphocyte reaction (MLR) supernatant) (Cambier and Lehman, 1989). These results suggest that the combination of signals delivered by antigen (or anti-Ig) and IL-4 may induce quiescent B cells to process antigen for presentation to T helper cells, rather than stimulate proliferation and differentiation. In typical co-stimulation assays with high dose anti-Ig and cytokines, this important antigen-presenting step is not taken into account.

Activation of B cells with IL-4 results in increased MHC class II expression (Noelle *et al.*, 1984; Rousset, 1988), which may enhance cognate interactions with T cells. Surface IgM expression is also greatly increased (10-fold) on human B cells activated with IL-4 (Shields *et al.*, 1989). Of particular interest is the dose of IL-4 required for this effect. Whereas 50% maximum expression of B cell surface CD23, and proliferation of B cells in co-stimulation assays with anti-IgM, was obtained with about 10 units ml^{-1} of IL-4, half maximal stimulation of surface IgM expression was obtained with less than one-tenth of this IL-4 dose (about 0.2 units ml^{-1}) (Callard *et al.*, 1990). This result shows that IL-4 can have a pronounced effect on B cells at doses too low for proliferation. Whether activation by low concentrations of IL-4 enhances B cell antigen presentation or whether it serves some other function has yet to be determined.

Cytokines in specific antibody responses

Most of what we know about the action of cytokines on B cells has come from studies with polyclonal activators such as anti-Ig, lipopolysaccharide (LPS), SAC or phorbol myristate acetate (PMA). As a result, very little is known about the function of cytokines in specific antibody responses. IL-5 is a T cell replacing factor (TRF) for specific antibody responses in mice (Takatsu *et al.*, 1988) whereas IL-2 (but not IL-5) is a TRF in man (Callard *et al.*, 1986; Delfraissy *et al.*, 1988). However, IL-2 is only a TRF for low/medium density B cells and is unable to restore antibody production by high density "resting" B cells (Callard and Smith, 1988). Overnight incu-

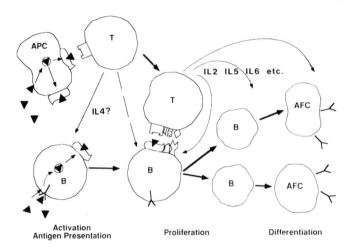

Figure 3 In antibody responses to T cell-dependent antigens, B cells first internalize, process, and re-express antigen in association with MHC class II antigens for presentation to T helper cells. This step may be regulated by IL-4. Subsequently, interaction with T cells and T cell derived cytokines (IL-2 in humans) results in proliferation and maturation into specific antibody-forming cells (AFC).

bation with antigen and T cells converted high-density B cells to IL-2 responders, suggesting that resting B cells stimulated with T-dependent antigens must receive a signal from T helper cells before they are able to respond to cytokines (in this case IL-2) and differentiate into antibody secreting cells.

Immunoglobulin production by human B cells stimulated with IL-2 and SAC was recently reported to be mediated by autocrine production of IL-6 (Xia *et al.*, 1989). Similarly, IL-6 has been shown to be essential for polyclonal Ig secretion in response to pokeweed mitogen (PWM) (Muraguchi *et al.*, 1988). In contrast to these findings, we have shown recently that although IL-6 sometimes enhances specific antibody responses to influenza virus by human tonsillar lymphocytes, a blocking IL-6 antibody had no effect showing that IL-6 is not required for this response (Callard *et al.*, 1990). In the mouse, IL-6 is required for production of specific antibody to influenza virus by naïve (unprimed) B cells but not by primed B cells (Hilbert *et al.*, 1989), which is consistent with our findings in human (primed) responses to influenza virus.

In humans at least, IL-2 seems sufficient for B cell proliferation and differentiation into antibody-forming cells after initial activation by antigen and T helper cells. This raises important questions about the function of other cytokines, such as IL-4, in specific antibody responses. In a recent study we have shown that IL-4 inhibits antibody production to influenza virus by human lymphocytes, and a blocking IL-4 antibody has little effect or slightly enhances the response (Callard *et al.*, 1990). These findings are consistent with the known ability of IL-4 to inhibit IL-2 induced B cell proliferation (Defrance *et al.*, 1988; Jelinek and Lipsky, 1988; Llorente *et al.*, 1989) and raise the possibility that IL-4 produced after T helper cell interaction with B cells may be involved in suppression.

Species differences in responses to cytokines

Because the underlying structure of the immune system in mice and humans is remarkably similar, it is common to assume that whatever immuno-regulatory mechanism is found in one will also hold for the other. Although this assumption is often correct, it should be remembered that the evolutionary lines giving rise to humans and mice diverged some 60 to 80 million years ago, and it is probable that selective pressures would have resulted in some differences in immunoregulation between the two species.

Several species differences in responses to cytokines have been reported. For example, IL-5 is a growth and differentiation factor for murine B cells, but in conventional assays has no activity on purified human B cells (Clutterbuck *et al.*, 1987). Human B cells do express IL-5 receptors, however, and it may be that the appropriate activation signal(s) required for B cell responses to IL-5 have not yet been identified in man. On the other hand, whereas IL-5 is a TRF for antigen-specific antibody responses in mice (Alderson *et al.*, 1987), only IL-2 and low molecular weight (LMW BCGF), and not IL-5, have TRF activity in man (Smith *et al.*, 1989). Another example of species differences can be found in the activation of B cells with IL-4. Pre-treatment of resting murine B cells with IL-4 increases their subsequent proliferation in response to mitogenic stimuli such as anti-IgM or LPS (Rabin *et al.*, 1985, 1986b). In contrast, human IL-4 fails to prepare B cells for a more vigorous response to subsequent stimulation with anti-IgM (Gordon *et al.*, 1988; Shields *et al.*, 1989) and has even been found to inhibit proliferation stimulated by mitogenic concentrations of anti-IgM (Gordon *et al.*, 1989).

Some of these differences may be due to the source of B cells (human tonsil and mouse spleen) and/or the experimental procedures employed. For example, IL-4 has been shown to signal human B cells by a novel pathway involving hydrolysis of phosphatidyl inositol bisphosphate (PIP_2) followed, after a brief lag period, by elevation of cAMP (Finney *et al.*, 1990). Neither PIP_2 hydrolysis nor cAMP elevation occur in mouse B cells

activated with IL-4. Although these results suggest that alternative signalling pathways may have evolved in the two species, there is now some
evidence to suggest that the preparation of mouse B cells by complement-
mediated lysis of T cells, rather than the negative selection by E-rosetting
used for human B cell preparations, may be responsible.

Although some of the differences in responses to cytokines may be due to
the experimental techniques used, the same cannot be said for IgG subclass
regulation in humans and mice. It is well established that IL-4 increases
IgG1 secretion by LPS-stimulated mouse B cells (Snapper *et al.*, 1988a) by
selective heavy chain switching (Esser and Radbruch, 1989). Similarly,
IFN-γ induces IgG2a secretion (Snapper *et al.*, 1988b). However, in studies
with human B cells, totally conflicting results have been obtained. Flores-
Romo *et al.* (1990) have shown that IL-4 increases IgG1-3 but not IgG4
secretion by B cells activated with phorbol dibutyrate (PdBu) and ionomycin. In contrast, IL-4 was shown in another study to increase the proportion
of PMA-activated B cells staining for cytoplasmic IgG4, with no effect on
IgG1 or IgG3 (Lundgren *et al.*, 1989). Others have found no reproducible
effect of IL-4 and have concluded that the particular result obtained is
dependent on the nature of the co-activating signal and the tissue from which
the B cells are prepared. The reason for this difference is most probably that
the IgG subclasses in humans and mice have arisen independently and at
different times in evolution (Wang *et al.*, 1980; Callard and Turner, 1990).
Under these circumstances it is extremely unlikely that the same regulatory
mechanisms would also have evolved in both species.

Conclusion

The cloning of cytokines active on B cells has for the first time allowed the
regulation of antibody responses to be put on a molecular basis. In this
sense, the work described in this book is only the beginning. The next
decade should see major advances in defining precisely which combination
of signals received at the B cell surface will determine a particular differentiation pathway. Cytokines of course are not the whole story, as cell
interaction molecules and other functional cell-surface antigens all interact
to determine the fate of any one B cell. Functionally distinct B cell
subpopulations must also be considered in the future, as these are likely to
be subject to different regulatory mechanisms. Ultimately, this molecular
approach will be combined with more holistic studies of cytokine production
and B cell responses *in vivo*, such as those recently described by Bosseloir *et
al.* (1989), MacLennan *et al.* (1988) and Liu *et al.* (1990), to yield a full
understanding of how antibody responses are regulated in the intact animal.

Acknowledgements

This work is supported by grants from the Leukaemia Research Fund and Action Research for the Crippled Child.

References

Alderson, M. R., Pike, B. L., Harada, N., Tominaga, A., Takatsu, K. and Nossal, G. J. V. (1987) *J. Immunol.* **139**, 2656–2660.

Bosseloir, A., Hooghe-Peters, E. L., Heinen, E., Cormann, N., Kinet-denoel, C., Vanhaelst, L. and Simar, L. (1989) *Eur. J. Immunol.* **19**, 2379–2381.

Brown, A. N., Thurstan, S. M. and Callard, R. E. (1989) In *Leucocyte Typing IV*, pp. 203–205. Ed. by W. Knapp *et al.* Oxford University Press, Oxford.

Brunswick, M., Finkelman, F. D., Highet, P. F., Inman, J. K., Dintzis, H. M. and Mond, J. J. (1988) *J. Immunol.* **140**, 3364–3372.

Brunswick, M., June, C. H., Finkelman, F. D., Dintzis, H. M., Inman, J. K. and Mond, J. J. (1989) *Proc. Natl. Acad. Sci. USA* **86**, 6724–6728.

Callard, R. E. and Smith, S. H. (1988) *Eur. J. Immunol.* **18**, 1635–1638.

Callard, R. E. and Turner, M. W. (1990) *Immunol. Today* **11**, 200–203 .

Callard, R. E., Smith, S. H., Shields, J. and Levinsky, R. J. (1986) *Eur. J. Immunol.* **16**, 1037–1042.

Callard, R. E., Smith, S. H., Scott,K. E. and Thurstan, S. M. (1990) In *Proceedings of the 1st International Conference on Cytokines*: *Basic Principles and Clinical Applications*. Serono Symposia Publications, in press.

Cambier, J. C. and Lehmann, K. R. (1989) *J. Exp. Med.* **170**, 877–886.

Claman, H. N., Chaperon, E. A. and Triplett, R. F. (1966) *Proc. Soc. Exp. Biol. Med.* **122**, 1167–1171.

Clutterbuck, E., Shields, J. G., Gordon, J., Smith, S. H., Boyd, A., Callard, R. E., Campbell, H. D., Young, I. G. and Sanderson, C. J. (1987) *Eur. J. Immunol.* **17**, 1743–1750.

Defrance, T., Aubry, J-P., Vanbervliet, B. and Banchereau, J. (1986) *J. Immunol.* **137**, 3861–3867.

Defrance, T., Vanbervliet, B., Aubry, J-P. and Banchereau, J. (1988) *J. Exp. Med.* **168**, 1321–1337.

Delfraissy, J.-F., Wallon, C. and Galanaud, P. (1988) *Eur. J. Immunol.* **18**, 1379–1384.

Esser, C. and Radbruch, A. (1989) *EMBO J.* **8**, 483–488.

Finney, M., Guy, G. R., Michell, R. H., Dugas, B., Rigley, K. P., Gordon, J. and Callard, R. E. (1990) *Eur. J. Immunol.* **20**, 151–156.

Flores-Romo, L., Millsum, M. J., Gillis, S., Stubbs, P., Sykes, C. and Gordon, J. (1990) *Immunology* **69**, 342–347.

Gordon, J., Millsum, M. J., Guy, G. R. and Ledbetter, J. A. (1988) *J. Immunol.* **140**, 1425–1430.

Gordon, J., Millsum, M. J., Flores-Romo, L. and Gillis, S. (1989) *Immunology* **68**, 526–531.

Gosselin, E. J., Tony, H-P. and Parker, D. C. (1988) *J. Immunol.* **140**, 1408–1413.

Gowans, J. L. and McGregor, D. D. (1965) *Progr. Allergy* **9**, 1–78.

Gowans, J. L. and Uhr, J. W. (1966) *J. Exp. Med.* **124**, 1017–1031.

Hilbert, D. M., Cancro, M. P., Scherle, P. A., Nordan, R. P., Van Snick, J., Gerhard, W. and Rudikoff, S. (1989) *J. Immunol.* **143**, 4019–4024.

Jelinek, D. F. and Lipsky, P. E. (1988) *J. Immunol.* **141**, 164–173.

Lanzavecchia, A. (1988) *EMBO J.* **7**, 2945–2951.

Liu, Y-J., Joshua, D. E., Williams, G. T., Smith, C. A., Gordon, J. G. and MacLennan, I. C. M. (1989) *Nature* **342**, 929–931.

Llorente, L., Crevon, M-C., Karray, S., Defrance, T., Banchereau, J. and Galanaud, P. (1989) *Eur. J. Immunol.* **19**, 765–769.

Lundgren, M., Persson, U., Larsson, P., Magnusson, C., Edvard Smith, C. I., Hammarstrom, L. and Severinson, E. (1989) *Eur. J. Immunol.* **19**, 1311–1315.

MacLennan, I. C. M., Oldfield, S., Liu, Y-J. and Lane, P. J. L. (1988) In *Cell Kinetics of the Inflammatory Reaction*, pp. 37–57. Ed. by O. H. Iverson, Springer-Verlag.

Miller, J. F. A. P. and Mitchell, G. F. (1968) *J. Exp. Med.* **128**, 801–820.

Mitchell, G. F. and Miller, J. F. A. P. (1968) *J. Exp. Med.* **128**, 821–837.

Muraguchi, A., Hirano, T., Tang, B., Matsuda, T., Horii, Y., Nakajima, K. and Kishimoto, T. (1988) *J. Exp. Med.* **167**, 332–344.

Noelle, R., Krammer, P. H., Ohara, J., Uhr, J. W. and Vitetta, E. S. (1984) *Proc. Natl. Acad. Sci. USA* **81**, 6149–6153.

Paul, W. E. and Ohara, J. (1987) *Ann. Rev. Immunol.* **5**, 429–459.

Rabin, E. M., Mond, J. J., Ohara, J. and Paul, W. E. (1986a) *J. Immunol.* **137**, 1573–1576.

Rabin, E. M., Mond, J. J., Ohara, J. and Paul, W. E. (1986b) *J. Exp. Med.* **164**, 517–531.

Rabin, E. M., Ohara, J. and Paul, W. E. (1985) *Proc. Natl. Acad. Sci. USA* **82**, 2935–2939.

Romagnani, S., Giudizi, M. G., Biagiotti, R., Almerigogna, F., Mingari, C., Maggi, E., Liang, C-M. and Moretta, L. (1986) *J. Immunol.* **136**, 3513–3516.

Rousset, F., Malefijt, R. de W., Slierendregt, B., Aubry, J-P., Bonnefoy, J-Y., Defrance, T., Banchereau, J. and De Vries, J. E. (1988) *J. Immunol.* **140**, 2625–2632.

Shields, J. G., Armitage, R. J., Jamieson, B. N., Beverley, P. C. L. and Callard, R. E. (1989) *Immunology* **66**, 224–227.

Smith, S. H., Shields, J. G. and Callard, R. E. (1989) *Eur. J. Immunol.* **19**, 2045–2049.

Snapper, C. M., Finkelman, F. D. and Paul, W. E. (1988a) *Immunol. Rev.* **102**, 51–75.

Snapper, C. M., Peschel, C. and Paul, W. E. (1988b) *J. Immunol.* **140**, 2121–2127.

Takatsu, K., Tominaga, A., Harada, N., Mita, S., Matsumoto, M., Takahashi, T., Kikuchi, Y. and Yamaguchi, N. (1988) *Immunol. Rev.* **102**, 107–135.

Tony, H-P. and Parker, D. C. (1985) *J. Exp. Med.* **161**, 223–241.

Valentine, M. A., Clark, E. A., Shu, G. L., Norris, N. A. and Ledbetter, J. A. (1988) *J. Immunol.* **140**, 4071–4078.

Wang, A-C., Tung, E. and Fudenberg, H. H. (1980) *J. Immunol.* **125**, 1048–1054.

Xia, X., Lee, H-K., Clark, S. C. and Choi, Y. S. (1989) *Eur. J. Immunol.* **19**, 2275–2281.

2
The physico-chemical properties of B cell growth and differentiation factors and their receptors

ROBIN E. CALLARD, ANDREW J. H. GEARING
AND RICHARD J. ARMITAGE

Introduction

This chapter describes the physico-chemical properties of cytokines known to regulate B cell responses. Only data derived from cDNA and gene cloning of human and murine cytokines and their receptors are included. Cross-species (human and mouse) reactivity is given in Table 1. Information on the

Table 1 Cross-species specificity (mouse–human) for different cytokines.

Cytokine	% Homology (amino acid sequence)	Cross-reactivity Human	Mouse
IL-1	26	←———————————→	
IL-2	60	No ———————————→	
IL-3	29	None	
IL-4	46	None	
IL-5	71	←———————————→	
IL-6	41	No ———————————→	
IL-7	60	←———————————→	
IFN-α	62	[a] Partial ←———→	
IFN-β	48	None	
IFN-γ	40	None	
NGF	90	←———————————→	
TNF-α	79	←———————————→	
TNF-β	74	←———————————→	
TGF-β_1	99	←———————————→	

[a] Mouse IFN-α_1 has no (<1%) activity on human cells but mouse IFN-α_2 has significant activity on human cells (about 20% compared with its activity on mouse cells) (Shaw et al., 1983).

CYTOKINES AND B LYMPHOCYTES
ISBN 0–12–155145–8

action of the different cytokines on B cells, and on the mechanism of signal transduction are discussed in other chapters.

Interleukin 1

Interleukin 1 (IL-1) has a wide range of biological activities on many different target tissues, including B cells, T cells, monocytes and many other cells outside of the immune system (reviewed by Dinarello, 1989; Fuhlbrigge *et al.*, 1989). There are two distinct molecular forms of IL-1 (IL-1α and IL-1β) which are derived from two different genes. Both human IL-1α and IL-1β (March *et al.*, 1985), and murine IL-1α (Lomedico *et al.*, 1984) and IL-1β (Gray *et al.*, 1986) have been cloned. Their biochemical properties are given in Table 2. Transcription of the *IL-1* gene(s) results in a precursor polypeptide with a M_r of about 31 K. Cleavage of the intracellular precursor gives rise to the active molecule. Interleukin 1α is mostly cell membrane associated whereas IL-1β is mostly secreted. Both forms are non-glycosylated globular proteins with six pairs of antiparallel β-strands but no disulphide bonds. Amino acid sequence homology between human and murine IL-1α is 62%, and between human and murine IL-1β is 68%. In contrast, homology between human IL-1α and IL-1β is only 20% and that between murine IL-1α and IL-1β is 23% (see for example Fuhlbrigge *et al.*, 1989). Despite the low sequence homology between IL-1α and IL-1β, biological assays have shown that these two molecules have very similar, if not identical, activities and bind to the same receptor (Dinarello *et al.*, 1989). Moreover, human IL-1 will act on mouse cells and vice versa. This seems to be due to short homologous sequences in the two molecules which bind to the receptor. The genes for IL-1α and IL-1β each comprise seven exons and are found on chromosome 2 in both humans and mice (Figure 1). In humans, the *IL-1α* gene is 12 kb and the *IL-1β* gene 9.7 kb long. Three glycosylation variants of an IL-1 inhibitor have recently been described and shown to bind to the IL-1 receptor (Hannum *et al.*, 1990). Cloning of the inhibitor has shown it to be structurally related to IL-1β (Eisenberg *et al.*, 1990). The IL-1 inhibitor is produced by the same cells that secrete IL-1 and is potentially a physiologically important regulator.

Figure 1 Genomic organization of human (h) cytokines. The scale shows the approximate size of each gene but the exons (numbered) are not drawn to scale. The *IL-7* gene spans approximately 33 kb (Lupton *et al.*, 1990). Exon V in the human *IL-7* gene is not found in the mouse gene and codes for an 18 amino acid insert in human IL-7. IFN-α and IFN-β have no introns and are not included in this figure.

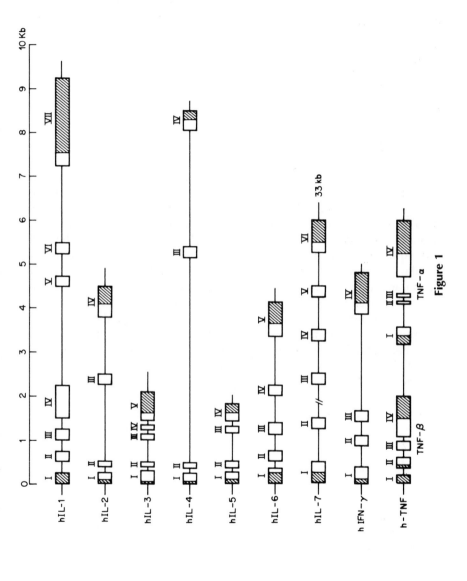

Figure 1

Table 2 Properties of interleukin 1.

Properties	Interleukin 1α		Interleukin 1β	
	Human	Mouse	Human	Mouse
pI	5.0	5.0	7.0	7.0
Amino acids—precursor	271	270	269	269
—mature	159	156	153	159
M_r (K)—expressed	17.5	17.4	17.3	17.5
Glycosylation sites	No	No	No	No
Disulphide bonds	No	No	No	No
Gene—chromosome	2q12-q21	2	2q13-q21	2
—exons	7	7	7	7

The IL-1 receptor is a glycosylated transmembrane protein with an M_r of 80–90 K. It is a member of the Ig super family with two β-pleated sheets and three disulphide bonds. The receptor binds both IL-1α and IL-1β mature proteins but only the IL-1α propeptide. The mouse IL-1 receptor on EL-4 thymoma cells has been cloned (Sims *et al.*, 1988) (Table 3). The core protein has 557 amino acids with a M_r of 65 K. This comprises an extra-cellular region of 319 amino acids with three Ig-like domains, a trans-membrane region of 21 amino acids and an intracellular region of 217 amino acids. Recent cloning of the human IL-1 receptor expressed by a T cell clone has shown a high degree of sequence homology (69%) with the mouse IL-1 receptor (Figure 2) (Sims *et al.*, 1989) (Table 3). An IL-1 receptor expressed in human dermal fibroblasts has also been cloned and found to be identical to the T cell IL-1 receptor. In transfection experiments, human IL-1 receptor cDNA resulted in the expression of high and low affinity receptors

Table 3 Interleukin 1 receptor[a].

Properties	Human	Mouse
Amino acids—precursor	569	576
—mature	552	557
M_r (K)—predicted	64.5	65
—expressed	80	80–90
Glycosylation sites	6N (5 conserved)	7N
Ig-like domains	3	3
Kinase activity	No	No
Phosphorylation sites	Yes	Yes
Signal transduction	Yes	Yes (by transfection)

[a] A separate M_r 60 K IL-1 receptor is also known to exist but no cloning information is yet available.

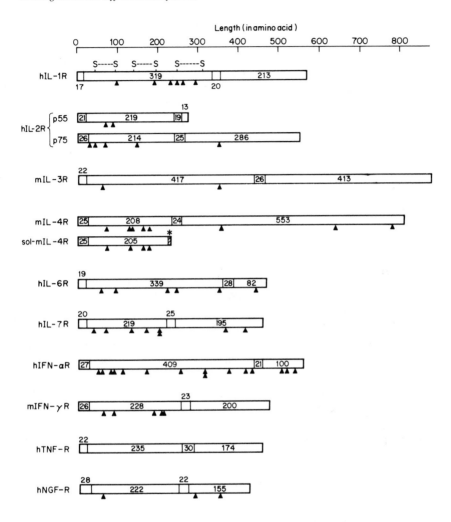

Figure 2 Structure of cytokine receptors. Each receptor is drawn to scale with respect to the number of amino acids. Reading from left (*N*-terminus) to right (*C*-terminus) are shown the signal peptide, extracellular, transmembrane, and intracellular domains. Putative *N*-linked glycosylation sites are indicated by triangles (▲). The positions of potential glycosylation sites for the TNF-R (2 *N* and 1 *O*) were not available at the time of going to press. For each cytokine, the human and murine receptors are very similar. For example, the murine IL-1R has 19, 319, 21 and 217 amino acids in the signal, extracellular, transmembrane and intracellular domains, respectively, compared with 17, 319, 20 and 213 amino acids in the human IL-1R. Note that the soluble form of the murine IL-4R has not yet been identified in man. * Last six amino acids of sol-mIL-4R are different to equivalent residues in intact receptor.

with dissociation constants indistinguishable from those determined for IL-1 receptors on the original T cell clone. These receptors bound IL-1 and were functional. An increase in phosphorylation of some cellular proteins in response to IL-1 has been reported, but there is no intracytoplasmic sequence with obvious homology to any known protein kinase. There may be a second chain to the IL-1 receptor with tyrosine kinase activity. There is also evidence for a second (M_r 60 K) IL-1 receptor present on B cells, granulocytes and macrophages (Bomsztyk et al., 1989). This is encoded by a separate gene (Chizzonite et al., 1989), but cloning information is not yet available.

Interleukin 2

IL-2 is a T cell derived cytokine which acts as a growth and differentiation factor for B cells as well as a growth factor for T cells and natural killer cells (reviewed by Smith, 1984; Smith, 1988). Both human (Taniguchi et al., 1983) and mouse (Kashima et al., 1985; Yokota et al., 1985) IL-2 cDNAs have been cloned. There is a single copy of the IL-2 gene consisting of four exons and three introns on chromosome 4 in humans. IL-2 is synthesized as a propeptide and processed into its mature form by removal of a signal peptide (Table 4). Post-translational modification results in O-glycosylation of the threonine residue at position 3 which is responsible for size and charge heterogeneity of the mature protein. Glycosylation is not necessary for biological activity. The molecule has been shown by X-ray crystallography to be a globular protein with antiparallel alpha helices held together by a single disulphide bond between residues 58 and 105. The tertiary structure is necessary for biological activity. From X-ray crystallographic studies it will soon be possible to identify the residues constituting the binding sites for both the p55 and p75 chains of the IL-2 receptor.

Table 4   Properties of interleukin 2.

Properties	Human	Mouse
Amino acids—precursor	153	169
—mature	133	149
M_r (K)—predicted	15.4	17.2
—expressed	15–20	15–30
Glycosylation sites	O-linked	O-linked
Cysteine residues[a]	3	3
Gene—chromosome	4q26–q27	?
—exons	4	4

[a] Tertiary structure maintained by a disulphide bond.

Table 5 Interleukin 2 receptor.

	p55 α-chain		p75 β-chain[a]	
Properties	Human	Mouse	Human	Mouse
Amino acids—precursor	272	268	551	539
—mature	251	247	525	513
M_r (K)—predicted	28.1	28	58	57
—expressed	55	50–65	75	75
Glycosylation sites	Yes (2 *N*)	Yes (4 *N*)	Yes (4 *N*)	Yes (6 *N*)
Ig-like domains	No	No	No	No
Kinase activity	No	No	No	No
Phosphorylation sites	Yes	Yes	Yes	Yes
Signalling	No	No	Yes	Yes
Gene—chromosome	10p15-p14	?	?	?
—exons	8	8?	?	?

[a] Information about human and mouse p75 chain was kindly supplied by Professor T. Taniguchi.

The IL-2 receptor is a complex of at least two distinct polypeptide chains. The α-chain, also known as Tac or p55, binds IL-2 with low affinity of 1.4×10^{-8} M and a short dissociation half-life of 1.7 s. The longer p75 β-chain binds IL-2 with intermediate affinity of 1.2×10^{-9} M and a long half-life of 46 min. The high affinity IL-2 receptor, with an equilibrium dissociation constant of 1.3×10^{-11} and a half-life of 50 min, is a heterodimer of the p55 and p75 chains. Both human (Cosman *et al.*, 1984; Leonard *et al.*, 1984) and mouse (Shimuzu *et al.*, 1985) p55 α-chains have been cloned (Table 5). The p55 α-chain has a short intracytoplasmic tail of 13 amino acids, including one phosphorylation site, but it seems unable to deliver any intracellular signal. The p75 β-chain has also been cloned (Hatakeyama *et al.*, 1989b) and its biochemical properties determined (Table 5). It has a long intracytoplasmic tail of 286 amino acids with a serine-rich region, an acidic region and a proline-rich region, which may be for association with another molecule (Figure 2). The p75 chain is essential for signal transduction (Hatakeyama *et al.*, 1989a). The α- and β-chains are thought to complex with other polypeptides including a 64 K phosphorylated protein. The means of signal transduction is not known.

Interleukin 3

IL-3 is a haemopoietic growth factor which has recently been shown to have some biological activity on B cells (Tadmori *et al.*, 1989; Ihle, 1989). The

Table 6   Properties of interleukin 3.

Properties	Human	Mouse
Amino acids—precursor	152	166
—mature	133	139/140
M_r (K)—predicted	15	16
—expressed	14–30	28
Glycosylation sites	Yes (2 N)	Yes (4 N)
Disulphide bonds	Yes	Yes (1)
Gene—chromosome	5q23-31	11
—exons	5	5

cDNA clones encoding murine (Fung *et al.*, 1984) and human (Yang *et al.*, 1986) IL-3 have been described (Table 6). The mature protein is derived from a propeptide after removal of a signal peptide. Human IL-3 has two *N*-linked glycosylation sites and a disulphide bond between residues 16 and 84. Mouse IL-3 has four potential *N*-linked glycosylation sites, of which the one at position 42 is probably the most important. Glycosylation is not necessary for biological activity. There are four cysteine residues in mouse IL-3 of which those at positions 43 and 106 are required for biological activity. Murine IL-3 binds to low and high affinity receptors. The receptor for IL-3 was initially described to have a M_r of 65–70 K, but cross-linking studies have indicated the presence of additional binding proteins of M_r 120 and 140 K. Signal transduction appears to involve a protein tyrosine kinase. The murine receptor for IL-3 has recently been cloned (Itoh *et al.*, 1990) (Table 7). Fibroblasts transfected with cDNA for the receptor bound IL-3 with low

Table 7   Interleukin 3 receptor.

Properties	Mouse
Amino acids—precursor	878
—mature	856
M_r (K)—predicted	94.7
—expressed	c. 120
Glycosylation sites	2 N
Cysteine residues	18 (8 conserved)[a]
Ig-like domains	No
Kinase activity	No
Phosphorylation sites	?
Signalling	No?

[a] Eight cysteine residues are conserved in two extracellular repeating motifs of the new receptor superfamily (IL-2R p75, IL-3R, IL-4R, IL-6R, etc. (see above and Itoh *et al.*, 1990).

affinity. No consensus sequence for a tyrosine kinase was present on the cytoplasmic domain, suggesting that another component may be required for functional high-affinity receptors. The IL-3 receptor has significant homology with several other cytokine receptors (erythropoietin, IL-4, IL-6, the β chain of the IL-2 receptor, etc.) and helps define a distinct receptor family (see below).

Interleukin 4

IL-4 is a pleiotropic cytokine derived from T cells with multiple biological effects on B cells (see reviews by Yokota *et al.*, 1988; Ohara, 1989; Banchereau, 1990). The cDNA for human (Yokota *et al.*, 1986) and mouse (Lee *et al.*, 1986; Noma *et al.*, 1986) IL-4 has been cloned and shown to code for proteins of 153 and 140 amino acids, respectively (Table 8). Removal of the signal peptide yields secreted proteins of 129 and 120 amino acids. The coding regions of human IL-4 from amino acid positions 1 to 90 and from positions 129 to 149 share approximately 50% homology with the corresponding regions of mouse IL-4. These regions and the 5' and 3' untranslated regions share about 70% homology. In contrast, the region of human IL-4 from positions 91 to 128 shares very little homology with the corresponding region of mouse IL-4 at either the amino acid or nucleotide sequence levels. The reason for this is unknown but, if the middle portion includes the receptor binding epitope, it could explain the lack of cross-reactivity between mouse and human IL-4, and possibly the difference in transmembrane signalling pathways utilized by IL-4 in the two species (Finney *et al.*, 1990).

The cDNAs encoding human (Idzerda *et al.*, 1990) and mouse (Mosley *et al.*, 1989) IL-4 receptors have now been cloned (Table 9). The receptors are single-chain transmembrane glycoproteins with long intracytoplasmic tails.

Table 8 Properties of interleukin 4.

Properties	Human	Mouse
Amino acids—precursor	153	140
—mature	129	120
M_r (K)—predicted	14	13
—expressed	15–19	15–19
Glycosylation sites	2 *N* sites	3 *N* sites
Disulphide bonds	Yes (6 Cys)	Yes (6 Cys)
Gene—chromosome	5q23-q31	11
—exons	4	4

Table 9 Interleukin 4 receptor.

Properties	Human	Mouse
Amino acids—precursor	825	810
—mature	800	785 (230)[a]
M_r (K)—predicted	87	85
—expressed	140	138–145 (32–41)[a]
Glycosylation sites	6 *N*	5 *N* + 3 *N*[b]
Cysteine residues	6	7
Ig-like domains	No	No
Kinase activity	No	No
Phosphorylation sites	No[c]	1 possible
Signalling	Yes (transfection)	?

[a] Secreted form of murine IL-4 receptor.
[b] Five extracellular *N*-linked glycosylation sites and three intracellular sites.
[c] Hypothetical PKC phosphorylation sites.

Transfection of the human IL-4 receptor into murine CT11-2 cells conveyed responsiveness to human IL-4. Two forms of mouse IL-4 receptor were identified, a membrane-bound receptor and a soluble receptor. The soluble receptor arises from a 114 bp insertion at nucleotide number 598, resulting in divergence nine amino acids upstream from the putative transmembrane region, adding six amino acids before termination. This gives rise to a secreted form of M_r 32–41 K. The secreted form of the IL-4 receptor is able to inhibit responses to mouse IL-4 and may serve as a regulatory protein for responses to IL-4. Probably the most interesting finding from the cloning of the mouse and human IL-4 receptors is the homology shown between the extracellular domains of this and other cytokine receptors (see Receptor families below). In addition, there is a high proportion of proline and acidic amino acids in the cytoplasmic region similar to that observed in the IL-2 receptor p75 β-chain.

Interleukin 5

Interleukin 5 is an eosinophil differentiation factor in mice and humans (Sanderson *et al.*, 1988) and a B cell growth and differentiation factor for mouse B cells but not for human B cells (Clutterbuck *et al.*, 1987). Natural mouse IL-5 is a heavily glycosylated homodimer secreted by T cells. Human T cells make IL-5 mRNA, but natural human IL-5 has not yet been purified. Both human (Campbell *et al.*, 1987; Yokota *et al.*, 1987) and mouse (Kinashi *et al.*, 1986) IL-5 cDNAs have been cloned (Table 10). The gene for IL-5 is

Table 10 Properties of interleukin 5.

Properties	Human	Mouse
Amino acids—precursor	134	133
—mature	115	113
M_r (K)—predicted	13	12.3
—expressed	45 (homodimer)	45–50 (homodimer)
Glycosylation sites	2 N	3 N
Cysteine residues	2	3
Gene—chromosome	5q23-q31	11
—exons	4	4

on human chromosome 5q23-31 and on mouse chromosome 11. In both cases it is closely linked to IL-3, IL-4, and granulocyte and macrophage colony stimulating factor (GM-CSF). In humans these four cytokines are found within a 500 kb segment and all have the same orientation suggesting they may be derived from a common ancestral gene. At the time of writing, the IL-5 receptor has not been cloned and little information about its properties is available. High- and low-affinity IL-5 binding sites have been reported and cross-linking studies have identified a protein of M_r 46.5 K that may constitute the low-affinity receptor (Mita *et al.*, 1989). A protein of M_r 114 K may be the high-affinity binding site, but whether this is a single peptide or a dimer (homo- or heterodimer) is not clear. Monoclonal antibodies to the IL-5 receptor that precipitate proteins of M_r 46, 130 and 140 K have also been reported, but it is not certain what relationship these have to high- and low-affinity receptors for IL-5.

Interleukin 6

Interleukin 6 is a pleiotropic cytokine made by a variety of different cell types, including T cells, B cells, macrophages, fibroblasts and endothelial cells. Like IL-1 and tumour necrosis factor (TNF), IL-6 gives non-lymphoid cells the potential to regulate the immune system. Secretion of IL-6 by many cells is induced by other cytokines such as IL-1, IL-4 and TNF, which often makes it difficult to determine which cytokine is responsible for a specific biological activity. The properties and biological activities of IL-6 are reviewed by Kishimoto (1989) and Kishimoto and Hirano (1988). Human IL-6 was discovered and cloned independently in six laboratories as a 26 K protein, a hybridoma growth factor, IFN-β_2, and a B cell stimulating factor 2 (BSF-2) (Hirano *et al.*, 1986). More recently, mouse IL-6 has also been cloned (Van Snick *et al.*, 1988). The physico-chemical properties of IL-6 are

Table 11   Properties of interleukin 6.

Properties	Human	Mouse
Amino acids—precursor	212	211
—mature	184	187
M_r (K)—predicted	20.7	21.7
—expressed	26	22–29
Glycosylation sites	2 N	0 N^a
Cysteine residues	4	4
Gene—chromosome	7p21-p14	5
—exons	5	5

[a] Some O-linked glycosylation.

given in Table 11. Interleukin 6 shares limited sequence homology with granulocyte colony stimulating factor (G-CSF); the positions of the four cysteine residues of IL-6 match those of G-CSF, suggesting that the genes for these cytokines may have evolved from a common ancestral gene, perhaps similar to the chicken myelomonocytic growth factor (Leutz et al., 1989).

The human (Yamasaki et al., 1988) and mouse (T. Kishimoto, personal communication) receptors for IL-6 have recently been cloned (Table 12). The receptor is a glycoprotein with an Ig-like domain between positions 20 and 110, a transmembrane region and an intracytoplasmic tail of about 82 amino acids (Figure 2). It is also a member of the new cytokine receptor

Table 12   Interleukin 6 receptor.

Properties	Human	Mouse
Amino acids—precursor	468	460
—mature	449	441
M_r (K)—predicted	c. 50	c. 50
—expressed	80	Not examined
Glycosylation sites	6 N^a	5 N^b
Cysteine residues	12	11
Ig-like domains	Yes	Yes
Kinase activity	No	No
Phosphorylation sites	No	No
Signalling	No	No

[a] Five extracellular N-linked glycosylation sites and one intracellular site.
[b] Four extracellular N-linked glycosylation sites and one intracellular site.

family (see below). The receptor binds IL-6 with high affinity but does not include any structure for signal transduction. Binding of IL-6 to the M_r 80 K receptor results in the association of a second non-IL-6 binding glycoprotein of M_r 130 K (gp130) which is required for signalling (Taga *et al.*, 1989).

Interleukin 7

Interleukin 7 is a stromal cell derived growth factor for pre B cells and T cells but not for myeloid cells, suggesting that it may act as a growth factor for a common lymphoid precursor (see review by Henney, 1989). Cloning of human (Goodwin *et al.*, 1989) and mouse (Namen *et al.*, 1988) IL-7 cDNA has recently been reported (Table 13). Mouse IL-7 is a M_r 25 K glycoprotein with two potential *N*-glycosylation sites and six cysteine residues. Reduction with 2-mercaptoethanol results in loss of biological activity, suggesting that tertiary structure dependent on disulphide bonds is required for function. Human IL-7 shares 60% amino acid sequence homology with mouse IL-7, with all six cysteine residues conserved; however, human IL-7 has a 19 amino acid insert at residues 96–114 as a result of an additional exon in the human gene. Not surprisingly, considering the high degree of homology between mouse and human IL-7, human IL-7 is active on human and mouse B cell progenitors. The receptors for both human and murine IL-7 receptors have been cloned (Goodwin *et al.*, 1990) and shown to be integral membrane glycoproteins with a M_r of about 70 K (Table 14, Figure 2). A soluble form of the IL-7 receptor has also been identified.

Table 13 Properties of interleukin 7.

Properties	Human	Mouse
Amino acids—precursor	177	154
—mature	152	129
M_r (K)—predicted	17.4	14.9
—expressed	20–28	25
Glycosylation sites	3 *N*	2 *N*
Cysteine residues	6	6 (conserved)
Gene—chromosome	8q12-q13	?
—exons	6[a]	5

[a] Exon five in human IL-7 codes for an 18 amino acid insert which has not yet been demonstrated in murine IL-7 (Lupton *et al.*, 1990).

Table 14   Interleukin 7 receptor[a].

Properties	Human	Mouse
Amino acids—precursor	459	459
—mature	439	439
M_r (K)—predicted	49.5	49.6
—expressed (approx.)	70	70
Putative glycosylation sites[a]	9 N	6 N
Cysteine residues	13	11
Ig-like domains	No	No
Kinase activity[b]	No	No
Phosphorylation sites[c]	1	1
Signalling	?	?
Chromosome	?	?

[a] 6 extracellular and 3 intracellular sites in human IL-7R; 3 extra cellular and 3 intracellular sites in the murine receptor.
[b] No tyrosine kinase consensus sequence.
[c] No tyrosine kinase sites, one for PKC.

Interferon α and β

Interferon α (IFN-α) is a family of homologous (approximately 90%) molecules with a range of biological activities including resistance to viral infections and regulation of immune function (Balkwill, 1989). More than 23 human IFN-α genes have been identified, at least 15 of which code for functional proteins (first cloned by Mantei *et al.*, 1980; reviewed by Zoon, 1987). Most of these are non-glycosylated 166 amino acid proteins, but some are 165 amino acids long (e.g. IFN-α_2) and at least three species have O-linked polysaccharides (Table 15). The molecule is mostly α-helix with no β-sheets. Mouse IFN-α is a similar family of closely related molecules. Data from cloning of murine IFN-α_1 and IFN-α_2 (Shaw *et al.*, 1983) is given in Table 15. These differ from most human IFN-α molecules by having an N-linked glycosylation site at position 78–80 which is also found in human IFN-β. Homology between human and mouse IFN-α is about 60%. Interestingly, mouse IFN-α_1 is inactive on human cells whereas mouse IFN-α_2 does cross-react. However, antibody to human IFN-α will neutralize mouse IFN-α and vice versa. Interferon β is related to IFN-α and the genes for these two cytokines are located on the same chromosome (chromosome 9 in humans). There is only one IFN-β (IFN-β_2 is now known to be IL-6). Both human (Taniguchi *et al.*, 1980a, 1980b) and mouse (Higashi *et al.*, 1983) IFN-β have been cloned (Table 15). Human IFN-β has one N-linked glycosylation site and three cysteine residues, and the functional unit may be

Table 15   Properties of interferons α and β.

Properties	IFN-α[a]		IFN-β	
	Human	Mouse	Human	Mouse
Number of species	⩾15	>4	1	1
Amino acids—precursor	189/188[b]	189/190[b]	187	182
—mature	166/165	166/167	166	161
M_r (K)—predicted	19.7/19.2	19.7/19.8	20	19.7
—expressed	16–27	20–24	20	26–40
Glycosylation sites	0[c]	1 N	1 N	3 N
Cysteine residues	4/5[d]	5	3[e]	1[f]
Gene—chromosome	9p22-p13	4	9p22	4
—exons[g]	—	—	—	—

[a] Many IFN-α species have been identified in humans and mice. The values given are for the two major groups in man and for α_1 and α_2 in mice.
[b] Includes a signal peptide of 23 amino acids.
[c] The majority of human IFN-α species are not glycosylated but at least three species have been shown to have some O-linked glycosylation.
[d] Most human IFN-α species have four conserved cysteine residues at positions 1, 29, 98/99, 138/139, but some species have an extra cysteine residue at position 86. Two disulphide bonds are formed which are important for biological activity.
[e] One disulphide bond.
[f] No disulphide bonds.
[g] No introns.

a dimer. Mouse IFN-β has three N-linked glycosylation sites and only one cysteine residue. There is only 48% homology between human and mouse IFN-β and there is no species cross-reactivity.

A single receptor binds both IFN-α and IFN-β which is distinct from the

Table 16   Human interferon α receptor.

Properties	Human
Amino acids—precursor	557
—mature	530
M_r (K)—predicted	60.5
—expressed	95–110
Glycosylation sites	15 N
Cysteine residues	11
Ig-like domains	No
Kinase activity	No (?)
Signalling	Yes
Chromosome	21q21-qter

IFN-γ receptor (reviewed by Langer and Pestka, 1988). It is an integral membrane glycoprotein with an estimated M_r of 110–140 K which binds IFN-α/β with high affinity (10^{-9} to 10^{-11} M). The human IFN-α receptor has been cloned (Uze et al., 1990) (Table 16 and Figure 2). In transfection experiments the receptor binds IFN-αB and is functional. The transfectants expressing the receptor did not however respond to other IFN-α species or to IFN-β, suggesting that accessory molecules may be required for signalling by IFN-α/β molecules other than IFN-αB. The finding of higher molecular weight complexes in cross-linking studies supports this conclusion.

Interferon γ

Interferon γ is a T cell derived cytokine with important immunoregulatory properties in addition to its anti-viral and anti-proliferative activity. These include stimulation of murine IgG2a production, induction of MHC class I antigen expression, and inhibition of B cell responses to IL-4. Purified natural human IFN-γ is a M_r 40–70 K aggregate of two molecular weight

Table 17 Properties of interferon γ.

Properties	Human	Mouse
Amino acids—precursor	166	155
—mature[a]	143	133
M_r (K)—predicted	17	16
—expressed	40–70 (20, 25)[b]	40–80[c]
Glycosylation sites	2 N	2 N
Cysteine residues[d]	2 (0)	3 (1)
Gene—chromosome	12q24.1	10
—exons	4	4

[a] The predicted sequence after removal of a signal peptide of 20 amino acids for human IFN-γ and 19 amino acids for mouse IFN-γ gives a mature protein of 146 amino acids for human IFN-γ and 136 amino acids for mouse IFN-γ (Gray et al., 1982; Gray and Goeddel, 1983). However, sequencing of natural human IFN-γ has shown that the three N-terminal residues (Cys-Tyr-Cys) have been removed yielding a mature protein of 143 amino acids (Rinderknecht et al., 1984). Removal of the same three residues from natural mouse IFN-γ yields a protein of 133 amino acids.
[b] Aggregate of two species (M_r 20 and 25 K) of IFN-γ which differ only in the degree and sites of N-linked glycosylation.
[c] Aggregated form.
[d] Number in parentheses is after removal of the N-terminal Cys-Tyr-Cys residues.

Table 18 Interferon γ receptor.

Properties	Human	Mouse
Amino acids—precursor	489	477
—mature	472	451
M_r (K)—predicted	52.5	49.8
—expressed	90–95	90–95
Glycosylation sites	5 N	5 N
Cysteine residues	11	10
Ig-like domains	No	No
Kinase activity	No	No
Phosphorylation sites	Possible	Possible
Signalling	No	No
Chromosome	6q23-q24	10

species of M_r 20 and 25 K (Rinderknecht *et al.*, 1984). These differ only in degrees of glycosylation. The 20 K species is glycosylated only on residue 25, whereas the 25 K species is glycosylated at residues 25 and 97. Both human (Gray *et al.*, 1982) and mouse (Gray and Goeddel, 1983) IFN-γ have been cloned and their properties are given in Table 17. Each is a single polypeptide with two potential N-linked glycosylation sites. The N-terminal three amino acids (Cys-Tyr-Cys) are removed from the mature protein, which excludes any possible disulphide bonds. The receptors for human (Aguet *et al.*, 1988; Schreiber *et al.*, 1989) and mouse (Gray *et al.*, 1989) IFN-γ have been cloned (Table 18). The receptor is a single chain transmembrane glycoprotein with a high content of serine and threonine in the intracytoplasmic tail (Figure 2). There are five extracellular N-linked glycosylation sites and 11 cysteine residues in the human receptor, with at least one disulphide bridge essential for function. In transfection experiments of mouse receptor into human cells, and human receptor into mouse cells, binding of the appropriate IFN-γ failed to stimulate. This suggests that there may be an associated species-specific protein necessary for receptor signalling. In humans, mapping experiments have indicated a requirement for a protein coded for by a gene on chromosome 21, whereas the receptor gene is located on chromosome 6 (reviewed by Langer and Pestka, 1988).

Tumour necrosis factors α and β

TNF-α (tumour necrosis factor) and TNF-β (lymphotoxin) are important cytokines in inflammation and they also regulate the function of many cell types, including B cells. TNF-β is made by T cells and TNF-α is made by macrophages, B cells and other cell types. Their major properties have been

Table 19 Properties of TNF-α (tumour necrosis factor) and TNF-β (lymphotoxin).

Properties	TNF-α		TFN-β	
	Human	Mouse	Human	Mouse
Amino acids—precursor	233	235	205	202
—mature	157	156	171	169
M_r (K)—predicted	17.4	17.3	18.7	18.5
—expressed[a]	34–140	15–150	60–70	18–34
Glycosylation sites	No	1 N	1 N	1 N
Cysteine residues	2[b]	2[b]	No	1
Gene—chromosome[c]	6p21.3	17	6p21.3	17
—exons	4	4	4	4

[a] A range of M_r estimates have been reported due to aggregation. Human TNF-α is commonly found as a homotrimer (3 × 17 K). Glycosylation may give rise to some M_r heterogeneity except for human TNF-α which has no N-linked glycosylation sites.
[b] Forms a disulphide bridge which is probably required for biological activity.
[c] TNF-α and -β genes are closely linked (1200 bp apart) and found within the MHC complex in humans and mice.

reviewed by Balkwill (1989), Tracey et al. (1989) and by Paul and Ruddle (1988). Human (Pennica et al., 1984) and mouse (Pennica et al., 1985) TNF-α have both been cloned (Table 19). The mature human and mouse proteins of 157 and 156 amino acids, respectively, are obtained after removal of a particularly long signal peptide (76 and 79 amino acids, respectively). The signal peptide includes a long hydrophobic region which may be used to anchor a membrane bound form of TNF-α. Both human and mouse TNF-α have two cysteine residues which probably form a disulphide bridge. Mouse TNF-α has a single N-linked glycosylation site but human TNF-α does not. Glycosylation does not seem to be required for biological activity. Monomeric TNF-α is inactive whereas trimeric TNF-α is active.

TNF-β (lymphotoxin) from human (Gray et al., 1984) and mouse (Li et al., 1987) has also been cloned (Table 19). There is about 35% homology between TNF-α and TNF-β amino acid sequences in both species. Human TNF-β has a M_r of 60–70 K by molecular sieving, due to aggregation. Under reducing conditions, two species secreted from RPMI 1788 have been identified with M_r 25 and 20 K. The 25 K molecule is the monomeric glycoprotein, whereas the 20 K molecule is missing the first 23 N-terminal amino acids. The smaller molecule is biologically active but may represent a degradation product. Both human and mouse TNF-β have a single N-linked glycosylation site and the natural forms of the molecule are glycosylated,

Table 20 Tumour necrosis factor receptor.

Properties	Human	
	Type I[a]	Type II
Amino acids—precursor	461	455
—mature	439	426
M_r (K)—predicted	46	47.5
—expressed	85	55
Glycosylation sites[b]	3 *N*, 1 *O*	4 *N*
Cysteine residues	Cysteine-rich extracellular domain	
Kinase activity	No	No
Phosphorylation sites	?[c]	Yes
Signalling	?	?

[a] Information about the TNF type I receptor from Smith *et al.* (1990).
[b] The type I receptor has two putative *N*-linked glycosylation sites in the extracellular region and one in the cytoplasmic region. There is also one *O*-linked site next to the transmembrane region on the extracellular side. The type II receptor has three extracellular and one intracellular *N*-linked sites.
[c] The cytoplasmic domain is serine-rich.

although glycosylation is not required for biological activity. Mouse TNF-β has one cysteine residue but human TNF-β has none.

In humans and mice, the TNF-α and TNF-β genes are very closely linked (separated by about 1200 bp) and are found within the major histocompatibility (MHC) complex. There is a high degree of homology between human and mouse TNF-α and also for TNF-β (about 75%) and each cytokine is active on cells from either species.

Both TNF-α and TNF-β compete for a high affinity receptor (K_d about 10^{-10} M) present on a variety of cell types, although monocytes appear to have low- and high-affinity receptors. The number of receptors per cell varies from 1,000 to 10,000. The receptor is a M_r 70 K glycoprotein which is internalized rapidly on binding of TNF and rapidly degraded. The mechanism of signal transduction is unknown. The cDNA for human TNF receptor has recently been cloned (C. Smith, personal communication) and shown to code for a 435 amino acid integral membrane glycoprotein (Table 20 and Figure 2). The extracellular domain is cysteine rich (like the NGF receptor) and defines a new receptor family. The receptor binds both TNF-α and -β but has no homology with the IL-1 receptor, despite many overlapping activities between IL-1 and TNF. A second TNF receptor (M_r 55 K) has also been cloned (Schall *et al.*, 1990; Loetscher *et al.*, 1990). This receptor also has a cysteine rich extracellular region with homology to the NGF receptor and CD 40. A soluble form of this receptor has also been described.

Transforming growth factor β

The type β transforming growth factors (TGF-β) are a family of small non-glycosylated polypeptides which are distinct from TGF-α and which use different receptors (reviewed by Cheifetz et al., 1987; Wahl et al., 1989; Hsuan, 1989). The TGF-βs are multifunctional molecules which regulate inflammation, tissue repair, and immune function. Biologically active TGF-βs are M_r 25 K dimers of disulphide-linked, 112 amino acid polypeptides. Three isomeric forms of the 112 amino acid polypeptide have been identified (TGF-β_1, TGF-β_2 and TGF-β_3) which can combine to form both homodimers and heterodimers, resulting in a number of different biologically active TGF-βs. Both human (Derynck et al., 1985) and mouse (Derynck et al., 1986) TGF-β_1 cDNAs have been cloned and shown to code for 391 amino acid and 390 amino acid precursor peptides for humans and mice, respectively (Table 21). The mature 112 amino acid TGF-β monomer is located at the C-terminus of the precursor peptide and is released by proteolytic cleavage. There are three N-linked glycosylation sites on the precursor but none on the mature protein. There are nine cysteine residues in the mature protein and an additional three in the precursor. The N-terminal sequence of the human and mouse precursor is highly conserved and contains a sequence of 16 hydrophobic amino acids that may be important for secretion. There is only one amino acid difference between the human and mouse 112 amino acid mature TGF-β_1 proteins. In addition to the TGF-β_1 protein, human TGF-β_2 (de Martin et al., 1987) and TGF-β_3 (Dijke et al., 1988) have also been cloned. Both of these are also 112 amino

Table 21   Properties of transforming growth factor β_1 (TGF-β_1).

Properties	Human	Mouse
Amino acids—precursor	391	390
—mature	112	112
M_r (K)—predicted	12.5	12.5
—expressed[a]	25 (2 × 12.5)	25 (2 × 12.5)
Glycosylation sites	No[b]	No[b]
Cysteine residues	9[c]	9[c]
Gene—chromosome	19q13.1	?
—exons	?	?

[a] The three major forms of natural TGF-β are disulphide linked dimers of two β_1 chains (TGF-β_1), two β_2 chains (TGF-β_2), and a heterodimer of one β_1 chain and one β_2 chain (TGF-$\beta_{1.2}$).
[b] There are no N-linked glycosylation sites on the 112 amino acid mature protein but there are three on the precursor peptide.
[c] There are three additional cysteine residues on the precursor peptide.

acid non-glycosylated proteins derived from 414 and 412 amino acid precursors, respectively. Homology between TGF-β_2 and TGF-β_1 is about 71% and between TGF-β_3 and TGF-β_1 and -β_2 about 80%. The nine cysteine residues are conserved between all three isoforms. The TGF-β_2 precursor has three N-linked glycosylation sites whereas the TGF-β_3 precursor has four. An N-terminal hydrophobic amino acid sequence is present in all three. The genes for the different isoforms are all on different chromosomes (TGF-β_1 is mapped to 19q13.1–13.2, TGF-β_2 to 1q41, and TGF-β_3 to 14q24). Three classes of TGF-β receptor have been described. Class I (M_r 65 K) and class II (M_r 85–110 K) both bind TGF-β_1 with higher affinity than TGF-β_2. The class III receptor is a disulphide linked proteoglycan (M_r about 600 K) which can be reduced to M_r 280–300 K and which binds TGF-β_1, TGF-β_2 and TGF-β_3 with similar efficiency. No TGF-β receptor has yet been cloned.

Nerve growth factor

Nerve growth factor (NGF) is a polypeptide that enhances the survival, growth and neurotransmitter biosynthesis of sympathetic and sensory neurones (Levi-Montalcini, 1987), recently NGF has been shown also to stimulate growth and differentiation of human B lymphocytes (Otten *et al.*, 1989). The cDNAs encoding mouse (Scott *et al.*, 1983) and human (Ulrich *et al.*, 1983) NGF precursors have been cloned (Table 22). The sequence

Table 22 Properties of nerve growth factor.

Properties	Human	Mouse
Amino acids—precursor[a]	307	307
—mature	118	118
M_r (K)—predicted	13	13
—expressed	26 (130)[b]	26 (130)[b]
Glycosylation sites	1 N	1 N
Cysteine residues	6	6
Gene—chromosome	1p13	?
—exons	2	2

[a] The cloned cDNA encodes an open reading frame of 307 amino acids known as the prepro NGF polypeptide. Cleavage of this precursor polypeptide gives rise to NGF which is sited towards the carboxy-terminus, and possibly three other peptides whose function is not known.
[b] Biologically active NGF is a homodimer which may be covalently linked by disulphide bonds. NGF is also found as a high molecular weight complex with two other proteins one of which has esteropeptidase activity and may be involved in processing the NGF precursor.

coding for the NGF protein is sited near the carboxy-terminus of the precursor and is flanked at the N-terminus by 187 amino acids which may be cleaved at dibasic residues to generate three peptides. Two additional amino acids at the carboxy-terminus are also removed. There is a high degree of homology between human and mouse NGF (90%). The six cysteine residues are conserved and form disulphide bonds which are important for tertiary structure and biological activity. NGF is found naturally as a dimer and as a complex with two other proteins (Table 22).

Two types of NGF receptors have been described, one low affinity (K_d 10^{-9} M) and one high affinity (K_d 10^{-11} M) known as the fast and slow receptor respectively. The fast receptor has a M_r of 83 K in the rat and 70–75 K in man whereas the slow receptor has a M_r of about 140 K. The human (Johnson et al., 1986) and rat (Radeke et al., 1987) fast receptors have been cloned (Table 23). Each is an integral membrane glycoprotein which binds dimeric NGF with a K_d of 10^{-9} M (Figure 2). The extracellular segment is very rich in cysteine residues, has one (human) or two (rat) N-linked glycosylation sites, and is very acidic. It contains four repeating elements in which the positions of the cysteine residues are highly conserved. Similar cysteine rich N-terminal domains are also found in receptors for TNF epidermal growth factor (EGF) and platelet derived growth factor (PDGF). In contrast, the intracellular domain has only three cysteine residues and is essentially neutral in charge. It also lacks the ATP binding site consensus sequence characteristic of both the tyrosine and serine or threonine kinases. The slow (high-affinity) receptor is a complex of the fast receptor and another M_r 60 K polypeptide which may have tyrosine kinase activity. Signal transduction may therefore depend on the association of the fast receptor with the M_r 60 K polypeptide in the high-affinity receptor. The

Table 23 Nerve growth factor receptor.

Properties	Human	Rat
Amino acids—precursor	427	425
—mature	399	396
M_r (K)—predicted	49.7	49.3
—expressed	70–75	83
Glycosylation sites	3 N[a]	2 N
Cysteine residues	28	29
Ig-like domains	No	No
Kinase activity	No	No
Phosphorylation sites	Yes	Yes
Signalling	?	?
Chromosome	17q21-q22	?

[a] One on the extracellular region and two on the intracellular region.

NGF receptor has significant sequence homology with the TNF receptor and the CD40 antigen found on B cells and some carcinomas (Stamenkowic *et al.*, 1989). Binding of CD40 monoclonal antibodies is known to deliver an activation and growth promoting signal to B cells.

Receptor families

Several groups of cell surface receptors can be identified by their shared structural features. Hormone receptors coupled to G-proteins typically have

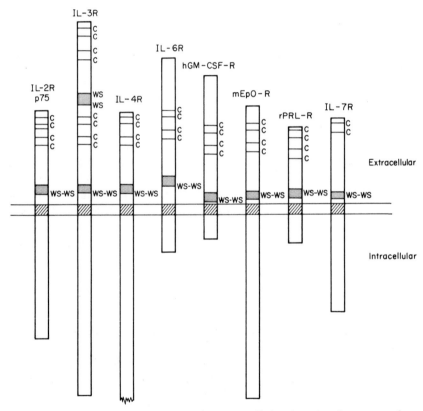

Figure 3 Cytokine receptor family. The extracellular domain of receptors for a number of cytokines including IL-4, IL-3, IL-6, Il-7, human GM-CSF, prolactin (PRL) and erythropoietin (EpO), and the p75 chain of the IL-2 receptor have been recently shown to have a similar structure defined by an *N*-terminal motif with four conserved cysteine residues (c), and a second motif at the proximal end of the extracellular domain based on the sequence Val-X-X-Arg-X_{6-11}-Trp-Ser-X-Trp-Ser, known as the WS–WS box (Bazan, 1989; Gearing, 1989).

multiple transmembrane domains whereas receptors for EGF and PDGF both have a single transmembrane domain and a tyrosine kinase as part of their large intracellular region. Others, such as the IL-1, MCSF and IL-6 receptors, have Ig-like domains in their extracellular regions and are members of the Ig superfamily. The recent cloning of receptor binding proteins for IL-3 and IL-4 has enabled a new superfamily to be defined. This family now includes the receptors for IL-3, IL-4, IL-6, IL-7, GM-CSF, erythropoietin, prolactin, growth hormone and the p75 (β) chain of the IL-2 receptor (Bazan, 1989; Gearing *et al.*, 1989; Idzerda *et al.*, 1990; Itoh *et al.*, 1990). Comparison of the extracellular domains of these receptors has identified two conserved motifs separated by a sequence of 90–100 unique amino acids (Figure 3). The first motif at the N-terminal end of the extracellular domain consists of about 60 amino acids and includes four absolutely conserved cysteine residues and one tryptophan residue. The cysteine residues probably form disulphide bridges important for tertiary structure in the shape of a compact N-terminal head (Bazan, 1989). The second motif of about 30 amino acids is located at the proximal end of the extracellular domain and may be in the form of β-strands. It is based on the sequence Val-X-X-Arg-X_{6-11}-Trp-Ser-X-Trp-Ser, called the WS–WS box (Gearing *et al.*, 1989). The extracellular domain of the IL-3 receptor has two sets of each motif. In addition, the cytoplasmic domains of the receptors for IL-3, IL-4, erythropoietin and the IL-2R p75 chain have a high content of proline and serine and may interact with a common intracellular protein required for signal transduction. The homologous extracellular motifs of these receptors suggest a common structural framework which may function as the cytokine binding site. Although the cytokines themselves do not share homologous amino acid sequences, there may be hidden symmetries in their tertiary structure.

Acknowledgements

We should like to thank Professor T. Kishimoto for information on the murine IL-6 receptor and Professor T. Taniguchi for information on the murine IL-2 receptor p75 chain. Dr R. Callard is supported by grants from the Leukaemia Research Fund and Action Research for the Crippled Child.

References

Aguet, M., Bembic, Z. and Merlin, G. (1988) *Cell* **55**, 273–280.
Balkwill, F. R. (1989) *Cytokines in Cancer Therapy*. Oxford University Press, Oxford.
Banchereau, J. (1990) In *Hematopoietic Growth Factors in Clinical Applications*.

Ed. by R. Mertelsmann, F. Friedhelm and Hermann. Marcel Dekker, New York, in press.

Bazan, J. F. (1989) *Biochem. Biophys. Res. Commun.* **164**, 788–795.

Bomsztyk, K., Sims, J. E., Stanton, T. H., Slack, J., McMahan, C. J., Valentine, M. A. and Dower, S. K. (1989) *Proc. Natl. Acad. Sci. USA* **86**, 8034–8038.

Campbell, H. D., Tucker, W. Q. J., Hort, Y., Martinson, M. E., Mayo, G., Clutterbuck, E. J., Sanderson, C. J. and Young, I. G. (1987) *Proc. Natl. Acad. Sci. USA* **84**, 6629–6633.

Cheifetz, S., Weatherbee, J. A., Tsang, M. L-S., Anderson, J. K., Mole, J. E., Lucas, R. and Massague, J. (1987) *Cell* **48**, 409–415.

Chizzonite, R., Truitt, T., Kilian, P. L., Stern, A. S., Nunes, P., Parker, K. P., Kaffka, K. L., Chua, A. O., Lugg, D. K. and Gubler, U. (1989) *Proc. Natl. Acad. Sci. USA* **86**, 8029–8033.

Clutterbuck, E., Shields, J. G., Gordon, J., Smith, S. H., Boyd, A., Callard, R. E., Campbell, H. D., Young, I. G. and Sanderson, C. J. (1987) *Eur. J. Immunol.* **17**, 1743–1750.

Cosman, D., Ceretti, D. P., Larsen, A., Park, L., March, C., Dower, S., Gillis, S. and Urdal, D. (1984) *Nature* **312**, 768–771.

Derynck, R., Jarrett, J. A., Chen, E. Y., Eaton, D. H., Bell, J. R., Assoian, R. K., Roberts, A. B., Sporn, M. B. and Goeddel, D. V. (1985) *Nature* **316**, 701–705.

Derynck, R., Jarrett, J. A., Chen, E. Y. and Goeddel, D. V. (1986) *J. Biol. Chem.* **261**, 4377–4379.

Dijke, P. T., Hansen, P., Iwata, K. K., Pieler, C. and Foulkes, J. G. (1988) *Proc. Natl. Acad. Sci. USA* **85**, 4715–4719.

Dinarello, C. A. (1989) *Adv. Immunol.* **44**, 153–205.

Dinarello, C. A., Clark, B. D., Puren, A. J., Savage, N. and Rosoff, P. M. (1989) *Immunol. Today* **10**, 49–51.

Eisenberg, S. P., Evans, R. J., Arend, W. P., Verderber, E., Brewer, M. T., Hannum, C. H. and Thompson, R. C. (1990) *Nature* **343**, 341–346.

Finney, M., Guy, G. R., Michell, R. H., Dugas, B., Rigley, K. P., Gordon, J. and Callard, R. E. (1990) *Eur. J. Immunol.* **20**, 151–156.

Fuhlbrigge, R. C., Hogquist, K. A., Unanue, E. R. and Chaplin, D. D. (1989) In *The Year in Immunology 1988: Immunoregulatory Cytokines and Cell Growth*, pp. 21–37. Ed. by J. M. Cruse and R. E. Lewis. Karger, Basel.

Fung, M. C., Hapel, A. J., Ymer, S., Cohen, D. R., Johnson, R. M., Campbell, H. D. and Young, I. G. (1984) *Nature* **307**, 233–237.

Gearing, D. P., King, J. A., Gough, N. M. and Nicola, N. A. (1989) *EMBO J.* **8**, 3667–3676.

Goodwin, R. G., Lupton, S., Schmierer, A., Hjerrild, K. J., Jerzy, R., Clevenger, W., Gillis, S., Cosman, D. and Namen, A. E. (1989) *Proc. Natl. Acad. Sci. USA* **86**, 302–306.

Goodwin, R. G., Friend, D., Ziegler, S. F., Jerzy, R., Falk, B. A., Gimpel, S., Cosman, D., Dower, S. K., March, C. J., Namen, A. E. and Park, L. S. (1990). *Cell* **60**, 941–951.

Gray, P. W. and Goeddel, D. V. (1983) *Proc. Natl. Acad. Sci. USA* **80**, 5842–5846.

Gray, P. W., Leung, D. W., Pennica, D., Yelverton, E., Najarian, R., Simonsen, C. C., Derynck, R., Sherwood, P. J., Wallace, D. M., Berger, S. L., Levinson, A. D. and Goeddel, (1982) *Nature* **295**, 503–508.

Gray, P. W., Aggarwal, B. B., Benton, C. V., Bringman, T. S., Henzel, W. J., Jarrett, J. A., Leung, D. W., Moffat, B., Ng, P., Svedersky, L. P., Palladino, M. A. and Nedwin, G. E. (1984) *Nature* **312**, 721–724.

Gray, P. W., Glaister, D., Chen, E., Goeddel, D. V. and Pennica, D. (1986) *J. Immunol.* **137**, 3644–3648.

Gray, P. W., Leong, S., Fennie, E. H., Farrar, M. A., Pingel, J. T., Fernandez-Luna, J. and Schreiber, R. D. (1989) *Proc. Natl. Acad. Sci. USA* **86**, 8497–8501.

Hannum, C. H., Wilcox, C. J., Arend, W. P., Joslin, F. G., Dripps, D. J., Heimdal, P. L., Armes, L. G., Sommer, A., Eisenberg, S. P. and Thompson, R. C. (1990) *Nature* **343**, 336–340.

Hatakeyama, M., Mori, H., Doi, T. and Taniguchi, T. (1989a) *Cell* **59**, 837–845.

Hatakeyama, M., Tsudo, M., Minamoto, S., Kono, T., Doi, T., Miyata, T., Miyasaka, M. and Taniguchi, T. (1989b) *Science* **244**, 551–556.

Henney, C. S. (1989) *Immunol. Today* **10**, 170–173.

Higashi, Y., Sokawa, Y., Watanabe, Y., Kawade, Y., Ohno, S., Takaoka, C. and Taniguchi, T. (1983) *J. Biol. Chem.* **258**, 9522–9529.

Hirano, T., Yasukawa, K., Harada, H., Taga, T., Watanabe, Y., Matsuda, T., Kashiwamura, S-I., Nakajima, A., Koyama, K., Iwamatsu, A., Tsunasawa, S., Sakiyama, F., Matsui, H., Takahara, Y., Taniguchi, T. and Kishimoto, T. (1986) *Nature* **324**, 73–76.

Hsuan, J. J. (1989) *Brit. Med. Bull.* **45**, 425–437.

Idzerda, R. L., March, C. J., Mosley, B., Lyman, S. D., VandenBos, T., Gimpel, S. D., Din, W. S., Grabstein, K. H., Widmer, M. B., Park, L. S., Cosman, D. and Beckman, M. P. (1990) *J. Exp. Med.* **171**, 861–873.

Ihle, J. N. (1989) In *The Year in Immunology 1988: Immunoregulatory Cytokines and Cell Growth*, pp. 59–102. Ed. by J. M. Cruse and R. E. Lewis. Karger, Basel.

Itoh, N., Yonehara, S., Schreurs, J., Gorman, D. M., Maruyama, K., Ishii, A., Yahara, I., Arai, K-I and Miyajima, A. (1990) *Science* **247**, 324–327.

Johnson, D., Lanahan, A., Buck, C. R., Sehgal, A., Morgan, C., Mercer, E., Bothwell, M. and Chao, M. (1986) *Cell* **47**, 545–554.

Kashima, N., Nishi-Takaoka, C., Fujita, T., Taki, S., Yamada, G., Hamuro, J. and Tanaguchi, T. (1985) *Nature* **313**, 402–404.

Kinashi, T., Harada, N., Severinson, E., Tanabe, T., Sideras, P., Konishi, M., Azuma, C., Tominaga, A., Bergstedt-Lindqvist, S., Takahashi, M., Matsuda, F., Yaoita, Y., Takatsu, K. and Honjo, T. (1986) *Nature* **324**, 70–73.

Kishimoto, T. (1989) *Blood* **74**, 1–10.

Kishimoto, T. and Hirano, T. (1988) *Ann. Rev. Immunol.* **6**, 485–512.

Langer, J. A. and Pestka, S. (1988) *Immunology Today* **9**, 393–400.

Lee, F., Yokota, T., Otsuka, T., Meyerson, P., Villaret, D., Coffman, R., Mosmann, T., Rennick, D., Roehm, N., Smith, C., Zlotnik, A. and Arai, K-I (1986) *Proc. Natl. Acad. Sci. USA* **83**, 2061–2065.

Leonard, W. J., Depper, J. M., Crabtree, G. R., Rudikoff, S., Pumphrey, J., Robb, R. J., Kronke, M., Svetlik, P. B., Peffer, N. J., Waldmann, T. A. and Greene, W. C. (1984) *Nature* **311**, 626–631.

Leutz, A., Damm, K., Sterneck, E., Kowenz, E., Ness, S., Frank, R., Gausepohl, H., Pan, Y-C. E., Smart, J., Hayman, M. and Graf, T. (1989) *EMBO J.* **8**, 175–181.

Levi-Montalcini, R. (1987) *Science* **237**, 1154–1162.

Li, C-B., Gray, P. W., Lin, P-F., McGrath, K. M., Ruddle, F. H. and Ruddle, N. H. (1987) *J. Immunol.* **138**, 4496–4501.

Loetscher, H., Pan, Y-C. E., Lahm, H. W., Gentz, R., Brockhaus, M., Tabuchi, H. and Lesslauer, W. (1990). *Cell* **61**, 351–359.

Lomedico, P. T., Gubler, U., Hellmann, C. P., Dukovich, M., Giri, J. G., Pan, Y-C. E., Collier, K., Semionow, R., Chua, A. O. and Mizel, S. B. (1984) *Nature* **312**, 458–462.

Lupton, S. D., Gimpel, S., Jerzy, R., Brunton, L. L., Hjerrild, K. A., Cosman, D. and Goodwin, R. G. (1990) *J. Immunol.* in press.

Mantei, N., Schwarzstein, M., Streuli, M., Panem, S., Nagata, S. and Weissmann, C. (1980) *Gene* **10**, 1–10.

March, C. J., Mosley, B., Larsen, A., Cerretti, D. P., Braedt, G., Price, V., Gillis, S., Henney, C. S., Kronheim, S. R., Grabstein, K., Conlon, P. J., Hopp, T. P. and Cosman, D. (1985) *Nature* **315**, 641–647.

Martin de, R., Haendler, B., Hofer-Warbinek, R., Gaugitsch, H., Wrann, M., Schlusener, H., Seifert, J. M., Bodmer, S., Fontana, A. and Hofer, E. (1987) *EMBO J.* **6**, 3673–3677.

Mita, S., Tominaga, A., Hitoshi, Y., Sakamoto, K., Honjo, T., Akagi, M., Kikuchi, Y., Yamaguchi, N. and Takatsu, K. (1989) *Proc. Natl. Acad. Sci. USA* **86**, 2311–2315.

Mosley, B., Beckmann, M. P., March, C. J., Idzerda, R. L., Gimpel, S. D., VandenBos, T., Friend, D., Alpert, A., Anderson, D., Jackson, J., Wignall, J. M., Smith, C., Gallis, B., Sims, J. E., Urdal, D., Widmer, M. B., Cosman, D. and Park, L. S. (1989) *Cell* **59**, 335–348.

Namen, A. E., Lupton, S., Hjerrild, K., Wignall, J., Mochizuki, D. Y., Schmierer, A., Mosley, B., March, C. J., Urdal, D., Gillis, S., Cosman, D. and Goodwin, R. G. (1988) *Nature* **333**, 571–573.

Noma, Y., Sideras, P., Naito, T., Bergstedt-Lindquist, S., Azuma, C., Severinson, E., Tanabe, T., Kinashi, T., Matsuda, F., Yaoita, Y. and Honjo, T. (1986) *Nature* **319**, 640–646.

Ohara, J-I. (1989) In *The Year in Immunology 1988: Immunoregulatory Cytokines and Cell Growth*, pp. 126–159. Ed. by J. M. Cruse and R. E. Lewis. Karger, Basel.

Otten, U., Ehrhard, P. and Peck, R. (1989) *Proc. Natl. Acad. Sci. USA* **86**, 10059–10063.

Paul, N. L. and Ruddle, N. H. (1988) *Ann. Rev. Immunol.* **6**, 407–438.

Pennica, D., Nedwin, G. E., Hayflick, J. S., Seeburg, P. H., Derynck, R., Palladino, M. A., Kohr, W. J., Aggarwal, B. B. and Goeddel, D. V. (1984) *Nature* **312**, 724–729.

Pennica, D., Hayflick, J. S., Bringman, T. S., Palladino, M. A. and Goeddel, D. V. (1985) *Proc. Natl. Acad. Sci. USA* **82**, 6060–6064.

Radeke, M. J., Misko, T. P., Hsu, C., Herzenberg, L. A. and Shooter, E. M. (1987) *Nature* **325**, 593–597.

Rinderknecht, E., O'Connor, B. H. and Rodriguez, H. (1984) *J. Biol. Chem.* **259**, 6790–6797.

Sanderson, C. J., Campbell, H. D. and Young, I. G. (1988) *Immunol. Rev.* **102**, 29–50.

Schall, T. J., Lewis, M., Koller, K. J., Lee, A., Rice, G. C., Wong, G. H. W., Gatanaga, T., Granger, G. A., Lentz, R., Raab, H., Kohr, W. J. and Goedd, D. V. (1990) *Cell* **61**, 361–370.

Schreiber, R. D., Calderon, J., Hershey, G. K. and Gray, P. W. (1989) In *Progress in Immunology VII*, pp. 641–648. Ed. by F. Melchers. Springer Verlag, Berlin.

Scott, J., Selby, M., Urdea, M., Quiroga, M., Bell, G. I. and Rutter, W. (1983) *Nature* **302**, 538–540.

Shaw, G. D., Boll, W., Taiva, H., Mantei, N., Lengyel, P. and Weissmann, C. (1983) *Nucleic Acids Res.* **11**, 555–573.

Shimuzu, A., Kondo, S., Takeda, S-I., Yodoi, J., Ishida, N., Sabe, H., Osawa, H., Diamantstein, T., Nikaido, T. and Honjo, T. (1985) *Nucleic Acids Res.* **13**, 1505–1516.

Sims, J. E., March, C. J., Cosman, D., Widmer, M. B., MacDonald, H. R., McMahan, C. J., Grubin, C. E., Wignall, J. M., Jackson, J. L., Call, S. M., Friend, D., Alpert, A. R., Gillis, S., Urdal, D. L. and Dower, S. K. (1988) *Science* **241**, 585–589.

Sims, J. E., Acres, B., Grubin, C. E., McMahan, C. J., Wignall, J. M., March, C. J. and Dower, S. K. (1989) *Proc. Natl. Acad. Sci. USA* **86**, 8946–8950.

Smith, C. A., Davis, T., Anderson, D., Solam, L., Beckmann, M. P., Jerzy, R., Dower, S. K., Cosman, D. and Goodwin, R. G. (1990). *Science* **248**, 1019–1023.

Smith, K. A. (1984) *Ann. Rev. Immunol.* **2**, 319–333.

Smith, K. A. (1988) *Science* **240**, 1169–1176.

Stamenkovic, I., Clark, E. A. and Seed, B. (1989) *EMBO J.* **8**, 1403–1410.

Tadmori, W., Feingersh, D., Clark, S. C. and Choi, Y. S. (1989) *J. Immunol.* **142**, 1950–1955.

Taga, T., Hibi, M., Hirata, Y., Yamasaki, K., Yasukawa, K., Matsuda, T., Hirano, T. and Kishimoto, T. (1989) *Cell* **58**, 573–581.

Taniguchi, T., Mantei, N., Schwarzstein, M., Nagata, S., Muramatsu, M. and Weissmann, C. (1980a) *Nature* **285**, 547–549.

Taniguchi, T., Ohno, S., Fujii-kuriyama, Y. and Muramatsu, M. (1980b) *Gene* **10**, 11–15.

Taniguchi, T., Matsui, H., Fujita, T., Takaoka, C., Kashima, N., Yoshimoto, R. and Hamuro, J. (1983) *Nature* **302**, 305–310.

Tracey, K. J., Vlassara, H. and Cerami, A. (1989) *Lancet* **i**, 1122–1125.

Ulrich, A., Gray, A., Berman, C. and Dull, T. J. (1983) *Nature* **303**, 821–825.

Uze, G., Lutfalla, G. and Gresser, I. (1990) *Cell* **60**, 225–234.

Van Snick, J., Cayphas, S., Szikora, J-P., Renauld, J-C., Van Roost, E., Boon, T. and Simpson, R. J. (1988) *Eur. J. Immunol.* **18**, 193–197.

Wahl, S. M., McCartney-Francis, N. and Mergenhagen, S. E. (1989) *Immunol. Today* **10**, 258–261.

Yamasaki, K., Taga, T., Hirata, Y., Yawata, H., Kawanishi, Y., Seed, B., Taniguchi, T., Hirano, T. and Kishimoto, T. (1988) *Science* **241**, 825–828.

Yang, Y-C., Ciarletta, A. B., Temple, P. A., Chung, M. P., Kovacic, S., Witek-Giannotti, J. S., Leary, A. C., Kriz, R., Donahue, R. E., Wong, G. G. and Clark, S. C. (1986) *Cell* **47**, 3–10.

Yokota, T., Arai, N., Lee, F., Rennick, D., Mosmann, T. and Arai, K-I. (1985) *Proc. Natl. Acad. Sci. USA* **82**, 68–72.

Yokota, T., Otsuka, T., Mosmann, T., Banchereau, J., Defrance, T., Blanchard, D., De Vries, J. E., Lee, F. and Arai, K-I. (1986) *Proc. Natl. Acad. Sci. USA* **83**, 5894–5898.

Yokota, T., Coffman, R. L., Hagiwara, H., Rennick, D. M., Takebe, Y., Yokota, K., Gemmell, L., Shrader, B., Yang, G., Meyerson, P., Luh, J., Hoy, P., Pene, J., Briere, F., Spits, H., Banchereau, J., De Vries, J., Lee, F. D., Arai, N. and Arai, K-I. (1987) *Proc. Natl. Acad. Sci. USA* **84**, 7388–7392.

Yokota, T., Arai, N., De Vries, J., Spits, H., Banchereau, J., Zlotnik, A., Rennick, D., Howard, M., Takebe, Y., Miyatake, S., Lee, F. and Arai, K-I. (1988) *Immunol. Rev.* **102**, 137–187.

3
Receptor signalling in B lymphocytes

KEVIN RIGLEY AND MARGARET HARNETT

Introduction

B lymphocytes represent one arm of the adaptive immune response in vertebrates. In the presence of antigen the appropriate clones of cells are activated, and induced to proliferate and to mature into antibody secreting plasma cells (Forni, 1985). This process of differentiation encompasses the production of antibody of a particular class and isotype; the generation of immunological memory and self/non-self discrimination. In addition to antigen, a plethora of antigen-non-specific soluble factors are intimately involved in the regulation of B lymphocyte activation (reviewed in O'Garra *et al.*, 1987b; Callard, 1989). At present the number of well-defined factors known to regulate human B cell activity include the interleukins IL-1, IL-2, IL-4, IL-5, IL-6, IL-7, low molecular weight B cell growth factor (BCGF low) interferons α and γ, and (TNF; see chapter 2). The picture that is emerging is that B cells, in common with other cell types, contain on their surface specific receptors through which these factors are able to elicit the production of intracellular second messengers, which ultimately results in transcriptional activation/inactivation and the induction of differentiation (Cambier and Ransom, 1987; Klaus *et al.*, 1987). Over the last few years a wealth of information has been obtained regarding the nature and number of signals controlling cell growth (Berridge and Irvine, 1989; Cyert and Thorner, 1989; Czech, 1989; Pelech and Vance, 1989). It is somewhat surprising that a relatively small number of second messengers (not discounting those that are undoubtedly awaiting discovery) appear to control cell growth and differentiation. It follows that the underlying complexities controlling cell growth lie not in the nature of the signals generated but in the manner in which these signals co-exist to determine an appropriate response.

CYTOKINES AND B LYMPHOCYTES
ISBN 0–12–155145–8

Whilst the elucidation of the various second messenger systems is of fundamental importance to our understanding of cellular pathways of activation, it is important to remember that the signals generated act ultimately within the nucleus, i.e. to induce transcription of a variety of genes that are involved in these growth processes (Herrlich and Ponta, 1989). The observation that mRNAs coding for the proto-oncogenes c-*myc*, c-*fos* and c-*jun* are transiently expressed in response to mitogenic stimulation provided the next piece of the jigsaw of the pathway leading to cell activation growth and differentiation (Cole, 1985; Herrlich and Ponta, 1989). In addition to these proto-oncogenes, it has become apparent that a considerable number of "anonymous" genes are transiently expressed in response to mitogens (Almendral *et al.*, 1988; Zipfel *et al.*, 1989). It is therefore essential that the second messengers and specific genes activated in response to these molecules should be identified, so that an understanding of the molecular pathways leading to cell growth and differentiation can be better appreciated. That many cytokines appear not to utilize any of the classically described pathways only adds to the frustration of our attempts at dissecting the complexities of B-cell immune regulation.

The main aim of this chapter is to review the mechanisms of signal transduction operative in the regulation of quiescent B-lymphocyte function. For the most part, this chapter describes the biochemistry of signal transduction in B cells, and focuses on signal transduction via surface immunoglobulin (sIg), Fc-receptors (FcR) and IL-4 receptors. Brief consideration is also given to signal transduction via the IL-1 and IL-2 receptors. Also, recent developments in the study of early-response genes will be discussed.

Receptor signalling: an overview

Much of what we now know about the mechanisms of signal transduction has been derived not from lymphocytes but from other non-haemopoietic cell types. There are at present four established second messenger systems: (a) the phosphoinositide (PI) pathway, (b) the adenylate cyclase system, (c) the cyclic GMP system and (d) tyrosine kinase activity (Berridge, 1984; Rozengurt, 1986; Sibley *et al.*, 1987; Berridge and Irvine, 1989). Whilst it is likely that each of these systems exists in B lymphocytes, only the phosphoinositide and adenylate cyclase systems have been firmly established in controlling the growth of these cells (reviewed in Klaus *et al.*, 1987; Cambier and Ransom, 1987; see Figure 1). A fundamental feature of these systems is that they all lead to the activation of various protein kinases. Since the activity of a considerable number of proteins is modulated by their state of phosphorylation (Cyert and Thorner, 1989) the elucidation of how these second messengers are generated and regulated, and how they interact with each other, should enhance our understanding of the underlying processes governing cell growth and differentiation. A detailed description of these pathways can be found elsewhere; only the salient features are described herein.

There are at least three protein components required for the efficient translation of external signals into the production of second messengers (Dolphin, 1987; Graziano and Gilman, 1987; Harnett and Klaus, 1988b; Neer and Clapham, 1988; and Figure 2). These include receptor, effector enzyme and a coupling protein that acts in such a way as to activate the effector enzyme in the presence of specific ligand. The coupling proteins operative in the activation of adenylate cyclase and the phosphoinositide-phosphodiesterase (PPI-PDE) are GTP-binding proteins (G proteins). It has been known for some time that activation of adenylate cyclase is regulated by two G proteins: Gs which is stimulatory and Gi which is inhibitory. Thus Gs and Gi provide a mechanism of positive and negative control of adenylate cyclase (Dolphin, 1987; Neer and Clapham, 1988). Identification of G proteins has been assisted by exploiting the ability of bacterial toxins to modify their function (Katada and Ui, 1982a,b). Hence, pertussis toxin and cholera toxin ADP-ribosylate Gi and Gs result in inactivation of Gi and activation of Gs, respectively. G proteins are typically heterotrimers consisting of three protein subunits termed α, β and γ. The current model of G protein activation is shown in Figure 2. Interaction of ligand with its appropriate receptor promotes an increase in the affinity of receptor for the $\alpha\beta\gamma$ complex and an increase in the binding of GTP to the GTP-binding α-subunit. This binding of GTP provokes dissociation of the α-GTP from the $\beta\gamma$ subunits. Free α-GTP then activates the effector enzyme until the intrinsic GTPase activity of the α-subunit hydrolyses the bound GTP. The resulting α-GDP subunit then re-associates, and the inactive $\alpha\beta\gamma$ heterotrimer is reformed.

More recently a GTP-binding protein (termed Gp) has been shown to be required for ligand activation of PPI-PDE in a number of cell types (Cockcroft and Gomperts, 1985; Gomperts *et al.*, 1987). Although this protein has not yet been fully characterized, there are at least two forms since PPI-PDE activity is inhibited by pertussis toxin in some cell types but not in others (reviewed in Harnett and Klaus, 1988b). Importantly, an equivalent of the inhibitory G protein (Gi) has not been found, indicating that different inhibitory circuits might be involved in the control of the PPI-PDE (see "FcR: inhibition of B cell activation", below).

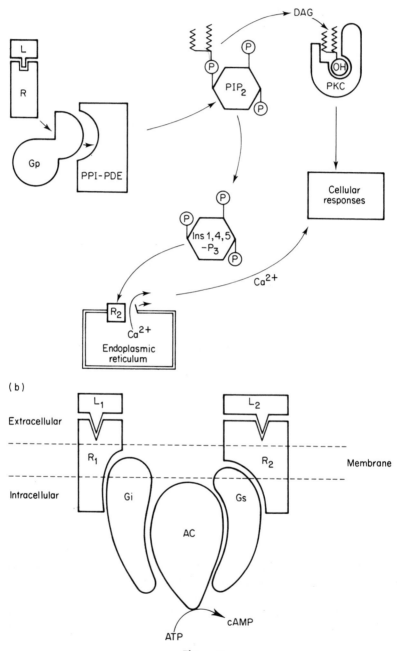

Figure 1

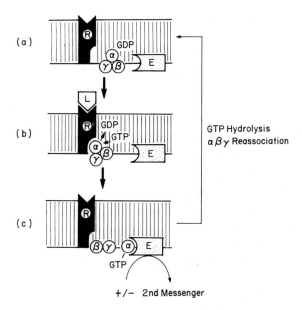

Figure 2 Model of G-protein coupling. (a) In the absence of ligand the $\alpha\beta\gamma$ G protein heterotrimer binds GDP and is inactive. (b) Ligand (L) binds to receptor (R) and promotes nucleotide exchange on the α-subunit of the heterotrimer. (c) The α-GTP complex dissociates from the $\beta\gamma$ dimer and activates the effector enzyme (E). The intrinsic GTPase activity of the α-subunit results in the reassociation of the inactive $\alpha\beta\gamma$-heterotrimer.

Figure 1 (a) The polyphosphoinositide pathway. Ligand/receptor (LR) binding stimulates a polyphosphoinositide-specific phosphodiesterase (PPI-PDE) via activation of a GTP-binding G protein (Gp). PPI-PDE provokes the hydrolysis of phosphatidylinositol 4,5-bisphosphate (PIP_2) into the second messengers diacylglycerol (DAG) and inositol 1,4,5-trisphosphate (Ins 1,4,5-P_3). DAG activates protein kinase C (PKC) and Ins 1,4,5-P_3 mediates the release of Ca^{2+} from endoplasmic reticulum. (b) The adenylate cyclase pathway. Ligand binding to receptor 1 (L_1R_1) and receptor 2 (L_2R_2) modulate adenylate cyclase (AC) activity via activation of the G proteins Gi and Gs, respectively. Gs stimulates AC to catalyse the formation of cAMP from ATP. Gi inhibits AC activity thus lowering levels of cAMP.

Surface immunoglobulin

The discovery that B lymphocytes carry on their surface clonally distributed immunoglobulin (sIg) formed the basis of a variety of theories attempting to explain essential features of B cell biology such as immunological tolerance and the generation of immunological memory. Initially, the role of sIg was thought to be passive, focusing antigen to an appropriate B cell clone (Coutinho and Moller, 1975). The proliferation and resulting differentiation of these cells was presumed to be a consequence of signals delivered via other mitogen receptors. More recently it has become clear that sIg acts not only to focus antigen but is in its own right able to transduce a mitogenic signal (Parker, 1975). Most of these studies have used anti-Ig antibodies as a polyclonal model of antigen-induced activation of B cells (Parker, 1975; Bijsterbosch et al., 1985a; Ransom et al., 1986). Using this model, it has been shown that anti-Ig provokes B cells to an increased expression of a variety of cell surface antigens (reviewed in Gordon and Guy, 1987; Klaus et al., 1987). Also, under certain conditions, anti-Ig provokes B cells to synthesize DNA (Parker, 1975). These studies left little doubt that sIg can transduce a physical signal across the plasma membrane. A major criticism of this model is that the concentrations of anti-Ig required to promote DNA synthesis were in the range 50–100 $\mu g \, ml^{-1}$, concentrations that are unlikely to be attained by antigen. To address this problem, Brunswick et al. (1988) used anti-Ig antibodies conjugated to high molecular weight dextran to stimulate B cells. Their findings show that this form of anti-Ig stimulates DNA synthesis in B cells at concentrations approximately 1,000-fold lower than its soluble counterpart. Importantly, this form of anti-Ig does not appear to significantly modulate sIg and so it could deliver repetitive signals to the B cell, perhaps explaining its mitogenic property (Brunswick et al., 1989).

Surface immunoglobulin: biochemical signalling

It is now clear from a variety of studies that sIg is coupled to the phospho-inositide pathway of signal transduction. This system has been reviewed extensively elsewhere (Cambier and Ransom, 1987; Klaus et al., 1987) and only the major features will be discussed here.

The molecular basis of signal transduction via sIg was first hinted at by Maino et al. (1975) who showed increased incorporation of ^{32}P into phosphatidylinositol following ligation of sIg by anti-Ig antibodies. More recently, increased phosphatidylinositol 4,5-biphosphate (PIP_2) turnover has been demonstrated in B cells stimulated with specific antigen. For example, dinitrophenyl (DNP)-ficoll binding to hapten (DNP)-purified antigen-specific B cells provokes an increase in inositol–phospholipid metabolism (Myers *et al.*, 1987).

Subsequently, it was shown that crosslinking of sIg promotes an increase in ^{32}P incorporation into phosphatidic acid, the phosphorylated derivative of diacylglycerol (DAG). Bijsterbosch *et al.* (1985a) used [^{3}H]inositol-labelled B cells to formally demonstrate that ligation of sIg provokes the release of inositol 1,4,5-trisphosphate (IP$_3$) followed by IP$_2$ and IP$_1$ leaving little doubt that sIg was coupled to the phosphoinositide pathway of signal transduction (see Figure 1). Importantly, the dose response relationships of IP$_3$ release and [^{3}H]thymidine incorporation were similar suggesting that the activation of PKC and release of inositol phosphates leads to DNA synthesis. Later studies showed that IP$_3$ mobilizes Ca^{2+} from endoplasmic reticulum (Ransom *et al.*, 1986) and that the profile of Ca^{2+} increase was made up of both intracellular and extracellular stores (Bijsterbosch *et al.*, 1986).

One method of showing G-protein involvement in receptor activation of the PPI-PDE is to demonstrate PIP$_2$ hydrolysis by adding a combination of agonist and a non-hydrolysable GTP analogue, such as GTPγS to permeabilized cells (Harnett and Klaus, 1988a) or to membrane preparations (Gold *et al.*, 1987). In the last year these groups, working independently and using these techniques, have demonstrated the requirement for a GTP-binding protein in the hydrolysis of PIP$_2$ provoked by anti-Ig antibodies. Furthermore, it is likely that both sIgD and sIgM share a common G protein. Thus it would seem that sIg utilizes the same mechanism of PIP$_2$ hydrolysis as other better-defined calcium mobilizing receptors. Whilst it is clear that both anti-Ig and antigen are able to provoke PIP$_2$ hydrolysis, it is more difficult proving a causal link between this hydrolysis and B cell activation.

Perhaps the most compelling evidence for a causal link between receptor-mediated increases in [Ca^{2+}]$_i$, PKC translocation and B cell activation, is the use of pharmacological agents that either mimic or interfere with the phosphoinositide pathway of signal transduction. Using this approach, it has been shown that activation of B cells with a combination of phorbol ester (which directly activates PKC) and calcium ionophore (which elevates intracellular calcium) stimulates these cells to synthesize DNA (Clevers *et al.*, 1985; Klaus *et al.*, 1985, 1986). In addition, pre-treatment of B cells with a calcium chelator (which ablates the rise in Ca^{2+}) or with staurosporin (an inhibitor of PKC) inhibits anti-Ig induced upregulation of Ia antigens and DNA synthesis, respectively. Furthermore, B cells from·mice carrying the *xid* defect are unable to synthesize DNA in response to normally mitogenic concentrations of anti-Ig (Wicker and Scher, 1986). This non-responsiveness correlates with the known severe impairment in the ability of anti-Ig antibodies to provoke the release of inositol phosphates in these cells (Rigley et al., 1989b).

Since B cells are provoked to synthesize DNA by anti-Ig antibodies in the absence of T-cell help, it has been proposed that this polyclonal activator mimics the action of T-cell independent antigens (TI-Ags). TI-Ags are typically composed of multimeric epitopes and so it can be envisaged that (like anti-Ig antibodies) they will cause extensive crosslinking of sIg and consequently high and persistent activation of the phosphoinositide pathway. Indeed, it has been suggested that a threshold of crosslinked sIg must occur before a mitogenic signal is received by the B cell (Dintzis et al., 1976). On the other hand T-dependent (TD) Ags are usually devoid of a multiplicity of repeating epitopes and consequently are unable to crosslink sIg. Despite this lack of repeating epitopes, TD antigens do induce some changes in B cell biology, including increased expression of Ia antigens (Snow and Noelle, 1987). This suggests that TD antigens activate B cells in the absence of extensive sIg crosslinking. Given that Fab fragments of anti-Ig antibodies do not provoke hydrolysis of PIP_2 (emphasizing the necessity for receptor crosslinking), it is reasonable to assume that TD antigens activate B cells via a pathway other than that addressed by activation of phosphoinositide hydrolysis.

The question of alternative pathways has recently been addressed. Mond et al. (1987) first down-regulated endogenous B-cell PKC activity by pretreating with phorbol-esters. These PKC-depleted B cells are provoked to increased expression of Ia antigens and retain full mitogenic responsiveness to anti-Ig antibodies if cultured in the presence of 8-mercaptoguanisine, suggesting that sIg can address a PKC-independent pathway. These experiments contain a major drawback in that the method used to deplete PKC also delivers a potent activating signal via this enzyme. More recently, Brunswick et al. (1989) have shown that low concentrations of anti-Ig-dextran (see above) that are fully mitogenic for B cells do not provoke accumulation of inositol-phosphates or release of $[Ca^{2+}]_i$. This suggests that the transient early rise in $[Ca^{2+}]_i$ observed in response to mitogenic doses of soluble anti-Ig might not be essential for B cell growth promoted via the B cell antigen-receptor.

These studies attempt to stimulate B cell activation in the absence of significant phosphoinositide hydrolysis. An alternative strategy is to demonstrate normal second messenger production in the absence of a concomitant biological response. One such example utilized the B cell lymphoma CH33 transfected with sIgD receptor (Ales-Martinez et al., 1988). Wild-type CH33 cells are growth arrested by anti-IgM antibodies and are thought to represent B cells of immature phenotype and thus provide a model of tolerance induction. In this study it was found that ligation of transfected sIgD provoked essentially the same degree of PIP_2 hydrolysis, as did crosslinking of sIgM. However, whilst the anti-IgM antibodies inhibited the growth of these cells, the anti-IgD antibodies did not, providing further evidence that sIg can address another pathway of signal transduction (Ales-Martinez *et al.*, 1988). In addition, it has recently been shown that anti-Ig stimulates a WEHI-231 mutant to increase $[Ca^{2+}]_i$ to levels observed in wild-type cells in the apparent absence of inositol phosphate release (Monroe *et al.*, 1989). This important finding suggests that sIg-generated Ca^{2+} signals might not be entirely due to inositol phospholipid hydrolysis. This view is supported by data from Nanberg and Rozengurt (1989) who find that increased calcium flux occurs before release of IP_3 in 3T3 cells. In the light of this finding it is possible that the "normal" Ca^{2+} flux observed in response to intact anti-Ig (see below) is generated not by the transient release of IP_3 but via another, unknown mechanism. The molecular mechanism underlying these observations might reside with the "CD3-like" phospho-proteins that have recently been shown to associate with sIgM and IgD (Campbell and Cambier, 1990; Weinands *et al.*, 1990). Given the short cytoplasmic tail of sIg heavy chains, the presence of additional proteins could explain the ability of sIg to couple to GTP binding proteins (Gold *et al.*, 1987; Harnett and Klaus, 1988a,b; Rigley *et al.*, 1989a,b).

Taken together, the studies documented above strongly indicate that sIg is coupled to a mitogenic pathway other than the phosphoinositide pathway. This is consistent with the already well established fact that other B cell mitogens such as lipopolysaccharide (LPS) and Epstein Barr Virus (EBV) stimulate DNA synthesis in B cells via a currently unidentified signal transduction pathway.

FcR: inhibition of B cell activation

Fc receptors for IgG (FcRII) are present on a variety of cell types including B cells, T cells, macrophages and neutrophils (reviewed in Unkeless *et al.*, 1988). It is known that these receptors are involved in a wide range of functions including the release of activated oxygen metabolites and mediators of inflammation, such as leukotrienes in neutrophils and macrophages. In contrast, these changes are not observed following ligation of FcRII on B-cells. The basis of this difference has been partly elucidated following the cloning of three cDNAs encoding the three isoforms of murine FcγR termed FcRII-A, -B1 and -B2.

FcRII-B2 is found predominantly on macrophages and mediates function in these cells whereas its FcRII-B1 counterpart, which is expressed on B cells, does not. This difference in function is thought to be due to an insertion of 47 amino acids into the cytoplasmic tail of FcRII-B1. A role for

FcRII-B1 in the regulation of B cell activation via the antigen receptor has been known for some years (reviewed in Sinclair and Panoskaltsis, 1987). Early studies demonstrated that the inhibition of specific antibody responses by antigen/antibody immune complexes is brought about by co-ligation of the FcRII-B1 and sIg. Later studies utilized anti-Ig antibodies to address the role of FcRII-B in B cell activation. To this end, Phillips and Parker (1984) have shown that whilst $F(ab')_2$ fragments of polyclonal rabbit IgG induce significant DNA synthesis in B cells, their intact counterparts do not. This is because intact anti-Ig binds simultaneously to sIg and FcRII-B1. It should be noted, however, that the inhibitory effect of intact-Ig is not complete since this form of anti-Ig provokes B cells to be activated to a transitional activation state (G_1T), between G_0 and G_1 proper, characterized by the expression of high levels of Ia antigen (Hawrylowicz *et al.*, 1984).

The biochemical basis of these FcRII-B1-dependent inhibitory effects of intact anti-Ig has been partly elucidated. Bijsterbosch and Klaus (1985b) showed that while $F(ab')_2$ anti-Ig provokes a sustained release of IP_3, its intact counterpart causes only a transient increase in PPI-PDE activity that is markedly diminished after some 30 s. Moreover, intact anti-Ig profoundly inhibits the release of IP_3 provoked by the mitogenic $F(ab')_2$ anti-Ig antibodies. This suggests that control of the PPI-PDE could be an important regulatory step in antigen-induced B cell activation. The mechanism by which co-crosslinking sIg and FcRII-B1 brings about the suppression of PIP_2 hydrolysis has recently been addressed. The introduction of non-hydrolysable GTP analogues such as $GTP\gamma S$ into permeabilized B cells enables the components of the (PI) pathway to be dissected. Using this system it has been shown that the abortive activation of PPI-PDE activity brought about by intact anti-Ig is mediated by the uncoupling of sIg from Gp (Rigley *et al.*, 1989a; Figure 3).

Although the mechanism leading to this uncoupling is unknown, one possibility is that engaging FcR could disrupt receptor:Gp contact by modifying the receptor contact site with Gp, perhaps by phosphorylation (Rall and Harriss, 1987; Sullivan *et al.*, 1987). Alternatively, it has been shown previously that capping of sIg also leads to the co-capping of FcRII-B1, suggesting that the uncoupling might be brought about by physical dissociation. In this context it is tempting to speculate that co-capping of sIg and FcR might disrupt the non-covalent binding of sIg to the "CD3-like" protein complex (Campbell and Cambier, 1990; Wienands *et al.*, 1990).

The inhibitory effect of intact anti-Ig can be overcome by T cell derived lymphokines including IL-4 (O'Garra *et al.*, 1987a). The mechanism by which IL-4 mediates its mitogenic effect in the presence of intact anti-Ig has not been elucidated, but IL-4 does not overcome the inhibition of PIP_2 hydrolysis in murine B cells (O'Garra *et al.*, 1987a). The FcRII-B1/sIg

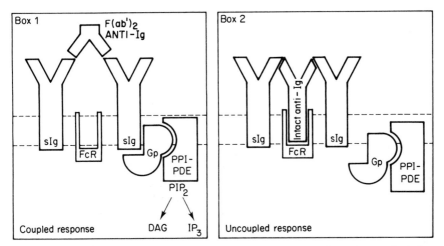

Figure 3 FcR-Induced uncoupling of sIg from Gp. (a) Crosslinking of sIg by F(ab')$_2$ anti-Ig brings about the coupling of Gp to the PPI-PDE and consequently provokes the sustained release of IP$_3$ and DAG. (b) Intact anti-Ig binds to sIg and FcR simultaneously. This co-crosslinking leads to the uncoupling of Gp from the PPI-PDE and as a result the hydrolysis of PIP$_2$ is inhibited.

complex therefore provides an attractive way of fine-tuning B cell responses, brought about by the summation of positive signals (generated by activation of sIg and lymphokine receptors) and negative signals (emanating from FcRII-B1).

Lymphokine receptors

It has been known for many years that soluble factors are able to elicit biological responses in B cells (reviewed in Arai *et al.*, 1987; Callard, 1988). However, early studies used conditioned medium from activated T lymphocytes to show that soluble factors were required in many B cell responses (Pure *et al.*, 1981; Swain *et al.*, 1981). More recently it has been recognized that these conditioned media were molecular soups containing a considerable number of cytokines. The availability of many of these cytokines in recombinant form has been a major force in dissecting out the nature of T cell "help". It has become apparent that all of the factors cloned thus far exert diverse effects on multiple cell types (reviewed in O'Garra *et al.*, 1987b). Although the biological effects of these factors are well documented, little is known of the signal transduction mechanisms that are used to convey information from activated interleukin receptors to the interior of the cell.

Of the interleukins that are known to elicit biological effects on B cells, information on the mechanism of signal transduction has been obtained for IL-2, IL-1 and IL-4 (see below).

Interleukin 4

The activity attributed to interleukin 4 (IL-4, formerly called B-cell stimulatory factor-1) was first identified in the supernatants of phorbol myristate acetate (PMA) stimulated thymoma cells (Howard *et al.*, 1982). It is a 20 kD glycoprotein which under reducing conditions binds to [^{14}C]iodoacetamide, indicating the existence of disulphide bonds in the intact molecule (Ohara *et al.*, 1986). The biological effects of IL-4 on B lymphocytes have been extensively reviewed elsewhere (Paul and Ohara, 1987). Both murine and human IL-4 are involved in the activation of B cells (Noelle *et al.*, 1984; Rousset *et al.*, 1989; Shields *et al.*, 1989). It has been shown that IL-4 will provoke quiescent B cells to increased cell volume and to expression of certain cell surface antigens such as Ia, sIgM, LFA-1, LFA-3 and CD23. IL-4 induces B cells to exit the G_0 phase of the cell cycle and to enter G_1, but does not alone provoke resting B cells to synthesize DNA. However, when added together with sub-mitogenic doses of anti-Ig (Howard *et al.*, 1982), or antigen (Stein *et al.*, 1986), IL-4 co-stimulates resting B cells to proliferate.

Receptors for IL-4

It has been shown previously that the receptor(s) for IL-4 are found on a variety of cell types (Park *et al.*, 1987; Lowenthal *et al.*, 1988). In common with other cytokine receptors, IL-4R are expressed at low frequency on the cell surface of most cell types. Binding studies have mostly suggested that only one class of receptor exists (Lowenthal *et al.*, 1988), although a recent report indicates that there are at least two IL-4 binding proteins of high (K_d 100 pM) and low affinity (30 nM) (Foxwell *et al.*, 1989). More recently, Mosley *et al.* (1989) have isolated two murine cDNA clones coding for an IL-4 binding protein. Interestingly, the difference between the isolated clones lies in the ability of one form to be secreted from the cell. Furthermore, these authors provide data indicating that the secreted form is able to neutralize IL-4 activity in some *in vitro* assays. The potential regulatory role of the secreted IL-4R remains to be explored but is of obvious importance.

Signalling via the IL-4 receptor

As discussed above, IL-4 can elicit activation of B cells and under certain circumstances can play a rôle in their proliferation and differentiation. Accordingly, it is likely that IL-4 can deliver signals at each stage of B cell activation. However the nature of the signal has until recently remained elusive.

Early attempts at elucidating the molecular mechanism of signal transduction via this important lymphokine used murine B cells. One study has suggested that IL-4 induces membrane phosphorylation of a 44 kD membrane-associated protein independently of PKC-activation (Justement *et al.*, 1986). Importantly, it has been reported in a variety of centres that IL-4 does not induce activity of PPI-PDE, Ca^{2+} mobilization, translocation of PKC, membrane depolarization or activition of adenylate cyclase, nor does it promote the production of arachidonic acid metabolites (Justement *et al.*, 1986; O'Garra *et al.*, 1987a; Mizuguchi *et al.*, 1986; Rigley, unpublished observation). In short, IL-4 does not address any of the classically defined second messenger pathways in murine B cells.

The situation in human B cells is quite different. Data from three laboratories indicate that human IL-4 couples to both the phosphoinositide and adenylate cyclase pathways of signal transduction in a unique fashion (Finney *et al.*, 1990; see Figure 4). These results show that following exposure of high density B cells to IL-4, an increase in IP_3 is observed. However, unlike anti-Ig antibodies which promote a sustained release of IP_3 (Bijsterbosch *et al.*, 1985a,b), activation of PPI-PDE observed in the presence of IL-4 is transient, lasting only 15–30 s before returning to the levels observed in unactivated B cells. This brief activation of the PPI-PDE is unusual amongst other calcium-mobilizing receptors (Klaus *et al.*, 1987; Gardner, 1989). A corollary to IP_3 release is a concomitant increase in levels of $[Ca^{2+}]_i$. Confirmation that IL-4 provokes an increase in intracellular calcium came from the demonstration that this lymphokine provoked a transient Ca^{2+} increase in indo-1 loaded resting B cells. The initial magnitude of this rise was comparable to that induced by anti-Ig antibodies, but the levels of $[Ca^{2+}]_i$ stimulated by IL-4 returned to basal levels within 1 min. Importantly, these biochemical changes were not observed in the presence of a neutralizing anti-IL-4 antibody, indicating that IL-4 is indeed responsible for the production of these second messengers.

The transient nature of the IL-4 induced release of IP_3 seemed unlikely to account for many of the biological effects attributed to this lymphokine. This was confirmed by the observation that IL-4 also provoked an increase in $[cAMP]_i$. Of particular interest was the timing of this increase: 8–10 min after the IL-4 induced PIP_2 hydrolysis. This was not a peculiarity of the

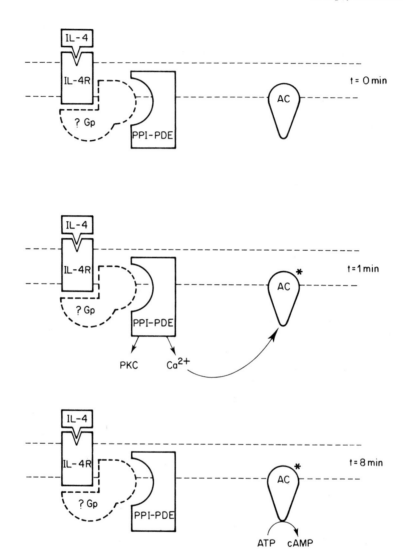

Figure 4 IL-4 activates the polyphosphoinositide-specific phosphodiesterase (PPI-PDE) and adenylate cyclase (AC) in a unique fashion. (a) In the absence of IL-4 both the PPI-PDE and AC are inactive. (b) IL-4 binding to its receptor activates the PPI-PDE to hydrolyse PIP_2 and provokes an increase in $[Ca^{2+}]_i$. (c) After a lag period of some 8 min an increase in cAMP is observed. This IL-4 invoked activation of AC is dependent on the prior elevation in $[Ca^{2+}]_i$.

adenylate cyclase (AC) in B cells since forskolin (which directly activates AC) elevated cAMP without any measurable delay. It is noteworthy that the dose response curves for the accumulation of IP_3, Ca^{2+} and cAMP parallel those required for the anti-Ig plus IL-4 induced co-stimulation of DNA synthesis.

One method of dissecting the molecular mechanism by which IL-4 addresses both the phosphoinositide and cAMP pathways of signal transduction is to specifically inhibit one or more components of these pathways. For instance, by pre-treating cells with the calcium chelator BAPTA it was possible to determine the role of this metal in the subsequent rise in cAMP. Experiments of this nature showed that whilst the IL-4 induced rise in cAMP was abolished, the accumulation in response to forskolin compared favourably to those increases seen in cells which did not receive BAPTA. It would appear, then, that the IL-4 induced Ca^{2+} flux is required for the subsequent elevation in cAMP. The mechanism underlying the Ca^{2+}-dependent rise in cAMP is not known, although it can be envisaged that an intermediate protein activated by the increased availability of Ca^{2+} subsequently activates adenylate cyclase. Alternatively. it is possible that binding of IL-4 promotes the Ca^{2+}-dependent release of an autocrine factor which is responsible for the increase in cAMP.

As described earlier, IL-4 provokes resting B cells to increased expression of CD23 and sIgM. It follows that if the sequence of second messengers described above accurately reflects the molecular mechanism by which IL-4 transduces a signal to the interior of the cell, then the induction of CD23 (the low affinity receptor for IgE) and sIgM should be induced by the appropriate pharmacological agents that mimic these second messengers. To test this hypothesis, we recently conducted a series of experiments in which resting B cells were stimulated for brief periods with phorbol dibutyrate (PDB) together with ionomycin. After removal of these agents by extensive washing, the cells were stimulated with dibutyryl-cAMP for a prolonged period. Interestingly, CD23 but not sIgM was upregulated in response to this treatment (Rigley, unpublished observations). There are at least two possible explanations for this result. Firstly, in addition to the novel signal transducing pathway detailed above, it is possible that the IL-4R is coupled to another as yet unidentified pathway. Secondly, it is possible that there are two IL-4 binding proteins which deliver biochemically distinct signals responsible for the independent regulation of sIgM and CD23 expression. There is circumstantial evidence to support the notion that IL-4 is coupled to two signalling pathways provided by the inhibitory action of the pan-B cell antigen, CD19. Crosslinking of this surface antigen inhibits the induction of DNA synthesis in B cells promoted by a combination of anti-Ig and IL-4.

Moreover, anti-CD19 antibodies inhibit the ability of IL-4 to induce CD23 expression but have no effect on the induction of sIgM (Callard, Rigley and Shields, in prep.). This observation is complicated by the fact that tonsil B cell preparations comprise not only the characteristic naïve phenotype (sIgD^{high} sIgM^{low}) but also cells that are sIgM, sIgG double-positive and sIgG single-positive. It is not yet known whether the upregulation of sIgM and CD23 occurs on the same B cell sub-population. Experiments designed to answer these questions are currently underway.

The discovery of this IL-4 inducible signal transduction pathway in human B cells is enigmatic; why has the same pathway not been described in mouse B cells? One obvious explanation is that the exact cell equivalents have not been used—spleen has been used for mouse and tonsil for human. Although this explanation cannot be ruled out, it is also possible that IL-4 utilizes a different biochemical pathway in the two species. This view is supported by some of the distinctly different responses exhibited by the two species' B cells to polyclonal stimulators. For example, human B cells proliferate in response to phorbol esters, whereas mouse B cells require the presence of a calcium ionophore. Furthermore, unlike human B cells, mouse B cells do not increase expression of sIgM in response to IL-4 (O'Garra et al., 1987a). The apparent discrepancy between the two species could also result from the different methods of cell selection used to obtain B cells. Mouse T cells are typically removed by complement lysis, whereas human T cells are removed by rosetting with sheep erythrocytes. It is not implausible that lysis of T cells leads to a massive release of pre-formed cytokines as well as deposition of complement fragments that are likely to affect B cell function.

Signalling via other lymphokine receptors

The activities of many of the recombinant interleukins were first described in non-B cells and, as a result, the biochemical consequences of binding of these factors has more often than not been elucidated in non-B cells. Although very little is known of the mechanisms by which these important molecules transduce a signal across the plasma membrane, some headway has been made.

Signalling via the IL-2 receptor

There are at least two IL-2 binding proteins, the p55 and p75 (reviewed in Smith, 1984; Smith, 1988). Each of these chains can exist independently of each other and still bind IL-2. IL-2 binds with low affinity to the p55 α-chain, and with intermediate affinity to the p75 β-chain. Importantly, the α-β

heterodimer binds IL-2 with high affinity (Robb *et al.*, 1987; Teshigawara *et al.*, 1987). It is currently thought that the p75 chain is the signal transducing molecule and that the p55 chain helps to focus IL-2 onto the plasma membrane. This conclusion has been reached from studies in which the amount of IL-2 required to invoke DNA synthesis in T cells pre-treated with anti-Tac antibodies (which block binding of IL-2 to the p55 chain but not to the p75 chain thus disrupting high affinity binding), was found to be a hundred times higher than that required to induce proliferation of untreated cells.

There is little (if any) expression of IL-2R on resting human B cells, although it is found on activated B cells (Tsudo *et al.*, 1984; Prakash *et al.*, 1985; Susuki and Cooper, 1985). We have recently found that both IL-4 and IL-2 alone invoke minimal expression of Tac. However, when B cells are co-cultured with either of these cytokines in the presence of anti-Ig a five- to ten-fold increase in Tac expression is observed (Rigley, unpublished observations). This suggests that resting human B cells must receive an activating signal via the antigen receptor and that IL-2 delivers a "progression" signal resulting in B cell proliferation. Interestingly, IL-4 and IL-5 co-ordinately regulate expression of the p55p75 on murine B cells which then become IL-2 responsive (Loughan and Nossal, 1989). At present no effect of IL-5 on human B cells has been observed (Clutterbuck *et al.*, 1988). In addition, IL-2 is a potent T-cell replacing factor in the specific antibody response to influenza (Callard *et al.*, 1986; Callard and Smith, 1988).

The nature of signals generated via the IL-2R is unclear. It is documented that binding of IL-2 to activated T cells results in the stimulation of an amiloride-sensitive Na^+/H^+ antiport and induces rapid alkalinization, but the mode of signal transduction that mediates this effect remains controversial (reviewed in Smith, 1988). It has been reported that IL-2 provokes the rapid release of inositol phosphates in IL-2 dependent, murine T cell lines (Bonvini *et al.*, 1987). In contrast, Mills *et al.* (1986) failed to detect any IL-2 promoted PIP_2 hydrolysis in either human or murine T-cells. In a later study IL-2 was shown not to trigger the release of inositol-phosphates, but rather to stimulate an increase in the production of cAMP (Wickremasinghe *et al.*, 1987). It is worth noting that the kinetics of cAMP accumulation seen in response to IL-2 parallels that observed in response to IL-4 in B cells (see above). Therefore there is an intriguing possibility that IL-2 utilizes a signal transduction pathway of which part is similar to the pathway(s) invoked by IL-4. More recently, it has been found that IL-2 induces tyrosine phosphorylation of a number of T cell proteins, one of which might be the p75 chain of the IL-2 receptor (Tigges *et al.*, 1989). The recent finding that PPI-PDE can be activated by tyrosine phosphorylation (Margolis *et al.*, 1989; Meisenhelder *et al.*, 1989), provides a rationale within which IL-2 can promote inositol phosphate release.

Signalling via the IL-1 receptor

Interleukin 1 is produced at high levels during an inflammatory response. There are two forms of this cytokine, both of which bind to high affinity receptors on T cells, B cells, mesangial cells and fibroblasts (Kilian *et al.*, 1986; Uhl *et al.*, 1989; reviewed by Dinarello *et al.*, 1989). *In vitro*, IL-1 is known to activate immunocompetent B cells and to induce kappa light chain synthesis in the pre-B cell line 70Z/3 (King *et al.*, 1988).

Little is known of the mechanism by which IL-1 transmits its signal. It has been reported by one group that IL-1 promotes an increase in cAMP via a pertussis toxin sensitive G protein (Shirakawa *et al.*, 1988). It has also been shown that IL-1 promotes an increase in the metabolism of phosphatidyl-ethanolamine (but not other phospholipids) in cultured rat mesangial cells (Kester *et al.*, 1989). Since hydrolysis of this phospholipid should generate DAG, it provides a mechanism of activating PKC in the absence of a concomitant calcium flux. Indeed, this biased activation of PKC has been suggested to be the mode of action of IL-3 (Cook *et al.*, 1989). It remains to be seen whether IL-1 does activate PKC in mesangial cells and whether the same mode of action is utilized by IL-1 receptors on B cells.

Control of gene expression

As described above, antigen alone or together with an assortment of growth factors initiates a complex set of intracellular events leading to either DNA synthesis and/or B cell differentiation. In the work discussed above, the biochemical changes measured in response to these stimuli have more often than not been measured over a period of minutes or hours. However, it is recognized that B cells begin to incorporate thymidine some 24 hours following exposure to mitogen and do not differentiate into antibody-secreting cells until days 5–7. The connection between the biochemical signals generated at the cell surface and the internal signals that must act within the nucleus is therefore of immediate importance. This poses the problem of attempting to uncover the order in which the early biochemical changes documented above initiate the specific gene transcription required for progression into and through the cell cycle.

There are a considerable number of receptors on any given cell type, yet the number of second messenger systems described thus far is relatively small; indeed, many of the receptor–ligand interactions result in the activation of common second messenger pathways. This paradigm of receptor action leaves us with the problem of explaining how ligand- and cell-specific responses are generated. Recent progress (mostly in cells other than B lymphocytes) has been made in this area by studying the expression of certain genes in response to ligand binding. It has become apparent that in many cell types the processes of proliferation and differentiation are characterized by rapid and often transient expression of mRNA transcripts. The most widely studied of these mRNAs include those that code for the proto-oncogenes c-*myc*, c-*fos* and c-*jun*, each of which are transiently expressed following receptor activation (Cole, 1985; Marshall, 1987; Katan and Parker, 1988). It is an attractive hypothesis that early and transient expression of these genes initiates a cascade of events that result in cell activation. If this is so, then dysregulation of these early response genes should lead to a profound effect on cell growth.

The approaches to these questions have been to either determine the effect of inserting the gene under consideration into a cell line or into a particular tissue in transgenic mice, or alternatively to use anti-sense RNA to interfere specifically with mRNA transcription. Using these techniques, a variety of studies have shown that over-expression of c-*myc*, for example, leads to tissue-specific tumours (Adams *et al.*, 1985; Langdon *et al.*, 1986; Spanopoulou *et al.*, 1989). Also, the addition of anti-sense c-*myc* inhibits cell entry into S phase but has no effect on the exit of these cells from G_0 of the cell cycle (Heikkila *et al.*, 1987). These studies suggest that c-*myc* is important later on in the cell cycle. A corollary to this is that the rôle played by the early rise in c-*myc* expression in cell-cycle progression should be reconsidered.

Studies addressing the activation of these proto-oncogenes and their rôle in B cell activation are still in their infancy. It has been shown that increased c-*myc* and c-*fos* expression is provoked by a variety of agonists including anti-Ig antibodies and IL-4. Moreover, non-mitogenic, intact anti-Ig inhibits the accumulation of c-*myc* provoked by its mitogenic $F(ab')_2$ counterpart, prompting Phillips *et al.* (1988) to suggest a rôle for c-*myc* in the exit of B cells from quiescence. This conclusion is complicated by the finding that IL-4 co-stimulates DNA synthesis in B cells exposed to intact anti-Ig, but does not overcome the inhibition of c-*myc* expression.

More recently, it has become apparent that the proto-oncogenes represent only a small proportion of genes that are expressed early after cell stimulation. By using cDNA cloning methods it has been shown that a considerable number of novel genes (in addition to the proto-oncogenes) are rapidly expressed following receptor stimulation. This family of genes (early response genes; ERGs) have been identified in fibroblasts and T cells, where conservative estimates indicate that at least 100 distinct genes are expressed (Almendral *et al.*, 1988; Zipfel *et al.*, 1989). Whilst these data indicate great complexity of control, it should be possible to identify those genes that are involved in proliferation *per se* and those that are involved in cell-specific differentiation. It is easy to imagine that those genes required for the initiation of DNA synthesis will be found in a variety of cell types, whilst those that are involved in Ig class switching, for instance, will be restricted to cells of the B cell lineage. Although this is a simplistic approach, it should be possible to identify specific regulatory genes that are induced by the various lymphokines known to be involved in an immune response.

Indeed, this strategy has met with some success in the study of PMA-induced plasmacytoid differentiation of B chronic lymphocytic leukaemia (B-CLL) cells (Murphy and Norton, 1990). On the basis of morphology and antigenic profiles, it is generally agreed that these cells represent a stage of arrested differentiation somewhere between pre-B cell and mature immunocompetent B cells. Furthermore, these cells can be induced to differentiate into Ig-secreting cells by a variety of agents including PMA, IL-2 and alpha-IFN (Gordon *et al.*, 1984; Ostlund *et al.*, 1986; Emilie *et al.*, 1988), providing an attractive model of B cell differentiation. It has been shown that, in common with other cell types including normal resting B cells, activation of B-CLL cells results in an early and transient expression of the proto-oncogenes c-*fos*, c-*jun* and c-*myc*. In addition to proto-oncogene expression, Murphy *et al.* (1990) have isolated some 25 "anonymous" cDNA probes from a cDNA library constructed from PMA-activated B-CLL cells. Interestingly, PMA-stimulation of B-CLL cells invokes first the expression of proto-oncogenes and then, some hours later, the ERGs. Importantly, some of these ERGs appear to be B cell specific. Although their function is not yet known they are likely to provide an attractive resource for mapping different regulatory pathways.

Concluding remarks

It is now well established that in addition to antigen an assortment of growth factors can initiate a complex set of intracellular signals leading to the modulation of B cell growth and differentiation. In recent years a considerable number of laboratories attempted to elucidate the biochemical and molecular basis of these signals in the expectation that the ensuing information would enhance our understanding of both normal and aberrant B cell growth.

From these studies it has emerged that sIg utilizes the phosphoinositide signal transduction pathway and perhaps another, as yet undescribed, pathway. Indeed, it would appear that control of the PPI-PDE is a potent mechanism by which antigen-driven B cell growth can be regulated. It is also encouraging that the modes of signal transduction utilized by the various cytokines are beginning to be understood. There are, however, numerous questions that remain unanswered. For instance, it is becoming increasingly obvious that more than one cytokine will influence B cell growth at any one time; moreover it is known that cytokines such as interferon or IL-4 can be either stimulatory or inhibitory, depending on how they are assayed. How do these signals interact? Which genes do they switch on and off? How do different antigens induce particular isotype secretion? These are just a few of the important questions that have to be addressed. If progress in this field occurs at the same rate as it has done over the last few years it will not be long before these answers will arrive, no doubt provoking different, but no less important, questions. Clearly, the next few years will produce some exciting research in this field of immunology.

Acknowledgements

We would like to thank Gerry Klaus and Martin Bijsterbosch for introducing us to the complexities of B lymphocyte signal transduction. Kevin Rigley is supported by a grant from Action Research for the Crippled Child.

References

Adams, J. M., Harris, A. W., Pinkert, C. A., Corcoran, L. M., Alexander,W. S., Cory, S., Palmiter, R. D. and Brinster, R. L. (1985) *Nature* **318**, 533–538.
Ales-Martinez, J. E., Warner, G. L. and Scott, D. W. (1988) *Proc. Natl. Acad. Sci. USA* **85**, 6919–6923.
Almendral, J. M., Sommer, D., Macdonald-Bravo, H., Burckhardt, J., Perera, J. and Bravo, R. (1988) *Mol. Cell Biol.* **8**, 2140–2148.
Arai, K., Yokota, T., Miyajima, A., Arai, N. and Lee, F. (1987) *BioEssays* **5**, 166–171.
Berridge, M. J. (1984) *Biochem. J.* **220**, 345–360.
Berridge, M. J. and Irvine, R. F. (1989) *Nature* **341**, 197–205.
Bijsterbosch, M. K. and Klaus, G. G. B. (1985b) *J. Exp. Med.* **162**, 1825–1836.
Bijsterbosch, M. K., Meade, C. J., Turner, G. A. and Klaus, G. G. B. (1985a) *Cell* **41**, 999–1006.
Bijsterbosch, M. K., Rigley, K. P. and Klaus, G. G. (1986) *Biochem. Biophys. Res. Commun.* **137**, 500–506.
Bonvini, E., Ruscetti, F. W., Ponzoni, M., Hoffman, T. and Farrar, W. L. (1987) *J. Biol. Chem.* **262**, 4160–4164.
Brunswick, M., Finkelman, F. D., Highet, P. F., Inman, J. K., Dintzis, H. M. and Mond, J. J. (1988) *J. Immunol.* **140**, 3364–3372.
Brunswick, M., June, C. H., Finkelman, F. D., Dintzis, H. M., Inman, J. K. and Mond, J. J. (1989) *Proc. Natl. Acad. Sci. USA* **86**, 6724–6728.
Callard, R. E. (1989) *Brit. Med. Bull.* **45**, 371–388.
Callard, R. E. (1988) In *Developments in Biological Standardisation. Cytokines:*

laboratory and clinical evaluation. Ed. by A. J. H. Gearing and W. Hennessen. Karger, vol. 69, pp. 43–49.

Callard, R. E. and Smith, S. H. (1988) *Eur. J. Immunol.* **18**, 1635–1638.

Callard, R. E., Smith, S. H., Shields, J. and Levinsky, R. J. (1986) *Eur. J. Immunol.* **16**, 1037–1042.

Cambier, J. C. and Ransom, J. T. (1987) *Ann. Rev. Immunol.* **5**, 175–199.

Campbell, K. S. and Cambier, J. C. (1990) *EMBO J.* **9**, 441–448.

Clevers, H. C., Versteegen, J. M. T., Logtenberg, T., Gmelig-Meyling, F. H. J. and Ballieux, R. E. (1985) *J. Immunol.* **135**, 3827–3830.

Clutterbuck, E., Shields, J. G., Gordon, J., Smith, S. H., Boyd, A., Callard, R. E., Campbell, H. D., Young, I. G. and Sanderson, C. J. (1987). *Eur. J. Immunol.* **17**, 1743–1750.

Cockroft, S. and Gomperts, B. D. (1985) *Nature* **314**, 534–536.

Cole, M. D. (1985) *Nature* **318**, 510–511.

Cook, N., Dexter, T. M., Lord, B. I., Cragoe, E. J. and Whetton, A. D. (1989) *EMBO J.* **8**, 2967–2974.

Coutinho, A. and Muller, G. (1975) *Adv. Immunol.* **21**, 113–236.

Cyert, M. S. and Thorner, J. (1989) *Cell* **57**, 891–893.

Czech, M. P. (1989) *Cell* **59**, 235–238.

Dinarello, C. A., Clark, B. D., Puren, A. J., Savage, N. and Rosoff, P. M. (1989) *Immunol. Today* **10**, 49–51.

Dintzis, H. M., Dintzis, R. Z. and Vogelstein, B. (1976) *Proc. Natl. Acad. Sci. USA* **73**, 3671–3675.

Dolphin, A. C. (1987) *TINS* **10**, 53–58.

Emilie, D., Karray, S., Merle-Beral, H., Debre, P. and Galanaud, P. (1988) *Eur. J. Immunol.* **18**, 1479–1483.

Finney, M., Guy, G. R., Michell, R. H., Dugas, B., Rigley, K. P., Gordon, J. and Callard, R. E. (1989) *Eur. J. Immunol.* **20**, 151–156.

Forni, L. (1985) *Scand. J. Immunol.* **22**, 235–243.

Foxwell, B. M. J., Woerly, G. and Ryffel, B. (1989) *Eur. J. Immunol.* **19**, 1637–1641.

Gardner, P. (1989) *Cell* **59**, 15–20.

Gold, M. R., Jakway, J. P. and DeFranco, A. L. (1987) *J. Immunol.* **139**, 3604–3613.

Gomperts, B. D., Cockcroft, S., Howell, T. W., Nusse, O. and Tatham, P. E. (1987) *Biosci. Rep.* **7**, 369–381.

Gordon, J. and Guy, G. R. (1987) *Immunol. Today* **8**, 339–344.

Gordon, J., Mellstedt, H., Aman, P., Biberfeld, P. and Klein, G. (1984) *J. Immunol.* **132**, 541–547.

Graziano, M. P. and Gilman, A. G. (1987) *TIPS* **8**, 478–481.

Harnett, M. M. and Klaus, G. G. B. (1988a) *J. Immunol.* **140**, 3135–3139.

Harnett, M. M. and Klaus, G. G. B. (1988b) *Immunol. Today* **9**, 315–320.

Hawrylowicz, C. M., Keeler, K. D. and Klaus, G. G. B. (1984) *Eur. J. Immunol.* **14**, 244–250.

Heikkila, R., Schwab, G., Wickstrom, E., Loke, S. L., Pluznik, D., H., Watt, R. and Neckers, L. M. (1987) *Nature* **328**, 445–449.

Herrlich, P. and Ponta, H. (1989) *TIG* **5**, 112–115.

Howard, M., Farrar, J., Hilfiker, M., Johnson, B., Takatsu, K., Hamaoka, T. and Paul, W. (1982) *J. Exp. Med.* **155**, 914–923.

Justement, L., Chen, Z., Harris, L., Ransom, J., Sandoval, V., Smith, C., Rennick, D., Roehm, N. and Cambier, J. (1986) *J. Immunol.* **137**, 3664–3670.

Katada, T. and Ui, M. (1982a) *Proc. Natl. Acad. Sci. USA* **79**, 3129–3133.
Katada, T. and Ui, M. (1982b) *J. Biol. Chem.* **257**, 7210–7216.
Katan, M. and Parker, P. J. (1988) *Nature* **332**, 203.
Kester, M., Simonson, M. S., Mene, P. and Sedor, J. R. (1989) *J. Clin. Invest.* **83**, 718–723.
Kilian, P. L., Kaffka, K. L., Stern, A. S., Woehle, D., Benjamin, W. R., Dechiara,T. M., Gubler, U., Farrar, J. J., Mizel, S. B. and Lomedico, P. T. (1986) *J. Immunol.* **136**, 4509–4514.
King, A. G., Wierda, D. and Landreth, K. S. (1988) *J. Immunol.* **141**, 2016–2026.
Klaus, G. G. B., Bijsterbosch, M. K. and Holman, M. (1985) *Immunology* **56**, 321–327.
Klaus, G. G. B., O'Garra, A., Bijsterbosch, M. K. and Holman, M. (1986) *Eur. J. Immunol.* **16**, 92–97.
Klaus, G. G. B., Bijsterbosch, M. K., O'Garra, A., Harnett, M. M. and Rigley, K. P. (1987) *Immunol. Rev.* **99**, 19–38.
Langdon, W. Y., Harris, A. W., Cory, S. and Adams, J. M. (1986) *Cell* **47**, 11–18.
Loughnan, M. S. and Nossal, G. J. V. (1989) *Nature* **340**, 76–79.
Lowenthal, J. W., Castle, B. E., Christiansen, J., Schreurs, J., Rennick, D., Arai, N., Hoy, P., Takebe, Y. and Howard, M. (1988) *J. Immunol.* **140**, 456–464.
Maino, V. C., Green, N. M. and Crumpton, M. J. (1975) *Biochem. J.* **146**, 247–252.
Margolis, B., Rhee, S. G., Felder, S., Mervic, M., Lyall, R., Levitski, A., Ullrich, A. and Zilberstein, A. (1989) *Cell* **57**, 1101–1107.
Marshall, C. J. (1987) *Cell* **49**, 723–725.
Meisenhelder, J., Suh, P., Rhee, S. G. and Hunter, T. (1989) *Cell* **57**, 1109–1122.
Mills, G. B., Stewart, D. J., Mellors, A. and Gelfand, E. W. (1986) *J. Immunol.* **136**, 3019–3024.
Mizuguchi, J., Beaven, M. A., Ohara, J. and Paul, W. E. (1986) *J. Immunol.* **137**, 2215–2219.
Mond, J. J., Feuerstein, N., Finkelman, F. D., Huang, F., Huang, K-P. and Dennis, G. (1987) *Proc. Natl. Acad. Sci. USA* **84**, 8588–8592.
Monroe, J. G., Seyfert, V. L., Owen, C. S. and Sykes, N. (1989) *J. Exp. Med.* **169**, 1059–1070.
Mosley, B., Beckmann, M. P., March, C. J., Idzerda, R. L., Gimpel, S. D., VandenBos, T., Friend, D., Alpert, A., Anderson, D., Jackson, J., Wignall, J. M., Smith, C., Gallis, B., Sims, J. E., Urdal, D., Widmer, M. B., Cosman, D. and Park, L. S. (1989) *Cell* **59**, 335–348.
Murphy, J. J. and Norton, J. D. (1990) *Biochem. Biophys. Acta* (in press).
Murphy, J. J., Tracz, M. and Norton, J. D. (1990) *Immunol.* **69**, 490–493.
Myers, C. D., Kriz, M. K., Sullivan, T. J. and Vitetta, E. S. (1987) *J. Immunol.* **138**, 1705–1711.
Nanberg, E. and Rozengurt, E. (1988) *EMBO J.* **7**, 2741–2747.
Neer, E. J. and Clapham, D. E. (1988) *Nature* **333**, 129–134.
Noelle, R., Krammer, P. H., Ohara, J., Uhr, J. W. and Vitetta, E. S. (1984) *Proc. Natl. Acad. Sci. USA* **81**, 6149–6153.
O'Garra, A., Rigley, K. P., Holman, M., McLaughlin, J. B. and Klaus, G. G. B. (1987a) *Proc. Natl. Acad. Sci. USA* **84**, 6254–6258.
O'Garra, A., Umland, S., Defrance, T. and Christiansen, J. (1987b) *Immunol. Today* **9**, 45–54.
Ohara, J., Coligan, J. E., Zoon, K., Malloy, W. L. and Paul W. E. (1987) *J. Immunol.* **139**, 1127–1134.

Ostlund, L., Einhorn, S., Robert, K-H., Juliusson, G. and Biberfeld, P. (1986) *Blood* **67**, 152–159.

Park, L. S., Friend, D., Sassenfeld, H. M. and Urdal, D. L. (1987) *J. Exp. Med.* **166**, 476–488.

Parker, D. C. (1975) *Nature* **258**, 361–363.

Paul, W. E. and Ohara, J. (1987) *Ann. Rev. Immunol* **5**, 429–459.

Pelech, S. L. and Vance, D. E. (1989) *TIBS* **14**, 28–30.

Phillips, N. E., Gravel, K. A., Tumas, K. and Parker, D. C. (1988) *J. Immunol.* **141**, 4243–4249.

Phillips, N. E. and Parker, D. C. (1984) *J. Immunol.* **132**, 627–632.

Prakash, S., Robb, R. J., Stout, R. D. and Parker, D. C. (1985) *J. Immunol.* **135**, 117–122.

Pure, E., Isakson, P. C., Takatsu, K., Hamaoka, T., Swain, S. L., Dutton, R. W., Dennert, G., Uhr, J. W. and Vitetta, E. S. (1981) *J. Immunol.* **127**, 1953–1958.

Rall, T. and Harris, B. A. (1987) *FEBS Lett.* **224**, 365–371.

Ransom, J. T., Harris, L. K. and Cambier, J. C. (1986) *J. Immunol.* **137**, 708–714.

Rigley, K. P., Harnett, M. M. and Klaus, G. G. B. (1989a) *Eur. J. Immunol.* **19**, 481–485.

Rigley, K. P., Harnett, M. M., Phillips, R. J. and Klaus, G. G. B. (1989b) *Eur. J. Immunol.* **19**, 2081–2086.

Robb, R. R., Rusk, C. M., Yodoi, J. and Greene, W. C. (1987) *Proc. Natl. Acad. Sci. USA* **84**, 2002–2006.

Rousset, F., Billaud, M., Blanchard, D., Figdor, C., Lenoir, G. M., Spits, H. and De Vries, J. E. (1989) *J. Immunol.* **143**, 1490–1498.

Rozengurt, E. (1986) *Science* **234**, 161–166.

Shields, J. G., Armitage, R. J., Jamieson, B. N., Beverley, P. C. L. and Callard, R. E. (1989) *Immunology* **66**, 224–227.

Shirakawa, F., Yamashita, U., Chedid, M. and Mizel, S. B. (1988) *Proc. Natl. Acad. Sci. USA* **85**, 8201–8205.

Sibley, D. R., Benovic, J. L., Caron, M. G. and Lefkowitz, R. J. (1987) *Cell* **48**, 913–922.

Sinclair, N. R. S. and Panoskaltsis, A. (1987) *Immunol. Today* **8**, 76–79.

Smith, K. A. (1984) *Ann. Rev. Immunol.* **2**, 319–333.

Smith, K. A. (1988) *Immunol. Today* **9**, 36–37.

Snow, E. C. and Noelle, R. J. (1987) *Immunol. Rev.* **99**, 173–192.

Spanopoulou, E., Early, A., Elliott, J., Crispe, N., Ladyman, H., Ritter, M., Watt, S., Grosveld, F. and Kioussis, D. (1989) *Nature* **342**, 185–189.

Stein, P., Dubois, P., Greenblatt, D. and Howard, M. (1986) *J. Immunol.* **136**, 2080–2089.

Sullivan, K. A., Miller, R. T., Masters, S. B., Beiderman, B., Heideman, W. and Bourne, H. R. (1987) *Nature* **330**, 758–760.

Suzuki, T. and Cooper, M. D. (1985) *J. Immunol.* **134**, 3111–3119.

Swain, S. L. (1985) *J. Immunol.* **134**, 3934–3943.

Swain, S. L. and Dutton, R. W. (1977) *J. Immunol.* **119**, 1179–1186.

Swain, S. L., Dennert, G., Warner, J. F. and Dutton, R. W. (1981) *Proc. Natl. Acad. Sci. USA* **78**, 2517–2521.

Teshigawara, K., Wang, H-M., Kato, K. and Smith, K. A. (1987) *J. Exp. Med.* **165**, 223–238.

Tigges, M. A., Casey, L. S. and Koshland, M. E. (1989) *Science* **243**, 781–786.

Tsudo, M., Uchiyama, T. and Uchino, H. (1984) *J. Exp. Med.* **160**, 612–617.

Uhl, J., Newton, R. C., Giri, J. G., Sandlin, G. and Horuk, R. (1989) *J. Immunol.* **142**, 1576–1581.

Unkeless, J. C., Scigliano, E. and Freedman, V. H. (1988) *Ann. Rev. Immunol.* **6**, 251–281.

Wicker, L. S. and Scher, I. (1986) *Curr. Topics Microbiol. Immunol.* **24**, 87–97.

Wickremasinghe, R. G., Mire-Sluis, A. R. and Hoffbrand, A. V. (1987) *FEBS Lett.* **220**, 52–56.

Wienands, J., Hombach, J., Radbruch, A., Riesterer, C. and Reth, M. (1990) *EMBO J.* **9**, 449–455.

Zipfel, P. F., Balke, J., Irving, S. G., Kelly, K. and Siebenlist, U. (1989) *J. Immunol.* **142**, 1582–1590.

4
Rôle of cytokines in the ontogeny, activation and proliferation of B lymphocytes

THIERRY DEFRANCE AND JACQUES BANCHEREAU

Introduction

Lymphocytes represent one of the important functional units of the immune system and billions of them are produced daily from the maturation and multiplication of haemopoietic multipotential and lineage-restricted progenitor cells of the bone marrow. B cells represent the effector cells of the humoral limb of immunity as they are the only cells able to produce antibodies. Two decades ago, Dutton *et al.* (1971) and Schimple and Wecker (1972), showed that T-cell derived soluble factors play an important rôle in different aspects of B cell differentiation. Now, it is well established that the development of an haemopoietic multipotential stem cell into antigen-specific immunoglobulin-producing plasma cells requires numerous steps that involve collaboration of various cell types and their soluble-derived factors, collectively termed cytokines. The molecular characterization of cytokines consecutive to advances in molecular and cellular biology can be considered as one of the hallmarks of the cell biology of the 1980s.

The first step, the development of the stem cell into mature $IgM^+ IgD^+$ B cells is independent of antigens and occurs primarily in the bone marrow and/or foetal liver. It is characterized by (i) an orderly cascade of rearrangements of the immunoglobulin variable region genes that encode antibody specificity and (ii) polyclonal proliferation. The second step, from the mature resting B cell to plasma cells and memory B cells, is antigen-dependent as well as T cell dependent and occurs mostly in secondary lymphoid organs such as lymph nodes, tonsils, spleen and Peyer's patches. It is characterized by antigen driven proliferation, affinity maturation through somatic hypermutations of antibody variable region genes and isotype switching (Kocks and Rajewsky, 1989). In the present review, we will

CYTOKINES AND B LYMPHOCYTES
ISBN 0–12–155145–8

concentrate on the role of cytokines in antigen-independent B cell maturation process and in antigen-dependent B cell activation and proliferation. The participation of cytokines in the differentiation of B cells into immunoglobulin-producing cells, although tightly linked to B cell activation and proliferation, will not be covered herein as it is discussed in another chapter of the present book.

Cytokines and antigen-independent B cell development

In vitro *models of haemopoiesis and lymphopoiesis*

Significant progresses in understanding haemopoiesis and lymphopoiesis followed the development of long-term bone marrow culture techniques. First, Dexter *et al.* (1977) established conditions suitable for maintenance of multipotential stem cells and granulopoiesis. Subsequently, Whitlock and Witte (1982) adapted these methods for selective growth of B lymphocytes. In such culture systems, pre-B cells grow on a complex layer of adherent cells composed of macrophages and various cell types collectively designated as "stromal cells" and comprising endothelial cells, fat cells and fibroblasts. Stromal cell clones, which are suitable for sustaining growth of established precursor B cell lines and B cell clones, also permit B lymphopoiesis. These stromal cell clones have been shown to produce many different cytokines including macrophage colony stimulating factor (M-CSF), granulocyte CSF, GM-CSF, IL-6, transforming growth factor (TGFβ), IL-4 and IL-7 (Kincade *et al.*, 1989). From these studies, it may be concluded that various cytokines affect B lymphopoiesis.

Interleukin 3

The culture of nu/nu mouse spleen cells or foetal liver pre-B cells in the presence of IL-3 results in the generation of IL-3 dependent pro-B and pre-B cell lines (Palacios *et al.*, 1984; Kinashi *et al.*, 1988; McKearn *et al.*, 1985; Palacios and Steinmetz, 1985; Palacios *et al.*, 1987). The pre-B cell lines express rearranged heavy and light chain genes, whereas the pro-B cell lines display heavy and light chain genes in germ-line configuration. The pre-B cell lines differentiate into Ig-producing cells when cultured in the presence of lectin activated splenocytes or T cells and dendritic cells. It is noteworthy that dendritic cells and T cells from spleens stimulate IgM secretion, whereas cells isolated from Peyer's patches induce high levels of IgA and intermediate levels of IgG and IgM. The secreted isotype appears to be determined by the lymphoid tissue source of dendritic cells, not that of T cells (Spalding and Griffin, 1986). The rôle of cytokines in this differentiation process remains to be established. The pro-B cells can differentiate *in vivo* to a stage, where they can be stimulated *in vitro* to mature into antibody secreting cells (Palacios and Steinmetz, 1985; Palacios *et al.*, 1987). More recently, IL-3 responsive pre-B cell lines and clones were derived from Whitlock–Witte long term lymphocyte cultures (Rennick *et al.*, 1989). Optimal proliferation of these cells in the absence of stroma required both IL-3 and stromal cell conditioned medium.

In man, IL-3 as well as a purified preparation of low molecular weight B cell growth factor (LMW BCGF) could induce short-term proliferation of some $CD10^+$ progenitor B cells from foetal liver (Wörmann *et al.*, 1987; Uckun and Ledbetter, 1988). However, no-one has, up until now, been able to generate human IL-3 dependent precursor B cell lines.

Although the presence of IL-3 responsive B cell precursors is clearly demonstrated, the precise rôle of IL-3 in B lymphopoiesis is presently unclear. In this context, the first *in vivo* experiments based on continuous infusion of IL-3 to mice failed to show an increase of T and B cells in different organs, whereas a profound increase in other haemopoietic lineages could be observed (Metcalf *et al.*, 1986; Kindler *et al.*, 1987; Kimoto *et al.*, 1988). However, the parameters of these *in vivo* experiments may not have been appropriate to reveal the effects of IL-3 on the B cell compartment.

Interleukin 7

Stromal cell lines and clones isolated from long term Whitlock–Witte cultures have proven to produce soluble factors able to support the *in vitro* growth of precursor B cells. These observations allowed first the purification of what is now called IL-7 (Namen *et al.*, 1988a) and then the isolation of a specific cDNA (Namen *et al.*, 1988b). IL-7 is a potent growth factor for B cell progenitors (including pre-B $c\mu^+$ cells) from murine bone marrow, and the cellular target of its proliferative effect is likely to be the large population, more immature than the smaller cells (Lee *et al.*, 1989; Sudo *et al.*, 1989; Suda *et al.*, 1989). In semi-solid medium, IL-7 induces the formation of pre-B cell colonies composed of 25–2000 cells. Prolonged culturing in the presence of IL-7 results in a predominance of immature $c\mu^-$ lymphocytes. Human IL-7 induces proliferation of IL-7 dependent murine pre-B cell lines (Goodwin *et al.*, 1989). In human bone marrow assays, IL-7 induces only a minor proliferation of purified normal $CD34^+$ haemopoietic progenitors (S. Saeland and J. Banchereau, unpublished data). IL-7 is not lineage-specific, as it displays proliferative effects on thymocytes and lectin-stimulated peripheral T cells (Morissey *et al.*, 1989; Murray *et al.*, 1989; Takeda *et al.*,

Takeda et al., 1989; Welch et al., 1989). However, it does not appear to act on mature B cells. The in vitro effects of IL-7 on lymphoid cells were confirmed by in vivo studies. Infusion of IL-7 into mice induces an increase in the number of lymphoid cells in spleen and lymph nodes and an increase in the number of marrow pre-B cells (Henney, 1989).

Interleukin 4

Early experiments have shown that IL-4 suppresses the growth of pre-B cells in primary Whitlock–Witte cultures and in culture systems consisting of a cloned stromal cell line seeded with non adherent bone marrow cells (Rennick et al., 1987). IL-4 also inhibits in a reversible fashion the growth of stromal cell dependent pre-B cell lines (Rennick et al., 1987). This inhibition could be consistent with IL-4 inducing differentiation of pre-B cells into more mature B cells. In this context, it has been shown that the IL-3 dependent pro-B cell clones can differentiate in vitro into mature B cells, producing IgM and IgG by co-culture with bone marrow stromal cells (Kinashi et al., 1988) or with dendritic cells and T cells (Spalding and Griffin, 1986). The blocking effect of anti-IL-4 antibodies on the stromal cell-dependent maturation of these pro-B cell clones, suggests that IL-4 could be involved in this maturation process (Kinashi et al., 1988). Indeed stromal cell supernatants were found to induce maturation of mouse pre-B cells into sIgM$^+$ B cells, and this activity was blocked by an anti-IL-4 antibody (King et al., 1988). Furthermore, both murine and human recombinant IL-4 are able to induce pre-B cells to mature into sIgM-positive B cells (Hofman et al., 1988; King et al., 1988). Our own results (S. Saeland and J. Banchereau, unpublished observations) have shown that IL-4 could induce CD20 expression on normal human CD34$^+$ progenitors in the absence of any proliferation, whereas it failed to induce sIgM or CD21 expression which is associated with pre-B cell differentiation.

Others have suggested a rôle for IL-4 in the expansion of the precursor B cell compartment. IL-3 dependent pro-B cell clones were found to proliferate in response to IL-4, and bone marrow-derived long-term lymphoid cultures initiated in the presence of IL-4 resulted in the generation of very immature B cell precursors (Palacios et al., 1987; Peschel et al., 1989). This effect may, however, be indirect through the IL-4 induced release by stromal cells of a factor inducing proliferation of progenitor B cells. These precursors differentiate into B lineage cells when transferred on Whitlock–Witte stromal layers.

Taken together, the data collected by several groups suggest that IL-4 may induce proliferation of pro-B cells and induce the differentiation of late pro-B cells into early pre-B cells and that of late pre-B cells into immature

IgM$^+$ B cells. However, infusion of anti-IL-4 neutralizing antibodies did not result in an alteration of B cell numbers in lymphoid organs, whereas such treatment profoundly inhibits parasite or anti-IgD induced increase of serum IgE levels (Finkelman *et al.*, 1986; F. Finkelman, personal communication).

Interleukin 5

IL-3 dependent CD5$^+$ pro-B cell clones were initially found to proliferate in response to IL-5 (Palacios *et al.*, 1987). Following this initial observation, it was reported that bone marrow cells cultured for 4 weeks under Dexter type culture conditions proliferated in response to IL-5 in the presence of a stromal cell layer. Under Whitlock–Witte culture conditions, these cells yielded B lymphocytes and eosinophils (Tominaga *et al.*, 1989). Starting from Whitlock–Witte culture conditions, IL-5 dependent CD5$^+$ pre-B cell lines were obtained which showed Ig heavy chain gene rearrangement. The *in vivo* role of IL-5 in B cell lymphopoiesis has been studied using irradiated mice transplanted with bone marrow cells that had been infected with a recombinant retrovirus bearing the IL-5 coding sequence (Vaux *et al.*, 1989). Such mice displayed hypereosinophilia and, although no changes could be detected in the conventional B lymphocyte population, the peritoneum was repleted with B cells of the CD5$^+$ lineage. Thus, IL-5 may play an important rôle in the ontogeny of CD5$^+$ B cells that may represent a lineage different from the conventional B cell lineage (Hayakawa and Hardy, 1988). Accordingly, infusion of anti-IL-5 antibodies in mice, which blocks parasite induced hypereosinophilia, did not result in the depletion of the conventional B cell pool in peripheral lymphoid organs (Coffman *et al.*, 1989; F. Finkelman, personal communication).

Other cytokines acting on B lymphopoiesis

IL-1 is able to induce expression of sIg on precursor B cells, but it is not clear whether this effect is direct or whether it is indirect through release of IL-4 by stromal cells. A direct effect was, however, suggested by the IL-1 mediated induction of κ light chain expression on the pre-B tumour cell line 70Z/3 but such a model may not reflect the *in vivo* situation (Giri *et al.*, 1984). Interferon γ (IFN-γ) but not IL-4 is also able to induce κ chain on these cells.

Addition of IL-1 to Whitlock–Witte bone marrow cultures blocks B lymphopoiesis (Dorshkind, 1988). This effect may be indirect as IL-1 stimulates the production of myeloid colony-stimulating factors which

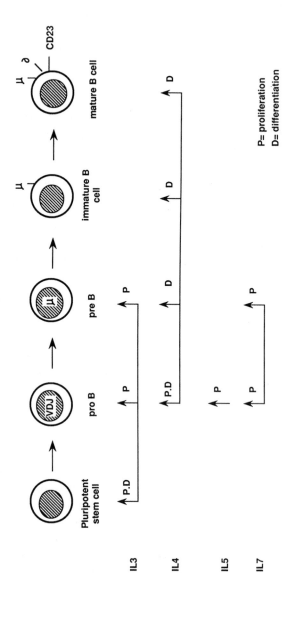

Figure 1 Schematic representation of the effects of cytokines on B cell ontogeny. Most of the results originate from murine studies except for the differentiation effects of IL-4, which were also found in human studies.

subsequently allow the expansion of myeloid cells versus lymphoid cells. However, according to recent studies, IL-1 would partially block the IL-7 dependent proliferation of precursor B cell lines (Lee *et al.*, 1989).

TGF-β, which displays antagonistic effects on many immune functions, also inhibits light chain expression on bone marrow-deprived pre-B cells, as well as on 70Z/3 cells (Lee *et al.*, 1987). TGF-β also blocks the IL-7 dependent proliferation of a subpopulation of pre-B cells (Lee *et al.*, 1989). Thus, lymphopoiesis is controlled by both agonist and antagonist factors. In this context, the absence of human B lymphopoiesis in *in vitro* models may be linked to an overproduction of such antagonists.

Cytokines and B lymphopoiesis: perspective

While it is now clear that the generation of B cells requires accessory cell types acting through the release of various cytokines (Figure 1), we are still at a very early stage in this field and many questions need to be addressed. What is the rôle of each of these cytokines in each of the stages of B cell lymphopoiesis? Are cytokines involved in the commitment of multipotential stem cells to lymphoid committed progenitor cells? Are cytokines involved in the T cells/dendritic cell-mediated maturation of B cell progenitors into Ig producing cells? The actual spectrum of cytokines involved in B lymphopoiesis is probably incomplete, as suggested by the study of Lemoine *et al.* (1988). Finally, there is now a need for establishing *in vitro* assays of human B lymphopoiesis to determine whether the initial observations made in the mouse model also apply to man (LeBien, 1989). Such information would help in understanding and controlling the development of leukaemic progenitor cells.

Antigen-dependent B cell activation and proliferation

T–B cell interactions and B cell activation

Maturation of B cells into antibody-secreting cells is a complex process that requires antigen and the collaboration between B cells, T cells and antigen-presenting cells. The demonstration by Chesnut and Grey (1981, 1986) and Lanzavecchia (1987) that B cells can also exert the function of antigen-presenting cells, introduced the novel concept that the cooperation between T and B cells could be sufficient to allow clonal expansion and differentiation of antigen-specific B cells (Jones, 1987).

According to this minimal model of T–B cell interactions, maturation of B cells into Ig secreting cells can be subdivided in two steps: (i) First, B cells specifically bind the thymus-dependent (TD) antigen, by means of their surface Ig receptors. After binding to surface Ig receptors, the antigen is internalized, processed, then re-expressed in association with major histo-compatibility complex (MHC) class II determinants and finally presented to the T helper cell. (ii) The second step is essentially under the control of T cell-derived soluble factors and permits expansion and differentiation of the antigen specific B cell clone. Triggering of cytokine release by T cells occurs following recognition by the T cell receptor of the processed antigen.

Because of their monovalent binding ability, TD antigens do not permit redistribution of surface Igs within the membrane and thus provide only minimal activation signal to B cells. In order to achieve the G_0 to G_1 transition and to acquire responsiveness to progression factors, B cells require additional stimuli that are provided by T cells. The T helper functions can occur via direct T–B cell contact through complementary structures expressed on both cell types, and via the release of cytokines.

Conversely, molecules presenting repeating motifs, such as certain bac-terial/fungal cell wall components, can induce cross-linkage of surface Ig receptors (Cambier and Monroe, 1984; Cambier *et al.*, 1987), thus providing a maximal activation signal. Such agents are designated as thymus-independent (TI) antigens, since they can induce proliferation and for some of them, differentiation of B cells into Ig-secreting cells without T cell help.

Polyclonal B cell activators

Due to the paucity of antigen-specific B cells in peripheral blood and in lymphoid organs, the study of B cell physiology has been primarily under-taken with *in vitro* culture systems allowing polyclonal activation of B cells. Most of the polyclonal B cell activators (PBA) used, both in mouse and human models, reproduce at a' larger scale the effects of thymus-independent antigens (Waldmann and Broder, 1982; Kehrl *et al.*, 1984; Jelinek and Lipsky, 1987a), and they can be subdivided into three groups.

(i) Agents binding to surface immunoglobulins, such as anti-Ig antibodies (anti-IgM, anti-IgD, anti-idiotypic mAb or immobilized particles of *Staphy-lococcus aureus*). These reagents induce crosslinking and redistribution of surface Ig receptors.

(ii) Agents binding to non-Ig-related surface receptors, such as lipopoly-saccharide (LPS) and dextran sulphate in the murine system or the Epstein–Barr virus (EBV) in the human system. Apart from their ability to initiate B cell activation, they can also induce their differentiation into Ig-secreting cells. Accumulating evidence has now demonstrated that non-Ig-related molecules, such as CD20, CD40 or Bgp95 (Clark and Ledbetter, 1989), can also deliver competence signals to human B cells. These antigens may constitute highly specialized B cell triggering structures binding to surface receptors expressed on T cells or accessory cells.

(iii) Agents bypassing surface receptors, such as phorbol esters often used in co-stimulation with a calcium ionophore. They act as direct agonists of protein kinase C, which plays a pivotal rôle in the cascade of events leading to B cell activation.

In vitro culture systems have also been designed in which B cells, selected on the basis of their antigenic specificity, are activated by their specific antigen.

Do accessory cells play a rôle in B cell activation?

The notion that polyclonal B cell activators could induce activation and proliferation of highly purified resting B cells in the absence of influences from other cell types has been challenged by the studies of Corbel and Melchers (1983). These authors reported that murine B cells lose their ability to respond to LPS or anti-Ig antibodies after extensive depletion of accessory cells. In the model proposed by Melchers and Anderson (1984), three restriction points control the cell cycle of activated murine B cells. The first restriction point occurs just after mitosis and progression to the second point of arrest in G_1 is controlled by the antigen (or anti-Ig antibodies). Progression from the second point, through S phase, up to the third point, in G_2, is under the dependence of macrophages (or α factors). T cells (or β factors) allow completion of the cell cycle by inducing mitosis.

Cytokines and B cell activation

Several molecularly defined cytokines, which were previously ascribed a rôle in later stages of B cell maturation, have now been demonstrated to be involved in the early B cell activation events.

Interleukin 4

IL-4 acts as a competence factor for mouse B cells. IL-4 was first defined as a B cell stimulatory factor for murine B cells on the basis of its capacity to co-stimulate with anti-Ig antibodies for induction of polyclonal B cell growth (Howard *et al.*, 1982). The possibility that IL-4 could act at an early stage, prior to anti-Ig stimulation was suggested by Oliver *et al.* (1985) and Rabin *et al.* (1985, 1986a) who showed that pretreatment of resting B cells with IL-4 increases their subsequent proliferative response to various mitogenic stimuli such as anti-IgM antibodies or LPS. Enhanced responsiveness of IL-4-stimulated B cells to subsequent progression signals is likely to be due to their accelerated entry into the cycle rather than to an enhanced proportion of cells recruited to proliferate. The priming effect of IL-4 is associated with a significant cell volume increase that affects the entire B cell population (Rabin et al., 1986b). In agreement with the notion that resting B lymphocytes constitute targets of IL-4, significant, albeit low, numbers of high-affinity receptors for IL-4 were detected on both mouse and human quiescent B cells (Ohara and Paul, 1987, Park et al., 1987; Zuber et al., 1990). In contrast, human IL-4 apparently fails to prepare resting human B cells for a more vigorous response to subsequent mitogenic stimuli (Gordon et al., 1988a; Shields et al., 1989) and has even been found to inhibit the growth signal delivered by mitogenic concentrations of anti-IgM antibodies (Gordon et al., 1989a).

IL-4 induces phenotypic alterations on quiescent B lymphocytes. A variety of surface markers, including sIgD, MHC class II molecules, Transferrin receptors, and IL-2 receptors, are modulated following *in vitro* activation of B cells with mitogenic substances (Kehrl et al., 1984). Similarly, IL-4 induces significant phenotypic alterations of resting B cells.

MHC class II antigens. Roehm et al. (1984) first reported that T cell-derived supernatants could increase the expression of MHC class II determinants on quiescent mouse B cells, independently of entry into G_2/M phase. Noelle et al. (1984, 1986) next demonstrated that IL-4 was responsible for this cytokine-mediated Ia increase. In contrast, IL-4 only poorly enhanced the expression of MHC class II antigens on normal human B cells (Diu et al., 1990; Defrance et al., unpublished results). The high density of MHC class II determinants constitutively expressed on resting human B cells prevents further upregulation by IL-4. In line with such an hypothesis, some Burkitt's lymphoma cell lines constitutively expressing low levels of MHC class II antigens have been shown to be inducible by IL-4 for DQ expression (Rousset et al., 1988).

CD23. CD23 the low affinity receptor for the Fc portion of IgE (FcεRII) (Yukawa et al., 1987; Bonnefoy et al., 1987), is expressed at low density on a subpopulation of human and mouse B cells. Surface expression of this antigen can be enhanced by polyclonal B cell activators, such as phorbol myristate acetate (PMA; Walker et al., 1986) or EBV (Thorley-Lawson et al., 1985) in man; LPS in mouse (Conrad et al., 1988); and most dramatically by IL-4 in both species (Defrance et al., 1987a; Hudak et al., 1987). Two species of CD23/FcεRII have been identified, FcεRIIa and FcεRIIb, which differ by the amino acid sequence of their N-terminal cytoplasmic portion and by their cellular distribution (Yokota *et al.*, 1988). Both forms of CD23 can be found on human B cells, but only FcεRIIa is constitutively expressed on B cells and B cell lines. Upon IL-4 stimulation, FcεRIIb is induced and the expression of FcεRIIa is increased. In human and mouse, CD23 (FcεRIIa) expression appears to be restricted to the mature virgin (sIgM$^+$, sIgD$^+$) B cell population (Kikutani *et al.*, 1986; Kehry and Hudak, 1989). CD23 is irreversibly lost after isotype switching and cannot be reinduced by IL-4 on memory B cells (Kikutani *et al.*, 1986; Armitage and Goff, 1988).

LFA1, LFA3, sIgM and CD40. IL-4 was found to specifically enhance leucocyte function adhesion antigen 1 and 3 (LFA-1 and LFA-3) expression on certain Burkitt's lymphoma cell lines characterized by a reduced or absent expression of these adhesion molecules (Rousset *et al.*, 1989). IL-4 enhances sIgM expression on mature human B cells without affecting expression of sIgD (Shields *et al.*, 1989). This appears not to be associated with an increased responsiveness of B cells to Ig-mediated signalling. In contrast, only modest IL-4 mediated increases of surface Igs are observed on murine B cells (Hudak *et al.*, 1987). IL-4 was found to enhance expression of CD40 on resting B cells (Gordon *et al.*, 1988a; Vallé *et al.*, 1989). CD40 is a 50 kD glycoprotein expressed on human B cells (Clark and Ledbetter, 1989), which delivers both competence (Gordon *et al.*, 1988a) and progression signals (Banchereau *et al.*, 1990) to human B cells.

Fcγ receptors. B lymphocyte receptors for the Fc portion of IgG (FcγRII/CD32) are involved in the regulation of immune responses since they are able to deliver inhibitory signals that control B cell activation (Kolsch *et al.*, 1980). Occupancy of these receptors by antigen–antibody complexes is likely to represent a natural mechanism of negative feedback control on Ig synthesis. Ligands which are able to bind simultaneously to surface Igs and FcγRII, such as intact anti-Ig antibodies, strongly inhibit activation, proliferation and differentiation of murine B cells (Bijsterbosch and Klaus, 1985). It has been demonstrated that IL-4 overcomes the negative signal delivered through FcγRII on mouse B cells by inducing both downregulation of FcγRII expression and a loss of their binding capacity (O'Garra *et al.*, 1987; Phillips *et al.*, 1988; Lazlo and Dickler, 1988).

IFN antagonizes IL-4-mediated activation of B cells. IFN-γ inhibits, both in mouse and human, IL-4 induced upregulation of MHC class II antigens and hyperexpression of CD23 (Mond *et al.*, 1986; Defrance *et al.* 1987a; Hudak *et al.*, 1987; Rousset *et al.*, 1988). In the murine system, IFN-γ also suppresses the IL-4 mediated cell volume enlargement and sensitization of resting B cells to accelerated DNA synthesis in response to mitogenic stimuli (Rabin *et al.*, 1986b).

Activation of B cells by IL-4: synthesis. The experimental findings described above suggest that IL-4 drives quiescent B cells to an intermediate state of activation (provisionally designated as G_0') between G_0 and G_1, which is characterized by several important functional and phenotypic modifications (see Table 1). The contribution of IL-4 to the early phase of B cell activation can be summarized in three points:

(i) IL-4 enhances the efficiency of antigen presentation by B cells. It upregulates expression of three sets of surface molecules involved either in binding (sIgM) or in presentation of the antigen (MHC class II molecules and CD23). The rôle of CD23/FcεRII in antigen presentation was recently suggested by Kehry and Yamashita (1989) who demonstrated that antigen-specific IgE bound by the mean of CD23 allows a 100-fold reduction in the concentration of antigen required for effective antigen presentation to antigen specific T cells.

(ii) IL-4 reinforces cellular interactions between T and B cells. As previously mentioned, T–B cell interactions occur via complementary structures on T and B cells. Apart from the B cell associated adhesion

Table 1 Phenotypic alterations associated with B cell activation.[a]

	IL-4 (G_0')		Polyclonal B cell activators (G_1)	
	Human	Mouse	Human	Mouse
sIgM	↑	→	→	→
sIgD	→	→	↓	↓
FcεRII/CD23	↑	↑	↑ [b]	↑ [b]
FcγRII	?	↓	?	↑
LFA-1, LFA-3	↑ [c]	?	?	?
MHC class II antigens	↑	↑	↑	↑
IL-2 receptor p55 chain	?	?	↑	↑
IL-2 receptor p70/75 chain	?	↑ [d]	↑	↑
CD5	↓ [e]	?	→ or ↑ [f]	?
CD40	↑	?	↑	?

[a] ↑ = upregulation; ↓ = downregulation; → = no effect; ? = not known.
[b] Enhancement of CD23 expression by PBA is moderate compared to that induced by IL-4.
[c] Enhanced expression of LFA-1, LFA-3 antigens is only detectable on certain Burkitt lymphoma cell lines.
[d] According to Loughnan and Nossal (1989).
[e] According to Defrance *et al.* (1989) and Freedman *et al.* (1989).
[f] Anti-Ig reagents do not alter CD5 expression on B cells, whereas PMA strongly upregulates its expression.

molecules described above (LFA-3, ICAM1), the MHC class II antigens are obviously important elements for T–B recognition since they can interact with two types of structures expressed on T cells, the T cell receptor complex and CD4. In this respect, IL-4 mediated upregulation of LFA-3 and MHC class II antigens probably contributes to strengthen the interactions necessary for effective collaboration between T and B cells. Additionally, the observation that the extracellular part of CD23 presents some homology with the lectin family (Gordon *et al.*, 1989b) leaves open the possibility that the high levels of CD23 induced by IL-4 stimulation could also be available for binding to surface molecules on the adjacent T helper cell. The notion that IL-4 reinforces T–B interactions has been elegantly demonstrated by Sanders *et al.* (1987), who showed that murine IL-4 augments the formation of T–B cell conjugates.

(iii) IL-4 prepares resting B cells for optimal expansion in response to growth factors. The IL-4 mediated optimization of B cell responses to growth factors can be related to its dual capacity to prime B cells for accelerated entry into cycle and to modulate expression of surface antigens that could potentially mediate proliferative signals. Five sets of membrane molecules (whose expression is affected by IL-4) may contribute to progression of B cells through S and G_2/M phases of the cell cycle:

(1) *sIgM*: A heightened expression of sIgM will increase the antigen binding capacity of B cells and subsequent signalling through sIgM.

(2) *MHC class II molecules*: Cambier and Lehmann (1989) recently demonstrated that murine B cells primed with anti-μ and IL-4 can undergo proliferation upon challenging with immobilized anti-Ia antibodies. Thus, it is tempting to speculate that concomitant triggering of B cells with IL-4 and antigen and subsequent crosslinking of Ia molecules by the T cell receptor/CD4 complex would provide reciprocal activation signals to both cell types and would allow B cell proliferation. In return, the release of B cell stimulating cytokines by the activated helper T cell would permit the maturation process of B cells.

(3) *CD40*: Increased levels of CD40 could amplify the progression signal delivered by its natural ligand.

(4) *CD23*: The intact form as well as the cleavage products of this molecule can stimulate growth of human B cells (Gordon *et al.*, 1989b). Interestingly, IL-4 not only upregulates surface expression of CD23 but also induces the shedding of its soluble products (Bonnefoy *et al.*, 1988; Delespesse *et al.*, 1989).

(5) *FcγRII/CD32*: The capacity of IL-4 to inactivate the negative signalling via FcγRII prevents inhibition of the B cell maturation process by antigen–antibody complexes.

Therefore, stimulation of resting B cells with IL-4 generates a multiplicity of cellular events which all contribute towards the B cell activation process initiated by binding of antigen to surface Ig receptors. The observation that IL-4 can stimulate virtually all B cells to achieve a certain level of activation might appear to conflict with the maintenance of the specificity of the immune response. It may be assumed that complete activation of bystander B cells is prevented by the fact that IL-4 only provides part of the activation signal necessary for responsiveness to progression and maturation factors, the other part being provided by cognate interactions with antigen and the antigen-specific T helper cell. However, polyclonal B cell responses could occur in situations in which antigen concentrations are massive, therefore allowing non-specific trapping of antigen molecules by B cells.

Interferon γ and interleukin 1

IFN-γ and IL-1 have both been described to prime human B cells for accelerated entry into cycle (Boyd et al., 1987; Freedman et al., 1988). According to Freedman et al. (1988), IL-1 would not modify the time course of the secondary response but would recruit more cells to undergo proliferation in response to mitogenic stimuli. Combinations of IL-1 and IFN-γ did not result in a potentiation of the priming effect exerted by each factor alone. The state of B cell activation induced by IFN-γ is not characterized yet, but, for IL-1, none of the early activation events attendant to anti-Ig stimulation (Ca^{2+} mobilization, cell volume increase, augmented RNA content) was affected. Similarly, none of the most characteristic phenotypic changes associated with IL-4 stimulation, namely upregulation of CD23 or MHC class II antigens, was found upon priming with IL-1 (Freedman et al., 1988).

Interleukin 5

Despite the fact that IL-5 is generally reported to be a late-acting factor (see paragraph on B cell proliferation), receptors for this cytokine are also expressed on quiescent mouse B cells. This was first demonstrated by Loughnan et al. (1987), who showed that IL-5 can induce expression of the p55 chain of the IL-2 receptor complex on resting mouse B cells, and this was further supported by Karasuyama et al. (1988), who showed that murine B cells directly mature into Ig-secreting cells upon exposure to IL-5. Moreover, according to Loughnan and Nossal (1989), expression of the p55 and p70/75 components of the IL-2 receptor complex would be under the control of IL-5 and IL-4, respectively; both cytokines being required to allow B cell proliferation in response to IL-2. This finding implies the existence of a novel B cell activation pathway in which B cells could be excited from their resting state and rendered responsive to progression factors, such as IL-2, by the sole combination of IL-4 and IL-5.

Complement fraction C3d

C3d is one of the proteolytic fragments of the third component of complement. Its surface receptor on B cells is CR2 (CD21), which has also been identified as a receptor for EBV in man. Antibodies directed against this antigen have been shown to stimulate proliferation of normal resting B cells (Clark and Ledbetter, 1989). According to Carter and Fearon (1989), C3d exerts a priming effect on human B cells. The proliferative response to mitogenic concentrations of anti-IgM is initiated 24 h earlier in resting B cells pretreated with polymerized C3d than in control cultures. Crosslinking of CD21 appears to be a requisite condition for priming since monomeric C3d was found to be inactive.

Cytokines and B cell proliferation

Interleukin 4

The nature of the activation stimulus is critical for the development of the growth promoting activity of IL-4.
Anti-Ig antibodies and immobilized particles of Staphylococcus aureus Cowan *(SAC).* Both murine and human IL-4 co-stimulate with anti-IgM antibodies to induce B cell proliferation (Howard *et al.*, 1982; Defrance *et al.*, 1987b). Whereas murine IL-4 would mostly act as a competence factor, human IL-4 rather acts as a progression factor, since it induces proliferation of B cells preactivated with anti-Ig antibodies (Defrance *et al.*, 1987b). Unlike IL-2, IL-4 fails to support DNA synthesis by human B cells co-stimulated with SAC (Jelinek and Lipsky, 1988; Defrance *et al.*, unpublished observations). However, a delayed addition of IL-4 to SAC-stimulated B cells results in an enhancement of B cell proliferation and, accordingly, SAC preactivated B cells proliferate in response to IL-4 (Defrance *et al.*, unpublished observations). The IL-4 induced proliferation of anti-Ig and SAC-stimulated B cells is short-lasting and probably involves only a subpopulation of B cells which remains to be identified.
Phorbol esters with or without calcium ionophore. The early addition of IL-4 to human B cells stimulated with mitogenic concentrations of phorbol

dibutyrate (PdBu) results in a consistent inhibition of the proliferative response elicited by this stimulating agent (Gordon *et al.*, 1988b). As observed with SAC, B cell growth is enhanced when addition of IL-4 to B cells activated with PdBu is delayed by 24 h (Gordon *et al.*, 1988b). Accordingly, IL-4 can also induce proliferation of human B cells pre-activated with combinations of PdBu and a calcium ionophore (Gordon *et al.*, 1987; Defrance *et al.*, unpublished data). No plausible explanation has been provided yet for the contrasting effects of IL-4 on PdBu driven proliferation of B cells.

LPS and dextran sulphate. Although LPS activated murine B cells can be induced by IL-4 to synthesize IgG1 and IgE, no enhancement of B cell proliferation is observed in B cell blasts obtained by pre-stimulation with LPS or LPS plus anti-Ig antibodies, upon exposure to IL-4 (Swain *et al.*, 1988). Unlike IL-5, IL-4 does not promote the proliferation of mouse B cells activated with dextran sulphate (Swain *et al.*, 1988).

Anti-CD40 antibodies. Monoclonal antibodies directed against the CD40 antigen display agonistic activities on human B cells (Clark and Ledbetter, 1986; Gordon *et al.*, 1988a; Vallé *et al.*, 1989) and combinations of IL-4 and anti-CD40 mAb are synergistic for maintaining DNA synthesis in pre-activated B cells (Gordon *et al.*, 1987). While soluble anti-CD40 antibodies are not mitogenic by themselves, we recently found that immobilized anti-CD40 antibodies induce a strong and long lasting proliferation of resting human B cells (Banchereau *et al.*, 1990). The induced proliferation is of greater amplitude than that observed with any other polyclonal B cell activator, in terms of both the proportion of cells recruited to enter into cycle and the duration of the response. IL-4 strongly enhances the anti-CD40 dependent B cell proliferation. Upon regular splitting of the cultures every 5–7 days, a cumulative expansion by 150 to 400-fold of the input B cells can be reached after 35 days. These factor-dependent cell lines are not transformed by EBV. This observation demonstrates that human IL-4 is a B cell growth factor.

Antigens. The relevance of the above findings obtained with polyclonally-activated B cells has been questioned by studies performed in antigen-driven systems. In a single cell assay system (Alderson *et al.*, 1987a), IL-4 was found to stimulate the clonal expansion of a single B cell activated by its specific TI-2 antigen. According to the studies of Stein *et al.* (1986), TD antigens used in association with IL-4 cannot promote B cell proliferation until carrier-specific T cells are provided.

Altogether, the experimental findings described above (summarized in Table 2) suggest that the effects of IL-4 on B cell proliferation depend upon the nature of the activation stimulus.

Table 2 IL-4 can induce or inhibit human B cell proliferation depending upon the mode of activation.

	Polyclonal B cell activators			
	SAC	Insolubilized anti-IgM antibodies	Phorbol esters	Immobilized anti-CD40 mAb
Co-stimulation assay[a]	No effect	Stimulatory	Inhibitory	Stimulatory
Re-stimulation assay[b]	Stimulatory	Stimulatory	Stimulatory	Stimulatory

[a] IL-4 resting B cells are cultured with the polyclonal B cell activator and IL-4.
[b] B cells are first cultured with the PBA, then with IL-4.

IL-4 and leukaemic B cells. Mature human B cell neoplasms have been shown to proliferate *in vitro* in response to several recombinant cytokines including IL-2 (Lantz *et al.*, 1985), tumour necrosis factor α (TNF-α; Digel *et al.*, 1989), IL-6 (Kawano *et al.*, 1988a; Yee *et al.*, 1989), IFN-γ (Östlund *et al.*, 1986) or LMW BCGF (Ford *et al.*, 1985a,b). In contrast, the vast majority of mature B cell leukaemia samples (B-CLL and non-Hodgkin's malignant lymphomas) failed to enter into cycle in response to combinations of IL-4 and anti-IgM or SAC (Karray *et al.*, 1988; Defrance *et al.*, unpublished results). This unresponsiveness is not due to a defect in their expression of functional IL-4 receptors, since IL-4 induces these cells to express CD23 (Karray *et al.*, 1988).

It is striking that IL-4 is able to stimulate DNA synthesis in leukaemic B cells activated with phorbol esters (PdBu/ionomycin) or immobilized anti-CD40 mAb (Defrance *et al.*, unpublished results). In the mouse, some but not all sublines of the murine BCL-1 tumour have been shown to proliferate in response to IL-4 (Swain *et al.*, 1988; O'Garra *et al.*, 1989).

Is the growth-promoting effect of IL-4 linked to the production of autocrine B cell stimulatory factors? Whether IL-4 exerts its growth-promoting activity via endogenous release of stimulatory molecules is presently a matter of debate. The most likely candidate for such an autocrine B cell growth factor activity would be a soluble form of FcεRII/CD23 as: (i) IL-4 specifically upregulates CD23 expression on B cells (Defrance *et al.*, 1987b; Hudak *et al.*, 1987) and stimulates the release of its soluble forms (Bonnefoy *et al.*, 1988; Cairns *et al.*, 1988); (ii) lymphoblastoid cell lines constitutively express high amounts of CD23 (Thorley-Lawson and Mann, 1985) and spontaneously produce truncated forms of this antigen (Thorley-Lawson *et al.*,

1986); (iii) the shed form of CD23, when purified to homogeneity, can act as a growth factor for EBV-transformed cell lines and normal B cells (Swende-man and Thorley-Lawson; 1987). However, the ability of soluble CD23 to support B cell growth could not be reproduced with the recombinant form of the molecule in B cell assays performed with anti-IgM antibodies (Uchi-bayashi *et al.*, 1989). According to Cairns and Gordon (personal communi-cation), the cleavage fragments of CD23 would be very labile and the intact form of the molecule could act as a membrane-anchored growth factor for human B cells. The possibility that other known cytokines could be involved in IL-4 dependent proliferation of B cells is suggested by the observation that IL-4 stimulates production of IL-6 (Smeland *et al.*, 1989; Denoroy *et al.*, 1990a) by normal human B cells and lymphoblastoid cell lines. Although IL-6 could not directly promote growth of normal human B cells (Defrance *et al.*, unpublished results), it cannot be excluded that combinations of IL-6, soluble CD23 and other B cell-derived regulatory molecules could account for the B cell growth activity of IL-4.

Interplay of IL-4 and other cytokines on B cell growth. Since several cytokines exert stimulatory effects on B cells, their combinations with IL-4 have been tested for induction of B cell proliferation (Tables 3 and 4) as follows;

(i) *IL-1*. The capacity of IL-1 to cooperate with IL-4, reported in the murine system (Howard *et al.*, 1983; Stein *et al.*, 1986) has not been demonstrated with human B cells. Stein *et al.* (1986) have shown, in an antigen-specific culture system, that the proliferative response of mouse B cells to TI-2 antigen and IL-4 is enhanced by IL-1. In contrast, studies performed in a single cell assay system (Alderson *et al.*, 1987a) did not confirm these data. Thus the synergy observed between IL-1 and IL-4 may involve participation of another cell type (a specific B cell subset, or a non-B cell population).

(ii) *IFN-γ*. In the mouse, IFN-γ suppresses the proliferative response of B cells elicited by IL-4 used in combination with anti-Ig antibodies (Mond *et*

Table 3 Human IL-4 can display antagonistic or additive effects on the B cell growth-promoting effect of IL-2.

Polyclonal B cell activators	Effect of IL-4 on IL-2 driven proliferation of B cells
SAC	Antagonism
Immobilized anti-IgM antibodies	Antagonism
Phorbol esters	Additivity
Immobilized anti-CD40 mAb	Additivity

Table 4   Interplay of IL-4 and other cytokines on B cell growth.[a]

	Mouse	Human
IL-1	↑	→
IL-2	↓	↑ or ↓ [b]
IL-3	?	→
IL-5	↑ [c]	→
IL-6	?	→
IL-7	?	→
IFN-γ	↓	↑
TNFα	?	↑
G-CSF	?	→
GM-CSF	?	→

[a] ↑ = stimulation; → = no effect; ↓ = inhibition; ? = not known.
[b] IL-4 potentiates or antagonizes the IL-2 driven proliferation of human B cells depending on the mode of B cell activation (see Table 3).
[c] On the BCL-1 lymphoma cell line.

al., 1985a) or antigen (Stein *et al.*, 1986). In contrast, in the human system IFN-γ, which can stimulate B cell growth by itself (Romagnani *et al.*, 1986a,b; Defrance *et al.*, 1986), enhances the growth promoting effect of IL-4 on B cells activated with anti-Ig reagents (Defrance *et al.*, 1987b) or immobilized anti-CD40 mAb (Rousset *et al.*, unpublished data). Since the inhibitory effect of IFN-γ on IL-4 driven proliferative responses of mouse B cells was observed with soluble, but not with insolubilized anti-Ig antibodies, it is likely that the discrepancies between mouse and human models might originate from differences in the assay systems.

(iii) *IL-2*. Combined additions of IL-4 and IL-2 to human B cells showed that IL-4 could also deliver inhibitory signals to B cells. IL-4 was found to antagonize IL-2 dependent proliferation of normal human B cells (Defrance *et al.*, 1988; Jelinek and Lipsky, 1988) and leukaemic human B cells, such as B-CLL (Karray *et al.*, 1988) and non Hodgkin's B lymphomas (Defrance *et al.*, 1990a) activated by anti-Ig reagents. Similar data were recently obtained with normal mouse B cells (Rolink *et al.*, 1989) and with the murine B lymphoma BCL-1 (Tigges *et al.*, 1989). The possibility that IL-4 might modulate expression of the IL-2 receptor complex has been explored by several investigators, but these studies reached different conclusions. According to Nakanishi *et al.* (1989) and Fernandez-Botran *et al.* (1989), IL-4 downregulates expression of high affinity IL-2 binding sites on B and T cells, whereas Tigges *et al.* (1989) conclude that IL-4 does not affect the IL-2 receptor in terms of number of binding sites and capacity to internalize IL-2.

IL-4 does not block the growth-promoting activity of IL-2 when human B cells are activated with phorbol esters (PdBu/ionomycin) (Carlsson *et al.*,

1989; Defrance *et al.*, unpublished results) or with an immobilized anti-CD40 mAb (Defrance *et al.*, unpublished results). In such culture systems, combinations of IL-4 and IL-2 display additive effects on proliferation of normal and leukaemic human B cells. The possibility that IL-4 could under certain conditions enhance the B cell growth-promoting activity of IL-2 is in accordance with the recent report of Loughnan and Nossal (1989) showing that murine IL-4 could specifically upregulate the p70 subunit of the IL-2 receptor complex. Altogether, these observations indicate that the outcome of IL-4 binding to its receptor on IL-2 responsiveness of B cells is dependent upon the nature of the activation stimulus. Since different sets of surface molecules can transduce activation signals to B cells (Clark and Ledbetter, 1989), it is tempting to speculate that the nature of the interactions between B cells and their microenvironment may govern the nature of the IL-4 effect (stimulatory or inhibitory).

Other cytokines. IL-4 has been consistently observed both in mice (Ennist *et al.*, 1987a,b) and in human B cells (Defrance *et al.*, 1987b) to cooperate with a partially purified preparation of a (12 kD) LMW BCGF (Ford *et al.*, 1981; Sharma *et al.*, 1987). However, the commercially available preparation of this product (Cellular Products, Buffalo, USA) was found to contain several cytokines including TNF-α, GM-CSF, M-CSF, IL-2, IL-1, IFN-γ and IL-3, which might participate in the observed results. Nevertheless, the cooperation between IL-4 and LMW BCGF has been confirmed using the recombinant material (S. Sharma, personal communication).

IL-4 and TNF-α cooperate to induce the proliferation of SAC activated B cells (B. Dugas, personal communication).

Human IL-3, IL-6, IL-7, GM-CSF and G-CSF fail to modulate the growth promoting activity of IL-4 on normal B cells (Defrance *et al.*, unpublished results). Although one report (O'Garra *et al.*, 1989) has suggested that IL-4 and IL-5 could cooperate in stimulating growth of the murine BCL-1 lymphoma cell line, no evidence for such an effect on normal murine B cell growth has been published.

Interleukin 2

Murine and human B cells display different activation requirements to acquire responsiveness to IL-2. The description of the expression of IL-2 receptors on B cells preceded the demonstration of the B cell growth-promoting effect of IL-2. The possibility that IL-2 could play a role in B cell functions was initially suggested by pioneering studies performed by Malek *et al.* (1983) and Tsudo *et al.* (1984), who demonstrated that antibodies directed against the murine or the human IL-2 receptor (Tac/CD25), respectively, could stain *in vitro* activated B cells. These initial observations were confirmed and extended and the B cell growth factor activity of IL-2 is now widely accepted. Several polyclonal B cell activators, including SAC, anti-IgM antibodies, phorbol esters or EBV, have been shown to induce expression of functional IL-2 receptors on human B cells and to allow their subsequent entry into cycle upon exposure to IL-2 (Jung *et al.*, 1984; Mingari *et al.*, 1984; Boyd *et al.*, 1985; Muraguchi *et al.*, 1985; Mittler *et al.*, 1985; Suzuki and Cooper, 1985). IL-2 recruits a larger proportion of anti-IgM activated human B cells to enter S and G_2/M phases than IL-4 (Defrance *et al.*, 1988). However, IL-2 displays only a weak growth-promoting effect on B cells stimulated with immobilized anti-CD40 mAb (Rousset *et al.*, unpublished results). Mouse B cells are less easily inducible for IL-2 receptor expression than human B cells, as LPS (Zubler *et al.*, 1984) or anti-Ig antibodies (Mond *et al.*, 1985b) do not allow B cells to respond to IL-2. Expression of functional IL-2 receptors on murine B cells necessitates at least two activation signals such as those provided by anti-Ig antibodies plus LPS (Zubler *et al.*, 1984) or LPS plus anti-Ig antibodies plus a source of α factors (Karasuyama *et al.*, 1988). Nakanishi *et al.* (1984) first showed that upon concomitant stimulation with anti-IgM antibodies, IL-4 and a T cell derived factor (B15-TRF), murine B cells could express determinants reacting with mAbs specific for the murine IL-2 receptor. The notion that cytokines could play a major rôle in modulation of expression of the IL-2 receptor in mouse was further supported by several studies demonstrating that IL-5 could induce IL-2 receptor expression on murine B cells (Harada *et al.*, 1985; Loughnan *et al.*, 1987; Nakanishi *et al.*, 1988; Loughnan and Nossal, 1989).

Consistent with a physiological rôle of IL-2 in B cell proliferation, Pike *et al.* (1984) showed that IL-2 can induce clonal expansion of murine B cells activated by antigen in a single cell assay system.

Effects of IL-2 on resting and in vivo *activated B cells.* The capacity of IL-2 to trigger proliferation of B cells in absence of an *in vitro* activation signal has been a matter of controversy. Bich Thuy and Fauci (1985, 1986) showed that normal human B cells can spontaneously proliferate and differentiate in response to high concentrations of IL-2. In agreement with the notion that certain B cell populations could spontaneously respond to IL-2, Mond *et al.* (1985b) reported that IL-2 could stimulate proliferation of large, presumably *in vivo* activated murine B cells, but these observations were challenged by Julius *et al.* (1987).

Recent data about the structure of the IL-2 receptor permit clarification of the issue. It is now admitted that the IL-2 receptor is composed of at least two proteins: the p55 chain (also known as Tac or CD25), which binds IL-2 with a low affinity and does not transduce intracellular signals, and the p70/75 chain, which binds IL-2 with an intermediate affinity and which is responsible for transduction of the mitogenic signals (Hatakeyama *et al.*, 1989). The non-covalent association of both proteins results in the formation of a high affinity receptor. The selective expression of the p70/75 IL-2 receptor protein on *in vivo* activated B cells (Tanaka *et al.*, 1988) correlates with their response to high concentrations of IL-2, and the proliferative response of *in vitro* activated B cells to low concentrations of IL-2 correlates with their expression of high affinity IL-2 receptors (Saiki *et al.*, 1988). It should be noted that the structure of functional IL-2 receptors might be more complex than the heterodimer (p55; p70/75) described above, since Saragovi and Malek (1987) have proposed a model of murine IL-2 receptor including three polypeptide chains.

IL-2 and leukaemic B cell proliferation. IL-2 has been shown to stimulate *in vitro* proliferation of a majority of chronic lymphocytic leukaemia B cell samples upon activation with anti-Ig reagents (Lantz *et al.*, 1985; Karray *et al.*, 1987) or phorbol esters (Kabelitz *et al.*, 1985). Other mature B cell neoplasms, such as non Hodgkin's B lymphomas (Defrance *et al.*, unpublished results), and hairy-cell leukaemias (Korsmeyer *et al.*, 1983) were also found to proliferate in response to IL-2 after polyclonal activation. Moreover, in a significant proportion of these leukaemias, spontaneous B cell growth could be observed upon exposure to IL-2, without requiring *in vitro* pre-activation (Karray *et al.*, 1987; Malkovska *et al.*, 1987; Murphy *et al.*, 1987). Expression of the IL-2 receptors on leukaemic B cells is very heterogeneous, but no correlation has been found between the clinical stage of the patient and the levels of spontaneous expression of Tac (Malkovska *et al.*, 1987). Thus, it is presently unlikely that IL-2 might be the key factor involved in the expansion of the leukaemic B cell clone. However, the possible triggering of leukaemic B cell proliferation should be taken into account in the treatment of malignant B cell tumours by high doses of IL-2.

Certain subclones of the murine B lymphoma cell line BCL-1 under defined *in vitro* culture conditions exhibit a proliferative response to IL-2 (Loughnan and Nossal, 1989; Tigges *et al.*, 1989).

Interplay of IL-2 and other cytokines on B cell growth.
IL-4 and IL-5. The regulatory functions exerted by IL-4 on IL-2 driven proliferation of human B cells has been discussed before (see above). However, it remains to be determined whether IL-4 and IL-2 act on different B cell subpopulations or whether they act at different stages of B cell activation. The great majority of mature B cell neoplasms have the capacity to proliferate *in vitro*, in response to IL-2, but not in response to IL-4, despite the fact that IL-4 can enhance CD23 expression and suppress the growth promoting effect of IL-2 on these cells (Karray *et al.*, 1988;

Defrance *et al.*, unpublished results). In this respect, the pattern of response of leukaemic B cells to IL-4 and IL-2 would argue in favour of the existence of at least two different B cell subsets: a B cell population (from which B-CLL would originate) proliferating in response to IL-2 and not to IL-4, but sensitive to the growth inhibitory effect of IL-4; and a second B cell population proliferating exclusively in response to IL-4. In the mouse, it has been shown that IL-2 and IL-4 are produced by two different types of helper T cells (T$_{H1}$ and T$_{H2}$) regulating different sets of immune responses (Mosmann and Coffman, 1989). Consequently, the inhibitory effect of IL-4 on IL-2 driven proliferation of B cells could be considered as a regulatory mechanism by which a T$_{H1}$ type mediated humoral response would be controlled at the B cell level by a specific T$_{H2}$ product.

Several lines of evidence suggest that IL-5 can modulate the response of B cells to IL-2. Indeed, it has been demonstrated in the mouse that IL-5 could induce IL-2 receptor expression on B cells (Harada *et al.*, 1987; Loughnan *et al.*, 1987; Nakanishi *et al.*, 1988) and render them responsive to the growth promoting effect of IL-2. According to Loughnan and Nossal (1989), IL-4 and IL-5 would stimulate expression of the p70/75 and p55 chains of the IL-2 receptor complex, respectively, and as such would both be required for induction of high affinity IL-2 receptors on mouse B cells.

Until now, no published data support the notion that human IL-5 shares with its murine homologue the capacity to potentiate the growth-promoting activity of IL-2. It remains that human IL-5 was found to increase p55 (Tac) expression on SAC pre-activated B cells (Brière *et al.*, 1990). Moreover, two different groups have described a 50 kD T cell derived factor able to stimulate p55 expression (Kawano *et al.*, 1987, 1988b; Vazquez *et al.*, 1987) and to cooperate with IL-2 for proliferation of human B cells, but the identity of this factor with IL-5 remains to be determined.

IFN-γ, TNF and LMW BCGF. A synergistic effect between IL-2 and IFN-γ (Jelinek *et al.*, 1986; Karray *et al.*, 1987; Jelinek and Lipsky, 1987b) and IL-2 and TNF-α (Jelinek and Lipsky, 1987c) for human B cell proliferation has been reported. It has also been suggested that IL-2 and the partially purified preparation of LMW BCGF could cooperate for B cell proliferation (Jelinek and Lipsky, 1987b). However, these experimental findings need to be reproduced with recombinant LMW BCGF.

Lack of effects of IL-2 in vivo. The recent results obtained with IL-2 *in vivo* failed to illustrate an effect on the B lymphocyte pool. *In vivo* administration of IL-2 to patients does not induce an increase in the absolute number of peripheral blood B lymphocytes, but rather results in a decrease in their relative numbers, as CD8$^+$ T cells and CD3$^-$ NK cell numbers increase (Favrot *et al.*, 1990). Accordingly, hybrid mice carrying both IL-2 and

Tac/CD25 transgenes display unusually high proportions of Thy 1^+/CD3$^-$ large granular lymphocytes with elevated NK activity (Ishida et al., 1989). This indicates either that IL-2 has no effect on the in vivo development of B cells in mice, or that the parameters of these in vivo experiments (e.g. lack of specific B cell activation) may not have been appropriate to reveal the effects of IL-2 on the B cell compartment.

Interleukin 5

BCGF-II and TRF-1 (T cell replacing factor) are interleukin 5. IL-5 (formerly BCGF-II/TRF-1/EDF) was originally described by Swain and Dutton (1982) as a growth factor for the murine BCL-1 lymphoma cell line. The pattern of reactivity of IL-5 in different biological assays clearly distinguishes it from IL-4. Interleukin 5 does not cause proliferation of normal mouse B cells co-stimulated with anti-Ig but stimulates the proliferation of normal B cells activated with dextran sulphate (Swain et al., 1983). BCGF-II was next found to be identical to TRF-1 (Hara et al., 1985) which was previously characterized as stimulating antigen-specific antibody responses from antigen-primed mice (Harada et al., 1985). Isolation of the cDNA encoding mouse TRF (Kinashi et al., 1986) definitively established that both BCGF-II activity and TRF activity were borne by the same molecular entity, for which the name interleukin 5 was proposed. Activities described as eosinophil differentiation factor (EDF) (O'Garra et al., 1986; Campbell et al., 1987), BCDFμ (Vitetta et al., 1984), and killer helper factor (KHF) (Takatsu et al., 1987) can also be attributed to IL-5.

IL-5 is a late-acting B cell growth factor. In most models of the growth requirements for murine B cells, IL-4 has been ascribed a role in the early phases of B cell activation, whereas IL-5 acts preferentially in the later steps. This is supported by the following observations:

(i) IL-5 is not active in co-stimulatory assays performed with anti-Ig antibodies which permit determination of the growth promoting activity of IL-4 (Swain et al., 1983; Harada et al., 1985; O'Garra et al., 1986). In contrast, conditions which stimulate cells to leave G_0 and progress through G_1 (such as pre-exposure of B cells to mitogenic concentrations of anti-Ig for 36–48 h) allow responsiveness to IL-5 (O'Garra et al., 1986; Müller et al., 1985);

(ii) IL-5 can promote spontaneous proliferation of large in vivo activated B cells, but is ineffective on small resting B cells (Nakajima et al., 1985; O'Garra et al., 1986);

(iii) According to Karasuyama et al. (1988), IL-5 behaves as a β factor acting late in the G_2 phase to allow completion of the cell cycle. Moreover,

Table 5 Effect of different activation protocols on the responsiveness of murine B cells to IL-5.[a]

Anti-Ig co-stimulation	→
Anti-Ig re-stimulation	↑
Phorbol ester + Ca^{2+} ionophore	→
Dextran sulphate	↑
LPS + anti-Ig + α factors	↑
Polyribitol ribosyl phosphate	↑
In vivo activation	↑

[a] → = no proliferative response; ↑ = stimulation of B cell growth.

as demonstrated for IL-4 and IL-2, IL-5 may act together with T-independent (TI-1) antigens to promote clone formation of single antigen specific B cells (Alderson *et al.*, 1987b). The stimuli necessary for murine B cells to proliferate in response to IL-5 are summarized in Table 5.

Is IL-5 a growth factor for human B cells? A few candidates for a human equivalent of murine BCGF-II were proposed before the cloning of the IL-5 specific cDNA. For example, Yoshizaki *et al.* (1983) have described a 40–50 kD T cell derived factor promoting the proliferation of chronic lymphocytic leukaemia B cells (B-CLL) activated with anti-idiotypic antibodies and able to synergize with a 17 kD BCGF for the growth of anti-IgM activated normal B cells. Similarly, Shimizu *et al.* (1985) reported an activity produced by HTLV-infected T cell lines with the following properties: (i) it was active in the murine BCGF-II assays, (ii) it could stimulate growth of *in vivo* activated human B cells, (iii) it failed to support proliferation of anti-Ig co-stimulated normal B cells. However, the recombinant human IL-5 molecule, although able to stimulate eosinophil differentiation and activation (Sanderson *et al.*, 1988), failed to demonstrate any activity in several human B cell proliferation assays (Clutterbuck *et al.*, 1987). We confirmed these data and found that IL-5 could not stimulate the growth of *in vitro* activated B lymphomas (Defrance *et al.*, 1990a). Several possibilities may account for the lack of growth activity of IL-5 on human B cells: (i) IL-5 is not a B cell growth factor for higher mammals; (ii) the suitable mode of activation to detect activity of IL-5 on human B cells (equivalent to dextran sulphate) has not been found yet; (iii) IL-5 selectively stimulates the proliferation of a B cell subset that might be poorly represented within the B cell populations studied in man.

Is the action of IL-5 restricted to a subpopulation of B cells? Certain studies have dealt with the possibility that CD5[+] B cells could be the preferential target of IL-5. CD5 (Ly-1) is a pan-T cell antigen, whose expression on certain murine B cells may delineate a B cell subset originating from progenitors distinct from those yielding the "conventional" CD5$^-$ B cell population (Hayakawa and Hardy, 1988). The first element which suggested a possible association between IL-5 and CD5$^+$ B cells was the observation that the BCL-1 lymphoma cell line (read-out system for IL-5 activity) constitutively expresses CD5 (Hardy et al., 1984). Furthermore, some autoimmune strains of mice (NZB) are characterized by an enhanced proportion of CD5$^+$ B cells with large lymphoblastoid morphology in the spleen. These cells mount a spontaneous proliferative response to IL-5 and are more sensitive to the growth promoting effect of IL-5 than the conventional CD5$^-$ population (Umland et al., 1989). Wetzel et al. (1989) reported that low-density peritoneal B cells isolated from normal mice, which are mainly constituted of CD5$^+$ B cells, express IL-5 receptors and undergo clonal expansion upon IL-5 stimulation. CD5$^-$ B cells were also found to respond to IL-5, although to a lesser extent. Finally, a positive correlation exists between in vivo expression of IL-5 and selective expansion of B cells belonging to the CD5$^+$ population, since irradiated mice transplanted with bone marrow cells infected with a retrovirus bearing the IL-5 coding sequence display an expansion of their peritoneal CD5$^+$ B cell pool (Vaux et al., 1989). In man, CD5$^+$ B cells, either normal, as isolated from tonsils and cord blood, or leukaemic, such as B-CLL, constantly failed to proliferate in response to IL-5 (Defrance et al., unpublished results).

A partially purified human T cell derived 50 kD BCGF was found to share some properties with mouse IL-5 as it could induce proliferation of B cells isolated from patients with systemic lupus erythematosus (Delfraissy et al., 1986) and stimulate growth of CD5$^+$ tonsil B cells (Richard et al., 1987). This factor remains to be molecularly identified and is likely to be different from IL-5 which fails to display the latter activity.

Interferons

Interferons have been classified into three major classes—α, β and γ—on the basis of cell source, antigenicity and biochemical properties (de Maeyer and de Maeyer-Guignard, 1988). These molecules were characterized early on by their antiviral, antiproliferative and immunomodulatory properties. Whereas growth-inhibitory effects of interferons on lectin and antigen induced lymphocyte proliferation have been widely documented (Siegel et al., 1986), their reported effects on B cell functions are diverse and conflicting. With respect to B cell proliferation, interferons have been shown to display stimulatory and inhibitory activities depending on (i) the species (mouse versus human), (ii) the nature of the B cell population (leukaemic B cells or virus infected B cells versus normal B cells) and (iii) the

Table 6 Effects of IFN-γ on the proliferation of human B cells activated with various polyclonal B cell activators.[a]

	Co-stimulation assays	Re-stimulation assays
Anti-IgM	↑	→
SAC	↑	→
PMA	↑ or →[b]	?
EBV	↓	→

[a] ↑ = enhancement of proliferation; → = no effect; ↓ = growth-inhibitory effect; ? = not known.
[b] Stimulation of growth of B PLL and inhibition of the PMA-induced proliferation of normal B cells.

activation protocol (co-stimulation versus re-stimulation assays) (see Table 6).

Interferons and normal B cells. IFN-γ was, after IL-2, the second recombinant cytokine shown to act as a growth factor for human B cells (Defrance *et al.*, 1986; Romagnani *et al.*, 1986a,b). In addition to its B cell growth stimulatory activity *per se*, IFN-γ can act as a cofactor for other B cell tropic cytokines, such as IL-4 (Defrance *et al.*, 1987b), IL-2 (Romagnani *et al.*, 1986a,b; Jelinek *et al.*, 1986; Karray *et al.*, 1987) and LMW BCGF (Xia and Choi, 1988). Both IFN-α (Morikawa *et al.*, 1987) and IFN-β (François *et al.*, 1988) share with IFN-γ the capacity to stimulate proliferation of normal B cells activated with anti-Ig reagents. As observed for their antiviral effects, combinations of α and γ interferons could synergize to amplify the proliferative response of anti-IgM activated human B cells (Morikawa *et al.*, 1987). Conversely, IFN-γ has been shown to antagonize the proliferation of murine B cells in response to soluble anti-Ig antibodies used alone or in combination with IL-4 (Mond *et al.*, 1985a), and to inhibit the priming effect of IL-4 on mouse resting B cells (Rabin *et al.*, 1986b).

Interferons and leukaemic B cells. The effects of interferons on leukaemic B cell proliferation are still conflicting. According to Östlund *et al.* (1986, 1989), chronic lymphocytic leukaemia B cells and B lymphomas can undergo some proliferation upon IFN-γ stimulation, whereas the study of Karray *et al.* (1987) led to opposite conclusions. The heterogeneity of mature B cell neoplasms might account for these discrepancies. Accordingly, Sauerwein *et al.* (1987) and Mongini *et al.* (1988), respectively, reported a stimulatory effect of IFN-γ on the proliferation of one clone of B prolymphocytic leukaemia and an inhibitory effect of IFN-γ on the proliferative response of one hairy cell leukaemia cell line.

Interferons are early acting factors in the human system. Several observations suggest that IFN-γ preferentially acts at a relatively early stage of the B cell response. While IFN-γ can stimulate B cell proliferation when added simultaneously with SAC or anti-IgM, it is ineffective on B cell blasts originating from preculture with the same polyclonal B cell activators (Nakagawa *et al.*, 1985; Defrance *et al.*, 1986; Romagnani *et al.*, 1986a,b; Morikawa *et al.*, 1987; François *et al.*, 1988; Xia and Choi, 1988). Moreover, when B cells are separated on the basis of their density, it appears that the B cell population responsive to IFN-γ is included within the high density fraction (Romagnani *et al.*, 1986b; Xia and Choi, 1988). This suggests that B cells, having already received an activation signal *in vivo*, are refractory to the growth-promoting effect of IFN-γ. Finally, as discussed above, IFN-γ could play a primary role in amplifying the early phases of the immune response. As has been demonstrated for IL-2, responsiveness of murine B cells to interferons might require a different timing of addition of the factor and/or a more stringent activation protocol than those necessitated for human B cells. The recent studies of Seyshab *et al.* (1989), showing that IFN-γ can act as a progression factor for murine B cells when added 36 h after stimulation with anti-IgM *plus* LPS, would favour such an hypothesis.

In vivo *effect of interferons on B cells.* Recombinant IFN-α has now been used for several years for the treatment of hairy cell leukaemias, non Hodgkin's B cell lymphomas and multiple myelomas (Balkwill, 1989). The functional basis for these therapeutic effects of interferons, observed after numerous clinical trials, remains unclear. Whereas some groups propose that IFN-α directly blocks the proliferation of the mature leukaemic clone, others suggest that IFN inhibits the differentiation or self-renewal of the leukaemic progenitor cells (Michalevicz and Revel, 1987). It is likely that IFN also acts indirectly through activation of the immune cells involved in immunosurveillance, such as T cells, NK cells and macrophages.

Low molecular weight B cell growth factor

The first human BCGF, originally identified by Maizel *et al.* (1982) and described as a low molecular weight molecule, had long been thought of as being the human homologue of murine IL-4. The isolation and characterization of a cDNA clone encoding LMW BCGF (Sharma *et al.*, 1987) established this factor as a new B cell tropic cytokine. Other LMW BCGFs derived from activated T cells have been described (Butler *et al.*, 1983; Yoshizaki *et al.*, 1983; Pathak *et al.*, 1985), but their molecular structure remains to be determined. LMW BCGF has been described to display multiple biological activities on B cells. However, it must be stressed that most of the work was performed with a semi-purified preparation of the factor (commercially available from Cellular Products, Buffalo, NY) which was shown to contain, among other B cell stimulatory cytokines, significant amounts of TNF-β. According to Kehrl *et al.* (1987a), 70% of the B cell growth-promoting activity could be blocked by specific neutralizing anti-TNF-β antibodies. Thus, although the B cell growth effect of the recombinant molecule was recently confirmed by Sharma *et al.* (personal communication), it remains to be established whether the recombinant material also displays the wide range of biological activities ascribed to the commercial preparation. Table 7 summarizes the characteristics of the growth-promoting activity of the semi-purified LMW BCGF. In contrast with IL-4, which is species specific, the semi-purified LMW BCGF was found to be active on murine B cells and to possess some of the biological properties ascribed to mouse IL-5 (Ennist *et al.*, 1987a,b).

Table 7   Characteristics of the B cell-growth promoting activity of LMW BCGF.

Human	Mouse
Induces growth of B cell blasts generated by PWM stimulation of B cells in the presence of irradiated T cells (Ford *et al.*, 1981)	Induces proliferation of resting B cells Induces growth of dextran sulphate-activated B cells
Stimulates growth of normal B cells activated with anti-IgM antibodies (Maizel *et al.*, 1983)	Promotes growth of *in vivo* activated B cells—cooperates with IL-5
Induces growth of long-term factor-dependent B cell lines (Maizel *et al.*, 1983)	Synergizes with IL-4 in co-stimulation with soluble anti-IgM
Stimulates proliferation of pre-B cell malignancies (Wörmann *et al.*, 1987; Uckun *et al.*, 1987)	Inhibits IL-5 dependent proliferation of the BCL-1 cell line (for all references see Ennist *et al.*, 1987a,b)
Stimulates proliferation of mature B cell neoplasms (Ford *et al.*, 1985a,b)	
Cooperates with IFN-γ (Xia and Choi, 1988), IL-2 (Jelinek and Lipsky, 1987b) and IL-4 (Defrance *et al.*, 1987b) for the growth of normal B cells	

Gordon et al. (1986, 1987) have proposed that CD23 or membrane molecules closely associated with this antigen could constitute the surface receptor for LMW BCGF. The growth-promoting effect of LMW BCGF would be mediated by the soluble products originating from the cleavage of the CD23 molecule initiated by binding of LMW BCGF to its receptor (Guy and Gordon, 1987; Swendeman and Thorley-Lawson, 1987). This hypothesis is presently questioned by two sets of data. First Uchibayashi et al. (1989) have shown that recombinant soluble CD23 molecule lacks BCGF activity. Second, according to Warrington et al. (1989) and Sharma et al. (personal communication), the loss of CD23 expression on human B cell lines is not associated with the disappearance of responsiveness to semi-purified or recombinant LMW BCGF. Finally, the presence of LMW BCGF mRNA in some malignant B cells (Sharma et al., personal communication) would suggest that this factor could be an essential component for autocrine growth of some B cell neoplasms. It is important to note that the LMW BCGF gene is located on chromosome 1 in q23-25, a region subject to translocation events in B cell leukaemias (S. Sharma et al., personal communication).

Interleukin 1, tumour necrosis factors and interleukin 6

Interleukin 1. The first description of the B cell stimulatory activity of IL-1 was originally made by Howard et al. (1983). They showed that IL-1 displays the dual capacity to directly promote murine B cell growth and to enhance the response of B cells to IL-4 under limiting culture conditions (low cell numbers or suboptimal concentrations of growth factor). Subsequently, IL-1 was shown to allow entry into cycle of both anti-Ig and dextran sulphate activated murine B cells (Booth and Watson, 1984; Chiplunkar et al., 1986). Demonstration that the growth-supporting effect of IL-1 was directly exerted on B cells came from Pike and Nossal (1985) who reported that IL-1 could act in synergy with antigen to promote growth and differentiation of single B cells. However, experiments performed in single assay systems failed to confirm the previously described synergy between IL-1 and IL-4 on B cell proliferation (Pike et al., 1987). In the human, early experiments had demonstrated that IL-1 could provide a modest growth stimulus for anti-Ig activated B cells (Falkoff et al., 1983), but we and others (Gordon et al., 1986; Jelinek and Lipsky, 1987c) failed to detect such an activity. However, IL-1 was found to enhance proliferation of human B cells co-stimulated with SAC and IL-2 (Jelinek and Lipsky, 1987c). Thus, the ability of IL-1 to modulate B cell proliferation could be dependent on the assays and/or on the B cell population studied. Moreover, the capacity of IL-1 to stimulate B cell entry into cycle remains marginal compared with other B cell stimulating factors such as IL-4 or IL-2. Numerous reports have described that EBV-transformed B cells release IL-1-like molecules that may be involved in their autocrine growth (Matsushima *et al.*, 1985; Gordon *et al.*, 1986; Wakasugi *et al.*, 1987; Vandenabeele *et al.*, 1988). The discrepancy between the virtual lack of responsiveness of normal human B cells to IL-1 and its stimulatory activity on EBV-transformed B cells, remains to be understood.

Interleukin 6. As do other cytokines, IL-6 mediates multiple functions on various cell types, as shown by the numerous names it was given before being designated IL-6 (IFN-β_2, hepatocyte stimulating factor, hybridoma growth factor, 26 kD protein and B cell stimulatory factor 2).

IL-6 is a growth factor for myeloma cells. In contrast to other previously described BCGFs, IL-6 is active on B cells displaying plasmacytoid or pre-plasmacytoid phenotype and therefore close to the final stage of B cell maturation. However, although it has been suggested that the Ig-secreting B cell populations could be actively cycling (Jelinek and Lipsky, 1983), there is no firm evidence that IL-6 could be involved in expansion of the pool of Ig-secreting cells generated in polyclonally activated cultures of normal B cells. Nevertheless, this molecule undoubtedly supports growth of transformed or malignant Ig-producing cells. The main targets of the growth-promoting activity of IL-6 are: B cell hybridomas and plasmacytomas in mouse (Poupart *et al.*, 1987; Van Snick *et al.*, 1987) and multiple myeloma cells in man (Kawano *et al.*, 1988a; Klein *et al.*, 1989; Shimizu *et al.*, 1989). Whether IL-6 induces expansion of myeloma cells in an autocrine or paracrine fashion is still presently a matter of debate. According to Kawano *et al.* (1988a) IL-6 can be detected both at the protein and mRNA levels in freshly isolated myeloma cells and in some established myeloma cell lines. Other authors (Klein *et al.*, 1989; Shimizu *et al.*, 1989) propose a paracrine mechanism in which the bone marrow environment would be the source of IL-6.

The exact maturation stage of the responsive B cell in multiple myeloma is still uncertain but it has been proposed by Klein *et al.* (1989) that the primary effect of IL-6 is the stimulation of the self-renewing and differentiating capacity of an immature precursor stem cell. In this respect, combinations of IL-6 and haemopoietic growth factors such as GM-CSF or IL-3 have been described to synergize for the growth of myeloma cells (Zhang *et al.*, 1990) or expansion of a pre-plasma cell present in freshly isolated peripheral blood lymphocytes (PBL) from multiple myeloma patients (Bergui *et al.*, 1989).

The activity of IL-6 is not species-restricted and murine hybridoma cell lines are widely used as sensitive and reliable bioassay systems for detection of both human and mouse IL-6 (O'Garra and Defrance, 1990).

Does IL-6 promote growth of normal B cells? In man, IL-6 repeatedly failed to induce cell-cycle entry of normal B cells when tested in a large range of

BCGF bioassays performed with anti-Ig reagents, or phorbol esters (Defrance *et al.*, unpublished results). In mouse, it was recently shown that purified natural IL-6 is poorly active by itself on normal B cell growth but that it could significantly stimulate anti-Ig and dextran sulphate induced proliferation of B cells when used in combination with IL-1 (Vink *et al.*, 1988). Two lines of evidence support the notion that IL-6 could act as a progression factor for non-plasmacytoid transformed B cells. The first one is the indication by Tosato *et al.* (1988) that IL-6 could induce proliferation of lymphoblastoid cell lines. The second one is the observation made by Yee *et al.* (1989) that cell lines established from non Hodgkin's B lymphomas can produce IL-6 and utilize it for their autocrine growth.

Tumour necrosis factors. TNF may induce lysis of malignant cells and cell lines and regression of some animal tumours. TNF-α and TNF-β (or lymphotoxin), although not structurally identical, interact with the same receptor. Their activity as proliferation-inducing factors in B cell cultures has been essentially documented in the human system. In contrast to IL-1 and IL-6, which do not display significant growth-promoting activity *per se* on normal B cells, both TNF-α and TNF-β can score in standard BCGF bioassays in man (Jelinek and Lipsky, 1987c; Kehrl *et al.*, 1987a,b). Like IL-1, TNF also behaves as a cofactor for various B cell tropic cytokines including IL-2 (Jelinek and Lipsky, 1987c; Kehrl *et al.*, 1987a,b; Zola and Nikoloutsopoulos, 1989), IFN-γ (Kehrl *et al.*, 1987b) and IL-4 (Zola and Nikoloutsopoulos, 1989; Dugas *et al.*, personal communication). Both TNF-α and TNF-β have been reported to spontaneously stimulate DNA synthesis from leukaemic B cells, namely B-CLL and HCL (Cordingley *et al.*, 1988; Digel *et al.*, 1989; Moberts *et al.*, 1989) and the TNF-dependent proliferation of these malignant B cells could be antagonized by IFN-α.

Can TNF be used as an autocrine B cell growth factor? The possibility that TNF could represent an autocrine growth factor for transformed B cells has been considered. Production of a TNF-like molecule by human lymphoblastoid cell lines was first reported by Williamson *et al.* (1983). Subsequently, it was described that TNF-β could be constitutively produced by lymphoblastoid cell lines and could support maintenance or growth of these cells (Seregina *et al.*, 1989).

It appears that IL-1, IL-6 and TNF play rather an ancillary role in proliferative responses of normal B cells. Nevertheless, since they are also released from activated normal B cells (Sung *et al.*, 1988, 1989; Bonnefoy *et al.*, 1989 Denoroy *et al.*, 1990a,b) they may participate individually or in a cooperative fashion to the autostimulatory activity detected in transformed B cell culture supernatants. Major characteristics of the growth supporting properties of these molecules are summarized in Table 8.

Table 8 Characteristics of the growth supporting activity of IL-1, IL-6 and TNF.

	IL-1		IL-6		TNF	
Stimulates B cell growth in standard BCGF bioassays	+ (mouse)	− (human)	−		? (mouse)	+ (human)
Acts as a cofactor for B cell tropic factors	+		+ (mouse)	− (human)	+	
Stimulates growth of plasmacytoid malignant B cells	−		+		−	
Stimulates growth of mouse hybridoma/ plasmacytoma cells	+[a]		+		+[a]	
Participates to the autocrine-growth of lymphoblastoid cell lines	+		+		+	

[a] According to Le *et al.* (1988).

Transforming growth factor β (TGF-β)

Originally detected in culture supernatants of transformed fibroblasts, TGF-β is in fact produced by many normal tissues. Among the several distinct forms of TGF-β which have been reported, TGF-β_1 and TGF-β_2 are the best studied. Both molecules are homodimers that present 70% sequence homology. They display equivalent biological activities, but bind to two different receptors on B cells (Kehrl *et al.*, 1989). TGF-β is often secreted as a biologically inert complex resulting from the association of one dimer of TGF-β and other proteins (Wakefield *et al.*, 1988). TGF-β can be activated upon mild acid treatment or by certain proteases (Keski-Oja *et al.*, 1987). This factor displays both growth-stimulatory and growth-inhibitory properties, depending on the cell target and the other growth factors present (Sporn and Roberts, 1988). TGF-β acts as a strong inhibitor of proliferation of normal activated human B cells, triggered by progression factors, such as IL-2 (Kehrl *et al.*, 1986, 1989) or semi-purified LMW-BCGF (Smeland *et al.*, 1987; Petit-Koskas *et al.*, 1988). In contrast with normal B cells, EBV-infected normal B cells, as well as EBV[+] Burkitt's lymphoma cell lines, are refractory to the growth-inhibitory effect of TGF-β (Blomhoff *et al.*, 1987). The unresponsiveness of EBV cell lines to the suppressive effect of TGF-β is not correlated with a loss of TGF-β receptors (Kehrl et al., 1989). Leu-kaemic B cells appear to be heterogeneous in terms of sensitivity to the suppressive effect of TGF-β. According to Petit-Koskas et al. (1988), TGF-β cannot inhibit the LMW BCGF induced proliferation of hairy cell leu-kaemias. In contrast, Smeland et al. (1987) report that the proliferative response of non Hodgkin's B lymphomas to LMW-BCGF and anti-Ig antibodies is suppressed by TGF-β. Transforming growth factor β would not interfere with the early steps of B cell activation (Ca^{2+} mobilization, cell volume increase, augmented RNA levels, c-*myc* transcription) triggered by anti-Ig reagents but would rather block the G_1/S transition (Smeland et al., 1987). Normal human B cells, activated via their surface Ig receptors can synthesize and produce TGF-β, as detected both at the protein and messen-ger levels (Kehrl et al., 1986). Although primarily released in an inactive form in B cell cultures, TGF-β is probably partly converted to its functional form, since addition of anti-TGF-β antibodies potentiates the proliferative response of B cells co-stimulated with anti-Ig antibodies and IL-2 (Kehrl et al., 1989). Thus, endogenous production of TGF-β by B cells could rep-resent an important negative-feedback control mechanism for regulation of B cell growth.

Complement fractions

Complement activation leads to the generation of multiple proteolytic fragments, which have been shown to modulate the immune response. Among those, C3b, C3d, Ba and Bb have been described to display B cell growth-promoting activity. In mice, according to the model proposed by Melchers et al. (1985), both C3b and C3d fragments presented in an immobilized form behave as α factors (see B cell activation), and, as such, control entry of activated B cells into S phase. In order to be active, C3b and C3d need to display a multivalent binding capacity to their surface receptors on B cells (Erdei et al., 1985; Melchers et al., 1985). In man, the capacity of the complement fragment C3d to stimulate B cell growth was substantiated by the following observations: (i) polymerized C3d fragments directly trigger proliferation of B lymphoblastoid cell lines cultured in serum-free conditions (Servis and Lambris, 1989) and that of normal B cells activated with PMA (Bohnsack and Cooper, 1988); and (ii) ligation of surface receptors for polyclonal C3d (CR2/CD21) by monoclonal and polyclonal antibodies deliver progression signals to B cells (Bohnsack and Cooper, 1988; Frade et al., 1985).

One of the activation fragments of complement factor B (Bb) has also been shown to enhance proliferation of SAC-stimulated human B cells (Peters et al., 1988). Interestingly, a strong antigenic and functional homology exists between Bb and a previously described high molecular weight BCGF (Ambrus *et al.*, 1985a,b), since antibodies directed against this latter factor recognize Bb and block its mitogenic effect on B cells.

It has been postulated that C3 could be required *in vivo* for induction and maintenance of immunologic memory (Klaus and Humphrey, 1986). Additionally, bacteria, virus and parasites have the capacity to directly activate complement and covalently bind some of its proteolytic fragments, such as C3d. Subsequent recognition of these pathogens by B cells, simultaneously via surface Ig receptors and CR2, might prompt B cells to an accelerated antibody response.

Cytokines and B cells: conclusions and perspectives

The present review has shown that many different cytokines are involved in B cell ontogeny, activation and differentiation and that a single cytokine can act at various stages of the development of a B cell (Figures 1 and 2). In spite of these numerous progresses, many questions remain to be addressed.

Are there yet other B cell tropic cytokines to be discovered?

Apart from the recombinant cytokines presented here, a multiplicity of B cell stimulatory factors have been described which still await molecular characterization. These include several high molecular weight BCGFs (Yoshizaki *et al.*, 1983; Ambrus and Fauci, 1985a,b; Dugas *et al.*, 1985) and also an activity called B cell activating factor (BCAF) which is characterized by the ability to induce the proliferation of resting B cells (Bowen *et al.*, 1986; Leclercq *et al.*, 1986; Diu *et al.*, 1987, 1990). In addition, many other molecularly defined cytokines remain to be tested for their effects on B cells. These include the recently isolated IL-8 (Baggiolini *et al.*, 1989), p40 (Van Snick *et al.*, 1989; Yang *et al.*, 1989) and cytokine synthesis inhibitory factor (CSIF; Fiorentino *et al.*, 1989). Furthermore, the effect on B lymphocytes of other apparently non-immunologically related polypeptidic hormones should be investigated. In this context, fibroblast growth factors have recently been shown to enhance proliferation of activated B cells induced by partially purified LMW BCGF (Genot *et al.*, 1989).

Neuroendocrine peptide hormones should also be considered for their effects on B cell development. One group (see Weigent and Blalock, 1987) has demonstrated that cells of the immune system can secrete such hormones including corticotropin (ACTH) and endorphins (both of which deriving from pro-opiomelanocortin), thyrotropin (TSH) and growth hormone. These polypeptides appear to alter *in vitro* immune responses, since

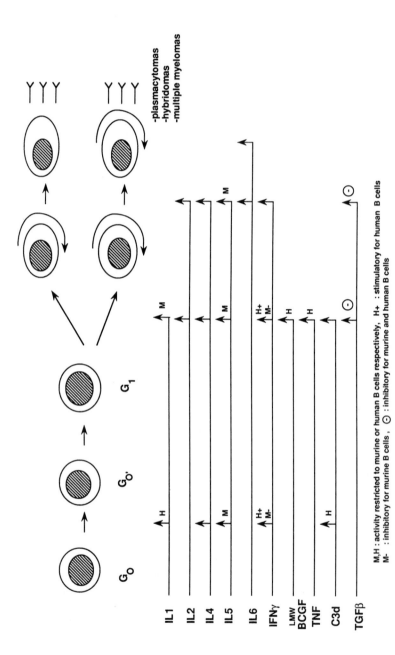

Figure 2 Schematic representation of the effects of cytokines on B cell activation, proliferation and differentiation.

M,H : activity restricted to murine or human B cells respectively,   H+ : stimulatory for human B cells
M- : inhibitory for murine B cells,   ⊙ : inhibitory for murine and human B cells

TSH strongly potentiates T-dependent and T-independent antibody production. In addition, neuropeptides such as substance P, somatostatin and vasoactive intestinal peptide have been shown to enhance or inhibit lymphocytic proliferation and immunoglobulin production (Stead *et al.*, 1987). Very recently, nerve growth factor has been shown to induce proliferation and differentiation of human B lymphocytes (Otten *et al.*, 1989).

What is the rôle of cell–cell contacts in B cell development?

Whereas the role for cell–cell interactions has been largely accepted in haemopoietic development, the role of cell–cell interactions in the antigen-driven B cell maturation process during *in vitro* studies has not been as seriously considered. The secondary lymphoid organs where immune responses take place are indeed organized structures (see Butcher and Weissman, 1989) which comprise B cell rich (follicles) and T cell rich areas. Primary B cell activation is thought to happen in the extrafollicular T cell rich areas in contact with interdigitating cells, whereas secondary B cell activation is happening in follicles in contact with follicular dendritic cells and some helper T cells (MacLennan and Gray, 1986; Szakal, 1989). In this context, it has been shown that activated T cells (Clement *et al.*, 1984) or their membranes (Brian, 1988) can activate B cells and induce them to proliferate. Furthermore, the activated EL-4 thymoma, in conjunction with cytokine rich supernatants, has been used to induce the expansion and differentiation of single human B cells (Zubler *et al.*, 1987). Therefore, the question arises as to whether these different B cell subpopulations (e.g. newly formed virgin B cells versus memory B cells) require different cell contacts and different cytokines for their activation.

What are the mechanisms underlying the agonistic and antagonistic effects of a single cytokine?

The possibility of a cytokine binding to two different receptors has been demonstrated for glucagon, which binds to high and low affinity receptors, respectively coupled to the phosphoinositides and to the cAMP pathways (Wakelam *et al.*, 1986). Upon binding to these different receptors, glucagon induces different physiological responses of hepatocytes. Preliminary data on B cell tropic cytokines are conflicting and a great deal of work remains to be done. For instance, we found that IL-4 induces CD23 expression on the Jijoye Burkitt's lymphoma B cell line without stimulating the phosphoinositides or the cAMP pathways (Galizzi *et al.*, 1988), whereas others have found that CD23 induction on normal B cells appears to be associated with activation of both phosphoinositides and cAMP pathways (Finney *et al.*,

1990). The activation pathways may be cell-specific, as IL-1 has been shown to bind to different receptors on T and B cells (Bomsztyk *et al.*, 1989; Chizzonite *et al.*, 1989; Scapigliati *et al.*, 1989). Therefore, it is expected that much information on the cascade of events involved in the transduction of the information from the cell surface to the nucleus will be sought within the next few years.

Do non-peptidic molecules alter cytokine responsiveness of B cells?

Whereas the inhibitory effects of prostaglandin E2 on immune responses were recognized relatively early (Chouaib and Bertoglio, 1988), recent experiments have shown that leukotriene B4 can stimulate human B lymphocytes (Yamaoka *et al.*, 1989) and that corticosteroids are necessary for IL-4 to induce chronic lymphocytic leukaemia B cells to secrete IgE (Sarfati *et al.*, 1989). Thus, the effects of these non-peptidic mediators on the different phases of B cell development must be carefully assessed.

What are the feedback mechanisms controlling B cell proliferation and differentiation?

All efforts aimed at understanding the development of B cells would be incomplete without attempting to understand the phenomena limiting B cell expansion. Is expansion of the B cell pool essentially passively limited via a tightly controlled production of B cell growth factors? Or, alternatively, is B lymphocyte proliferation actively controlled through inhibitory cytokines (e.g. TGF-β)? Finally, as the major rôle for B cells appears to be the production of Igs, it may be that Igs themselves play a rôle in controlling the expansion of the B cell pool. IgG immune complexes may inhibit B cell functions through binding to FcγR/CD32 (Ryan *et al.*, 1975; Morgan and Weigle, 1983). Similar mechanisms may occur for other isotypes such as IgE and IgA. It will be important to cover the retrocontrol of B cell development because alterations of these mechanisms may be involved in the development of leukaemias, myelomas and, possibly, autoimmune diseases.

How do in vitro experiments on highly purified B cells compare to what is really happening in vivo?

Understanding the *in vivo* phenomena controlling B cell development is obviously the ultimate goal for all investigators interested in B cells. Such questions can be addressed by infusing recombinant cytokines or cytokine-specific antibodies into animals. The first available data concerning B cell proliferation have been reported in this chapter. However, one should realize that these approaches may not be conclusive, as the delivery of these agents may not mimic physiological situations. Much of the important information should be obtained using animals expressing transgenes for cytokine or cytokine receptors or cytokine-induced intracellular proteins. Finally, the silencing of cytokine genes by homologous recombinations should provide a great deal of information about the *in vivo* relevance of cytokines in B cell development.

Acknowledgements

We thank Drs F. Rousset (Schering-Plough) and J. A. Waitz (DNAX) for helpful discussions and critical review of the manuscript. We also thank N. Courbière and M. Vatan for typing this manuscript, and B. Vanbervliet and B. Crouzet for helping with the final corrections.

References

Alderson, M. R., Pike, B. L. and Nossal, G. J. V. (1987a) *Proc. Natl. Acad. Sci. USA* **84**, 1389–1393.

Alderson, M. R., Beverley, L. P., Harada, N., Tominaga, A., Takatsu, K. and Nossal, G. J. V. (1987b) *J. Immunol.* **139**, 2656–2660.

Ambrus, J. L. and Fauci, A. S. (1985a) *J. Clin. Invest.* **75**, 7907–7911.

Ambrus, J. L., Jurgensen, C. H., Brown, E. J. and Fauci, A. S. (1985b) *J. Exp. Med.* **162**, 1319–1335.

Aoki, N. and Ohno, Y. (1987) *Immunology* **60**, 51–55.

Armitage, R. J. and Goff, L. K. (1988) *Eur. J. Immunol.* **18**, 1753–1760.

Baggiolini, M., Walz, A. and Kunkel, S. L. (1989) *J. Clin. Invest.* **84**, 1045–1049.

Balkwill, F. R. (1989) *The Lancet* i, 1060–1062.

Banchereau, J., de Paoli, P., Vallé, A., Garcia, E. and Rousset, F. (1990) Submitted.

Bergui, L., Schena, M., Gaidano, G., Riva, M. and Caligaris-Cappio, F. (1989) *J. Exp. Med.* **170**, 613–618.

Bich-Thuy, L. and Fauci, A. S. (1985) *Eur. J. Immunol.* **15**, 1075–1079.

Bich-Thuy, L. and Fauci, A. S. (1986) *J. Clin. Invest.* **77**, 1173–1179.

Bijsterbosch, M. K. and Klaus, G. G. B. (1985) *J. Exp. Med.* **162**, 1825–1836.

Blomhoff, H. K., Smeland, E., Mustafa, A. S., Godal, T. and Ohlsson, R. (1987) *Eur. J. Immunol.* **17**, 299–301.

Bohnsack, J. F. and Cooper, N. R. (1988) *J. Immunol.* **141**, 2569–2576.

Bomsztyk, K., Sims, J. E., Stanton, T. H., Slack, J., McMahan, C. J., Valentine, M. A. and Dower, S. K. (1989) *Proc. Natl. Acad. Sci. USA* **86**, 8034–8038.

Bonnefoy, J. Y., Aubry, J. P., Péronne, C., Wijdenes, J. and Banchereau, J. (1987) *J. Immunol.* **138**, 2970–2978.

Bonnefoy, J. Y., Defrance, T., Péronne, C., Ménétrier, C., Rousset, F., Pène, J., de Vries, J. E. and Banchereau, J. (1988) *Eur. J. Immunol.* **18**, 117–122.

Bonnefoy, J. Y., Denoroy, M. C., Guillot, O., Martens, C. L. and Banchereau, J. (1989) *J. Immunol.* **143**, 864–869.

Booth, R. J. and Watson, J. D. (1984) *J. Immunol.* **133**, 1346–1349.

Bowen, D. L., Ambrus, J. L. and Fauci, A. S. (1986) *J. Immunol.* **136**, 2158–2163.

Boyd, A. W., Fisher, D. C., Fox, D. A., Schlossman, S. F. and Nadler, L. M. (1985) *J. Immunol.* **134**, 2387–2392.

Boyd, A. W., Tedder, T. F., Griffin, J. D., Freedman, A. S., Fisher, D. C., Daley, J. and Naddler, L. M. (1987) *Cell. Immunol.* **106**, 355–365.

Brian, A. A. (1988) *Proc. Natl. Acad. Sci. USA* **85**, 564–568.

Brière, F., Chrétien, I., Pène, J., Rousset, F. and de Vries, J. E. (1990) Submitted.

Butcher, E. C. and Weissman, I. L. (1989) In *Fund. Immunol.*, pp. 117–136. Ed. by W. Paul. Raven Press, New York.

Butler, J. L., Muraguchi, A., Lane, H. C. and Fauci, A. S. (1983) *J. Exp. Med.* **157**, 60–68.

Cairns, J., Flores-Romo, L., Millsum, M. J., Guy, G. R., Gillis, S., Ledbetter, J. A. and Gordon, J. (1988) *Eur. J. Immunol.* **18**, 349–353.

Cambier, J. C. and Lehmann, K. R. (1989) *J. Exp. Med.* **170**, 877–886.

Cambier, J. C. and Monroe, J. G. (1984) *J. Immunol.* **133**, 576–581.

Cambier, J. C., Justement, L. B., Newell, M. K., Chen, Z. Z., Harris, L. K., Sandoval, V. M., Klemsz, M. J. and Ranson, J. T. (1987) *Immunol. Rev.* **95**, 37–57.

Campbell, H. D., Tucker, W. Q. J., Hort, Y., Martinson, M. E., Mayo, G., Clutterbuck, E. J., Sanderson, C. J. and Young, I. G. (1987) *Proc. Natl. Acad. Sci. USA* **84**, 6629–6633.

Carlsson, M., Sundström, C., Bengtsson, M., Tötterman, T. H., Rosen, A. and Nillson, K. (1989) *Eur. J. Immunol.* **19**, 913–921.

Carter, R. H. and Fearon, D. T. (1989) *J. Immunol.* **143**, 1755–1760.

Chesnut, R. W. and Grey, H. M. (1981) *J. Immunol.* **126**, 1075–1079.

Chesnut, R. W. and Grey, H. M. (1986) *Adv. Immunol.* **39**, 51–94.

Chiplunkar, S., Langhorne, J. and Kaufmann, S. H. E. (1986) *J. Immunol.* **137**, 3748–3752.

Chizzonite, R., Truitt, T., Kilian, P. L., Stern, A. S., Nunes, P., Parker, K. P., Kaffka, K. L., Chua, A. O., Lugg, D. K. and Gubler, U. (1989) *Proc. Natl. Acad. Sci. USA* **86**, 8029–8033.

Chouaib, S. and Bertoglio, J. H. (1988) *Lymphokine Res.* **7**, 237–245.

Clark, E. A. and Ledbetter, J. A. (1986) *Proc. Natl. Acad. Sci. USA* **83**, 4494–4498.

Clark, E. A. and Ledbetter, J. A. (1989) *Adv. Cancer Res.* **52**, 81–149.

Clement, L. T., Dagg, M. K. and Gartland, G. L. (1984) *J. Immunol.* **132**, 740–744.

Clutterbuck, E., Shields, J. G., Gordon, J., Smith, S. H., Boyd, A., Callard, R. E., Campbell, H. D., Young, I. G. and Sanderson, C. J. (1987) *Eur. J. Immunol.* **17**, 1743–1750.

Coffman, R. L., Seymour, B. W., Hudak, S., Jackson, J. and Rennick, D. (1989) *Science* **245**, 308–310.

Conrad, D. H., Keegan, A. D., Kalli, K. R., Van Dusen, R., Rao, M. and Levine, A. D. (1988) *J. Immunol.* **141**, 1091–1097.

Corbel, C. and Melchers, F. (1983) *Eur. J. Immunol.* **13**, 528–533.

Cordingley, F. T., Hoffbrand, A. V., Heslop, H. E., Turner, M., Bianchi, A., Reittie, J. E., Vyakarnam, A., Meager, A. and Brenner, M. K. (1988) *Lancet* ii, 969–971.

de Maeyer, E. and de Maeyer-Guignard, J. (1988) *Interferons and Other Regulatory Cytokines*, John Wiley & Sons, New York.

Defrance, T., Aubry, J. P., Vanbervliet, B. and Banchereau, J. (1986) *J. Immunol.* **137**, 3861–3867.

Defrance, T., Aubry, J. P., Rousset, F., Vanbervliet, B., Bonnefoy, J. Y., Arai, N., Takebe, T., Yokota, Y., Lee, F., Arai, K., de Vries, J. E. and Banchereau, J. (1987a) *J. Exp. Med.* **165**, 1459–1647.

Defrance, T., Vanbervliet, B., Aubry, J. P., Takebe, Y., Arai, N., Miyajima, A., Yokota, T., Lee, F., Arai, K., de Vries, J. E. and Banchereau, J. (1987b) *J. Immunol.* **139**, 1135–1141.

Defrance, T., Vanbervliet, B., Aubry, J. P. and Banchereau, J. (1988) *J. Exp. Med.* **168**, 1321–1337.

Defrance, T., Vanbervliet, B., Durand, I. and Banchereau, J. (1989) *Eur. J. Immunol.* **19**, 293–299.

Defrance, T., Fluckiger, A. C., Vanbervliet, B., Rossi, J. F., Sotto, J. J. and Banchereau, J. (1990a) Submitted.

Defrance, T., Vanbervliet, B. and Banchereau, J. (1990b) Submitted.

Delespesse, G., Sarfati, M. and Peleman, R. (1989) *J. Immunol.* **142**, 134–138.

Delfraissy, J. F., Wallon, C., Vazquez, A., Dugas, B., Dormont, J. and Galanaud, P. (1986) *Eur. J. Immunol.* **16**, 1251–1256.

Denoroy, M. C., Martens, C. L., Van Damme, J. and Banchereau, J. (1990a). Submitted.

Denoroy, M. C., Martens, C. L., Adolf, G. R. and Banchereau, J. (1990b) Submitted.

Dexter, T. M., Allen, T. D. and Lajtha, L. G. (1977) *J. Cell. Physiol.* **91**, 335–344.

Digel, W., Stefanic, M., Schöniger, W., Buck, C., Raghavachar, A., Frickhofen, N., Heimpel, H. and Porzsolt, F. (1989) *Blood* **73**, 1242–1246.

Diu, A., Gougeon, M.-L., Moreau, J.-L., Reinherz, E. L. and Thèze, J. (1987) *Proc. Natl. Acad. Sci. USA* **84**, 9140–9144.

Diu, A., Fevrier, M., Mollier, P., Charron, D., Banchereau, J., Reinherz, E. L. and Theze, J. (1990) *Cell. Immunol.* **125**, 14–28.

Dorshkind, K. (1988) *J. Immunol.* **141**, 531–538.

Dugas, B., Vazquez, A., Gerard, J. P., Richard, Y., Auffredou, M. T., Delfraissy, J. F., Fradelizi, D. and Galanaud, P. (1985) *J. Immunol.* **135**, 333–338.

Dutton, R. W., Falkoff, R., Hirst, J. A., Hoffman, M., Kappler, J. W., Kettman, J. R., Lesley, J. R. and Vann, P. (1971) *Prog. Immunol.* **1**, 355–368.

Ennist, D. L., Elkins, K. L., Cheng, S. C. and Howard, M. (1987a) *J. Immunol.* **139**, 1525–1531.

Ennist, D. L., Greenblatt, D., Coffman, R., Sharma, S., Maizel, A. and Howard, M. (1987b) *Cell Immunol.* **110**, 77–94.

Erdei, A., Melchers, F., Schulz, T. and Dierich, M. (1985) *Eur. J. Immunol.* **15**, 184–188.

Falkoff, R. J. M., Muraguchi, A., Hong, J.-X. H., Butler, J. L., Dinarello, C. A. and Fauci, A. S. (1983) *J. Immunol.* **131**, 801–805.

Favrot, M. C., Combaret, V., Negrier, S., Philip, I., Thiesse, P., Freydel, C., Bijmann, J. T., Franks, C. R., Mercatello, A. and Philip, T. (1990) *J. Biol. Resp. Modif.*, in press.

Fernandez-Botran, R., Sanders, V. M. and Vitetta, E. S. (1989) *J. Exp. Med.* **169**, 379–391.

Finkelman, F. D., Katona, I. M., Urban, J. F., Snapper, C. M., Ohara, J. and Paul, W. E. (1986) *Proc. Natl. Acad. Sci. USA* **83**, 9675–9678.

Finney, M., Guy, G. R., Michell, R. H., Gordon, J., Dugas, B., Rigley, K. P. and Callard, R. E. (1990) *Eur. J. Immunol.* **20**, 151–156.

Fiorentino, D. F., Bond, M. W. and Mosmann, T. R. (1989) *J. Exp. Med.* **170**, 2081–2095.

Ford, R. J., Mehta, S. R., Franzini, D., Montagna, R., Lachman, L. B. and Maizel, A. L. (1981) *Nature* **294**, 261–263.

Ford, R. J., Kouttab, N., Sahasrabuddhe, C. J., Davis, S. and Mehta, S. R. (1985a) *Blood* **65**, 1335–1341.

Ford, R. J., Yoshimura, L., Morgan, J., Quesada, J., Montagna, R. and Maizel, A. L. (1985b) *J. Exp. Med.* **162**, 1093–1098.

Frade, R., Crevon, M. C., Barel, M., Vazquez, A., Krikorian, L., Charriaut, C. and Galanaud, P. (1985) *Eur. J. Immunol.* **15**, 73–76.

François, D. T., Katona, I. M., Junc, C. H., Wahl, L. M. and Mond, J. J. (1988) *Clin. Immunol. Immunopath.* **48**, 297–306.

Freedman, A. S., Freeman, G., Whitman, J., Segil, J., Daley, J. and Nadler, L. M. (1988) *J. Immunol.* **141**, 3398–3404.

Freedman, A. S., Freeman, G., Whitman, J., Segil, J., Daley, J., Levine, H. and Nadler, L. M. (1989) *Eur. J. Immunol.* **19**, 849–855.

Galizzi, J.-P., Cabrillat, H., Rousset, F., Ménétrier, C., de Vries, J. E. and Banchereau, J. (1988) *J. Immunol.* **141**, 1983–1988.

Genot, E., Petit-Koskas, E., Sensenbrenner, M., Labourdette, G. and Kolb, J.-P. (1989) *Cell. Immunol.* **122**, 424–439.

Giri, J. G., Kincade, P. W. and Mizel, S. B. (1984) *J. Immunol.* **132**, 223–228.

Goodwin, R. G., Lupton, S., Schmierer, A., Hjerrild, K. J., Jerzy, R., Clevenger, W., Gillis, S., Cosman, D. and Namen, A. E. (1989) *Proc. Natl. Acad. Sci. USA* **86**, 302–306.

Gordon, J., Guy, G. and Walker, L. (1986) *Immunology* **57**, 419–423.

Gordon, J., Millsum, M. J., Guy, G. R. and Ledbetter, J. A. (1987) *Eur. J. Immunol.* **17**, 1535–1538.

Gordon, J., Millsum, M. J., Guy, G. R. and Ledbetter, J. A. (1988a) *J. Immunol.* **140**, 1425–1430.

Gordon, J., Cairns, J. A., Millsum, M. J., Gillis, S. and Guy, G. R. (1988b) *Eur. J. Immunol.* **18**, 1561–1565.

Gordon, J., Millsum, M. J., Flores-Romo, L. and Gillis, S. (1989a) *Immunol.* **68**, 526–531.

Gordon, J., Flores-Romo, L., Cairns, J. A., Millsum, M. J., Lane, P. J., Johnson, G. D. and MacLennan, I. C. M. (1989b) *Immunol. Today* **10**, 153–157.

Guy, G. R. and Gordon, J. (1987) *Proc. Natl. Acad. Sci. USA* **84**, 6239–6243.

Hara, Y., Takahama, Y., Murakami, S., Yamada, G., Ono, S., Takatsu, K. and Hamaoka, T. (1985) *Lymph. Res.* **4**, 243–249.

Harada, N., Kikuchi, Y., Tominaga, A., Takaki, S. and Takatsu, K. (1985) *J. Immunol.* **134**, 3944–3951.

Harada, N., Matsumoto, M., Koyama, N., Shimizu, A., Honjo, T., Tominaga, A. and Takatsu, K. (1987) *Immunol. Letters* **15**, 205–215.

Hardy, R. R. Hayakawa, K., Herzenberg, L. A., Morse, H. C. I. and Davidson, W. F. (1984) *Curr. Top. Microbiol. Immunol.* **113**, 231–236.

Hatakeyama, M., Tsudo, M., Minamoto, S., Kono, T., Doi, T., Miyata, T., Miyasaka, M. and Taniguchi, T. (1989) *Science* **244**, 551–556.

Hayakawa, K. and Hardy, R. R. (1988) *Ann. Rev. Immunol.* **6**, 197–218.
Henney, C. S. (1989) In *Progress in Immunology VII*, pp. 1272–1275. Ed. by F. Melchers. Springer Verlag.
Hofman, F. M., Brock, M., Taylor, C. R. and Lyons, b. (1988) *J. Immunol.* **141**, 1185–1190.
Howard, M., Farrar, J., Hilfiker, M., Johnson, B., Takatsu, K., Hamaoka, T. and Paul, W. E. (1982) *J. Exp. Med.* **155**, 914–923.
Howard, M., Mizel, S. B., Lachman, L., Ansel, J., Johnson, B. and Paul, W. E. (1983) *J. Exp. Med.* **157**, 1529–1543.
Hudak, S. A., Gollnick, S. O., Conrad, D. H. and Kehry, M. R. (1987) *Proc. Natl. Acad. Sci. USA* **84**, 4606–4610.
Ishida, T., Nishi, M., Taguchi, O., Inaba, K., Hattori, M., Minato, N., Kawaichi, M. and Honjo, T. (1989) *J. Exp. Med.* **170**, 1103–1115.
Jelinek, D. F. and Lipsky, P. E. (1983) *J. Immunol.* **130**, 2597–2604.
Jelinek, D. and Lipsky, P. E. (1987a) *Adv. Immunol.* **40**, 1–59.
Jelinek, D. F. and Lipsky, P. E. (1987b) *J. Immunol.* **139**, 1005–1013.
Jelinek, D. F. and Lipsky, P. E. (1987c) *J. Immunol.* **139**, 2970–2976.
Jelinek, D. F. and Lipsky, P. E. (1988) *J. Immunol.* **141**, 164–173.
Jelinek, D. F., Splawski, J. B. and Lipsky, P. E. (1986) *Eur. J. Immunol.* **16**, 925–932.
Jones, B. (1987) *Immunol. Rev.* **99**, 5–18.
Julius, M. H., Paige, C. J., Leanderson, T. and Cambier, J. C. (1987) *Scand. J. Immunol.* **25**, 195–202.
Jung, L. K. L., Hara, T. and Fu, S. M. (1984) *J. Exp. Med.* **160**, 1597–1602.
Kabelitz, D., Pfeffer, K., Von Steldern, D., Bartmann, P., Brudler, O., Nerl, C. and Wagner, H. (1985) *J. Immunol.* **135**, 2876–2881.
Karasuyama, H., Rolink, A. and Melchers, F. (1988). *J. Exp. Med.* **167**, 1377–1390.
Karray, S., Vazquez, A., Merle-Béral, H., Olive, D., Debré, P. and Galanaud, P. (1987) *J. Immunol.* **138**, 3824–3828.
Karray, S., Defrance, T., Merle-Béral, H., Banchereau, J., Debré, P. and Galanaud, P. (1988) *J. Exp. Med.* **168**, 85–94.
Kawano, M., Matsushima, K. and Oppenheim, J. J. (1987) *Cell. Immunol.* **108**, 132–149.
Kawano, M., Hirano, T., Matsuda, T., Taga, T., Horii, Y., Iwato, K., Asaoku, H., Tang, B., Tanabe, O., Tanaka, H., Kuramoto, A. and Kishimoto, T. (1988a) *Nature* **332**, 83–85.
Kawano, M., Matsushima, K., Masuda, A. and Oppenheim, J. J. (1988b) *Cell. Immunol.* **111**, 273–286.
Kehrl, J. H., Muraguchi, A., Butler, J. L., Falkoff, R. J. M. and Fauci, A. S. (1984) *Immunol. Rev.* **78**, 75–96.
Kehrl, J. H., Roberts, A. B., Wakefield, L. M., Jakowlew, S., Sporn, M. B. and Fauci, A. S. (1986) *J. Immunol.* **137**, 3855–3860.
Kehrl, J. H., Alvarez-Mon, M., Delsing, G. A. and Fauci, A. S. (1987a) *Science* **238**, 1144–1146.
Kehrl, J. H., Miller, A. and Fauci, A. S. (1987b) *J. Exp. Med.* **166**, 786–791.
Kehrl, J. H., Taylor, A. S., Delsing, G. A., Roberts, A. B., Sporn, M. B. and Fauci, A. S. (1989) *J. Immunol.* **143**, 1868–1874.
Kehry, M. and Hudak, S. A. (1989) *Cell. Immunol.* **118**, 504–515.
Kehry, M. R. and Yamashita, L. C. (1989) *Proc. Natl. Acad. Sci. USA* **86**, 7556–7560.

Keski-Oja, J., Lyons, R. M. and Moses, H. L. (1987) *J. Cell. Biochem.*, *Suppl.* **11A**, 60–70.

Kikutani, H., Suemura, M., Owaki, H., Nakamura, H., Sato, R., Yamasaki, K., Barsumian, E. L., Hardy, R. R. and Kishimoto, T. (1986) *J. Exp. Med.* **164**, 1455–1469.

Kimoto, M., Kindler, V., Higaki, M., Ody, C., Izui, S. and Vassalli, P. (1988) *J. Immunol.* **140**, 1889–1894.

Kinashi, T., Harada, N., Severinson, E., Tanabe, T., Sideras, P., Konishi, M., Azuma, C., Tominaga, A., Bergstedt-Lindqvist, S., Takahashi, M., Matsuda, F., Yaoita, Y., Takatsu, K. and Honjo, T. (1986) *Nature* **324**, 70–73.

Kinashi, T., Inaba, K., Tashiro, K., Palacios, R. and Honjo, T. (1988) *Proc. Natl. Acad. Sci. USA* **85**, 4473–4477.

Kincade, P. W., Lee, G., Pietrangeli, C. E., Hayashi, S.-I. and Gimble, J. M. (1989) *Ann. Rev. Immunol.* **7**, 111–143.

Kindler, V., Thorens, B. and Vassalli, P. (1987) *Eur. J. Immunol.* **17**, 1511–1514.

King, A. G., Wierda, D. and Landreth, K. S. (1988) *J. Immunol.* **141**, 2016–2026.

Klaus, G. G. B. and Humphrey, J. H. (1986) *Immunol. Today* **7**, 163–164.

Klein, B., Zhang, X.-G., Jourdan, M., Content, J., Houssiau, F., Aarden, L., Piechaczyk, M. and Bataille, R. (1989) *Blood* **73**, 517–526.

Kocks, C. and Rajewsky, K. (1989) *Ann. Rev. Immunol.* **7**, 537–559.

Kolsch, E., Oberbarnscheidt, J., Bruner, K. and Hever, J. (1980) *Immunol. Rev.* **49**, 61–78.

Korsmeyer, S. J., Greene, W. C., Cossman, J., Hsu, S. M., Jensen, J. P., Neckers, L. M., Marshall, S. L., Bakhshi, A., Depper, J. M., Leonard, W. J., Jaffe, E. S. and Waldmann, T. A. (1983) *Proc. Natl. Acad. Sci. USA* **80**, 4522–4526.

Lantz, O., Grillot-Courvalin, C., Schmitt, C., Fermand, J. P. and Brouet, J. C. (1985) *J. Exp. Med.* **161**, 1225–1230.

Lanzavecchia, A. (1987) *Immunol. Rev.* **99**, 39–51.

Laszlo, G. and Dickler, H. B. (1988) *J. Immunol.* **141**, 3416–3421.

Le, J., Reis, L. F. L. and Vilcek, J. (1988) *Lymphokine Res.* **7**, 99–105.

LeBien, T. W. (1989) *Immunol. Today* **10**, 296–298.

Leclercq, L., Cambier, J. C., Mishal, Z., Julius, M. H. and Theze, J. (1986) *J. Immunol.* **136**, 539–545.

Lee, G., Ellingsworth, L. R., Gillis, S., Wall, R. and Kincade, P. W. (1987) *J. Exp. Med.* **166**, 1290–1299.

Lee, G., Namen, A. E., Gillis, S., Ellingsworth, L. R. and Kincade, P. W. (1989) *J. Immunol.* **142**, 3875–3883.

Lemoine, F. M., Humphries, R. K., Abraham, S. D. M., Krystal, G. and Eaves, C. J. (1988) *Exp. Hematol.* **16**, 718–726.

Loughnan, M. S. and Nossal, G. J. V. (1989) *Nature* **340**, 76–79.

Loughnan, M. S., Takatsu, K., Harada, N. and Nossal, G. J. V. (1987) *Proc. Natl. Acad. Sci. USA* **84**, 5399–5403.

MacLennan, I. C. and Gray, D. (1986) *Immunol. Rev.* **91**, 61–85.

Maizel, A., Sahasrabuddhe, C., Mehta, S., Morgan, J., Lachman, L. and Ford, R. (1982) *Proc. Natl. Acad. Sci. USA* **79**, 5998–6002.

Maizel, A. L., Morgan, J. W., Mehta, S. R., Kouttab, N. M., Bator, J. M. and Sahasrabudde, C. J. (1983) *Proc. Natl. Acad. Sci. USA* **80**, 5047–5051.

Malek, T. R., Robb, R. J. and Shevach, E. M. (1983) *Proc. Natl. Acad. Sci. USA* **80**, 5694–5698.

Malkovska, V., Murphy, J., Hudson, L. and Bevan, D. (1987) *Clin. Exp. Immunol.* **68**, 677–684.

Matsushima, K., Tosato, G., Benjamin, D. and Oppenheim, J. J. (1985) *Cell. Immunol.* **94**, 418–426.

McKearn, J. P., McCubrey, J. and Fagg, B. (1985) *Proc. Natl. Acad. Sci. USA* **82**, 7414–7418.

Melchers, F. and Andersson, J. (1984) *Cell* **37**, 715–720.

Melchers, F., Erdei, A., Schulz, T. and Dierich, M. P. (1985) *Nature* **317**, 264–267.

Metcalf, D., Begley, C. G., Johnson, G. R., Nicola, N. A., Lopez, A. F. and Williamson, D. J. (1986) *Blood* **68**, 46–57.

Michalevicz, R. and Revel, M. (1987) *Proc. Natl. Acad. Sci. USA* **84**, 2307–2311.

Mingari, M. C., Gerosa, F., Carra, G., Accolla, R. S., Moretta, A., Zubler, R. H., Waldmann, T. A. and Moretta, L. (1984) *Nature* **312**, 641–643.

Mittler, R., Rao, P., Olini, G., Westberg, E., Newman, W., Hoffmann, M. and Goldstein, G. (1985) *J. Immunol.* **134**, 2393–2399.

Moberts, R., Hoogerbrugge, H., Van Agthoven, T., Löwenberg, B. and Touw, I. (1989) *Leukemia Res.* **13**, 973–980.

Mond, J. J., Finkelman, F. D., Sarma, C., Ohara, J. and Serrate, S. (1985a) *J. Immunol.* **135**, 2513–2517.

Mond, J. J., Thompson, C., Finkelman, F., Farrar, J., Schaefer, M. and Robb, R. J. (1985b) *Proc. Natl. Acad. Sci. USA* **82**, 1518–1521.

Mond, J. J., Carman, J., Sarma, C., Ohara, J. and Finkelman, F. (1986) *J. Immunol.* **137**, 3534–3537.

Mongini, P., Seremetis, S., Blessinger, C., Rudich, S., Winchester, R. and Brunda, M. (1988) *Blood* **72**, 1553–1559.

Morgan, E. L. and Weigle, W. O. (1983) *J. Immunol.* **130**, 1066–1070.

Morikawa, K., Kubagawa, H., Suzuki, T. and Cooper, M. D. (1987) *J. Immunol.* **139**, 761–766.

Morrissey, P. J., Goodwin, R. G., Nordan, R. P., Anderson, D., Grabstein, K. H., Cosman, D., Sims, J., Lupton, S., Agres, B., Reed, S. G., Mochizuki, D., Eisenman, J., Conlon, P. J. and Namen, A. E. (1989) *J. Exp. Med.* **169**, 707–716.

Mosmann, T. R. and Coffman, R. L. (1989) *Ann. Rev. Immunol.* **7**, 145–173.

Müller, L., Kühn, R., Goldmann, W., Tesch, H., Smith, F. I., Radbruch, A. and Rajewsky, K. (1985) *J. Immunol.* **135**, , 1213–1219.

Muraguchi, A., Kehrl, J. H., Longo, D. L., Volkman, D. J., Smith, K. A. and Fauci, A. S. (1985) *J. Exp. Med.* **161**, 181–197.

Murphy, J. J., Malkovska, V., Hudson, L. and Millard, R. E. (1987) *Clin. Exp. Immunol.* **70**, 182–191.

Murray, R., Suda, T., Wrighton, N., Lee, F. and Zlotnik, A. (1989) *Intern. Immunol.* **1**, 526–531.

Nakagawa, T., Hirano, T., Nakagawa, N., Yoshizaki, K. and Kishimoto, T. (1985) *J. Immunol.* **134**, 959–966.

Nakajima, K., Hirano, T., Takatsuki, F., Sakaguchi, N., Yoshida, N. and Kishimoto, T. (1985) *J. Immunol.* **135**, 1207–1212.

Nakanishi, K., Malek, T. R., Smith, K. A., Hamaoka, T., Shevach, E. M. and Paul, W. E. (1984) *J. Exp. Med.* **160**, 1605–1621.

Nakanishi, K., Yoshimoto, T., Katoh, Y., Ono, S., Matsui, K., Hiroïshi, K., Noma, T., Honjo, T., Takatsu, K., Higashino, K. and Hamaoka, T. (1988) *J. Immunol.* **140**, 1168–1174.

Nakanishi, K., Yoshimoto, T., Matsui, K., Hirose, S., Hiroishi, K., Hada, T. and Higashino, K. (1989) *Berlin, 7th International Congress of Immunology*, Abstract 63-40. VCH Publishers Inc, Florida.

Namen, A. E., Schmierer, A. E., March, C. J., Overell, R. W., Park, L. S., Urdal, D. L. and Mochizuki, D. Y. (1988a) *J. Exp. Med.* **167**, 988–1002.

Namen, A. E., Lupton, S., Hjerrild, K., Wagnall, J., Mochizuki, D. Y., Schmierer, A., Mosley, B., March, C. J., Urdal, D. G. S., Cosman, D. and Goodwin, R. G. (1988b) *Nature* **333**, 571–573.

Noelle, R., Krammer, P. H., Ohara, J., Uhr, J. W. and Vitetta, E. S. (1984) *Immunol.* **81**, 6149–6153.

Noelle, R. J., Kuziel, W. A., Maliszewski, C. R., McAdams, E., Vitetta, E. S. and Tucker, P. W. (1986) *J. Immunol.* **137**, 1718–1723.

O'Garra, A. and Defrance, T. (1990) *Bioassays for Interleukins*. Ed. by H. Zola, CRC Press, in press.

O'Garra, A., Warren, D. J., Holman, M., Popham, A. M., Sanderson, C. J. and Klaus, G. G. B. (1986) *Proc. Natl. Acad. Sci. USA* **83**, 5228–5232.

O'Garra, A., Rigley, K. P., Holman, M., McLaughlin, J. B. and Klaus, G. G. B. (1987) *Proc. Natl. Acad. Sci. USA* **84**, 6254–6258.

O'Garra, A., Barbis, D., Wu, J., Hodgkin, P. D., Abrams, J. and Howard, M. (1989) *Cell. Immunol.* **123**, 189–200.

Ohara, J. and Paul, W. E. (1987) *Nature* **325**, 537–540.

Oliver, K., Noelle, R. J., Uhr, J. W., Krammer, P. H. and Vitetta, E. S. (1985) *Proc. Natl. Acad. Sci. USA* **82**, 2465–2467.

Östlund, L., Einhorn, S., Robert, K. H., Juliusson, G. and Biberfeld, P. (1986) *Blood* **67**, 152–159.

Östlund, L., Einhorn, S., Robert, K. H., Christensson, B. and Einborn, S. (1989) *Blood* **73**, 2171–2181.

Otten, U., Ehrhard, P. and Peck, R. (1989) *Proc. Natl. Acad. Sci. USA* **86**, 10059–10063.

Palacios, R. and Steinmetz, M. (1985) *Cell* **41**, 727–734.

Palacios, R., Henson, G., Steinmetz, M. and McKearn, J. P. (1984) *Nature* **309**, 126–131.

Palacios, R., Karasuyama, H. and Rolink, A. (1987) *EMBO J.* **6**, 3687–3693.

Park, L. S., Friend, D., Sassenfeld, H. M. and Urdal, D. L. (1987) *J. Exp. Med.* **166**, 476–488.

Pathak, S. K., Tsang, K. Y., Cathcart, M. K., Arnaud, P., Boutin, B. and Fudenberg, H. H. (1985) *Immunol. Letters* **10**, 339–346.

Peschel, C., Green, I. and Paul, W. E. (1989) *J. Immunol.* **142**, 1558–1568.

Peters, M. G., Ambrus, J. L., Fauci, A. S. and Brown, E. J. (1988) *J. Exp. Med.* **168**, 1225–1235.

Petit-Koskas, E., Génot, E., Lawrence, D. and Kolb, J.-P. (1988) *Eur. J. Immunol.* **18**, 111–116.

Phillips, N., Gravel, K. A., Tumas, K. and Parker, D. C. (1988) *J. Immunol.* **141**, 4243–4249.

Pike, B. L. and Nossal, G. J. V. (1985) *Immunology* **82**, 8153–8157.

Pike, B. L., Raubitschek, A. and Nossal, G. J. V. (1984) *Proc. Natl. Acad. Sci. USA* **81**, 7917–7921.

Pike, B. L., Alderson, M. R. and Nossal, G. J. V. (1987) *Immunol. Rev.* **99**, 119–152.

Poupart, P., Vandenabeele, P., Cayphas, S., Van Snick, J., Haegeman, G., Kruys, V., Fiers, W. and Content, J. (1987) *EMBO J.* **6**, 1219–1224.

Rabin, E. M., Ohara, J. and Paul, W. E. (1985) *Proc. Natl. Acad. Sci. USA* **82**, 2935–2939.

Rabin, E. M., Mond, J. J., Ohara, J. and Paul, W. E. (1986a) *J. Exp. Med.* **164**, 517–531.

Rabin, E. M., Mond, J. J., Ohara, J. and Paul, W. (1986b) *J. Immunol.* **137**, 1573–1576.

Rennick, D., Yang, G., Muller-Sieburg, C., Smith, C., Arai, A., Takabe, Y. and Gemmel, L. (1987) *Proc. Natl. Acad. Sci. USA* **84**, 6889–6893.

Rennick, D., Jackson, J., Moulds, C., Lee, F. and Yang, G. (1989) *J. Immunol.* **142**, 161–166.

Richard, Y., Leprince, C., Dugas, B., Treton, D. and Galanaud, P. (1987) *J. Immunol.* **139**, 1563–1567.

Roehm, N. W., Leibson, H. J., Zlotnick, A., Kappler, J., Marrack, P. and Cambier, J. C. (1984) *J. Exp. Med.* **160**, 679–694.

Rolink, A. G., Andersson, J., Karasuyama, H. and Melchers, F. (1989) In *Topics in Immunology Ninth European Immunology Meeting*, Rome, pp. 118–124.

Romagnani, S., Giudizi, M. G., Biagiotti, R., Almerigogna, F., Mingari, M. G., Maggi, E., Liang, M. C. and Moretta, L. (1986a) *J. Immunol.* **136**, 3513–3516.

Romagnani, S., Giudizi, M. G., Almerigogna, F., Biagiotti, R., Alessi, A., Mingari, C., Liang, C., Moretta, L. and Ricci, M. (1986b) *Eur. J. Immunol.* **16**, 623–629.

Rousset, F., de Waal Malefijt, R., Slierendregt, B., Aubry, J. P., Bonnefoy, J. Y., Defrance, T., Banchereau, J. and de Vries, J. E. (1988) *J. Immunol.* **140**, 2625–2632.

Rousset, F., Billaud, M., Blanchard, D., Figdor, C., Lenoir, G. M., Spits, H. and de Vries, J. E. (1989) *J. Immunol.* **143**, 1490–1498.

Ryan, J. L., Arbeit, R. D., Dickler, H. B. and Henkart, P. A. (1975) *J. Exp. Med.* **142**, 814–826.

Saiki, O., Tanaka, T., Doi, S. and Kishimoto, S. (1988) *J. Immunol.* **140**, 853–858.

Sanders, V. M., Fernandez-Botran, R., Uhr, J. W. and Vitetta, E. S. (1987) *J. Immunol.* **139**, 2349–2354.

Sanderson, C. J., Campbell, H. D. and Young, I. G. (1988) *Immunol. Rev.* **102**, 29–50.

Saragovi, H. and Malek, T. R. (1987) *J. Immunol.* **139**, 1918–1926.

Sarfati, M., Luo, H. and Delespesse, G. (1989) *J. Exp. Med.* **170**, 1775–1780.

Sauerwein, R. W., Van der Meer, W. G. J. and Aarden, L. A. (1987) *Blood* **70**, 670–675.

Scapigliati, G., Ghiara, P., Bartalini, M., Tagliabue, A. and Borachi, D. (1989) *FEBS Lett.* **243**, 394–398.

Schimple, A. and Wecker, E (1972) *Nature* **237**, 15–17.

Seregina, T. M., Mekshenkov, M. I., Turetskaya, R. L. and Nedospasov, S. A. (1989) *Mol. Immunol.* **26**, 339–342.

Servis, C. and Lambris, J. D. (1989) *J. Immunol.* **142**, 2207–2212.

Seyschab, H., Friedl, R., Schindler, D., Hoehn, H., Rabinovitch, P. S. and Chen, U. (1989) *Eur. J. Immunol.* **19**, 1605–1612.

Sharma, S., Mehta, S., Morgan, J. and Maizel, A. (1987) *Science* **234**, 1489–1492.

Shields, J. G., Armitage, R. J., Jamieson, B. N., Beverley, P. C. L. and Callard, R. E. (1989) *Immunology* **66**, 224–227.

Shimizu, K., Hirano, T., Ishibashi, K., Nakano, N., Taga, T., Sugamura, K., Yamamura, Y. and Kishimoto, T. (1985) _J. Immunol._ **134**, 1728–1733.

Shimizu, S., Yoshioka, R., Hirose, Y., Sugai, S., Tachibana, J. and Konda, S. (1989) _J. Exp. Med._ **169**, 339–344.

Siegel, D. S., Junming, L. and Vilcek, J. (1986) _Cell. Immunol._ **101**, 380–390.

Smeland, E. B., Blomhoff, H. K., Holte, H., Ruud, E., Beiske, K., Funderud, S., Godal, T. and Ohlsson, R. (1987) _Exp. Cell Res._ **171**, 213–222.

Smeland, E. B., Blomhoff, H. K., Funderud, S., Shalaby, M. R. and Espevik, T. (1989) _J. Exp. Med._ **170**, 1463–1468.

Spalding, D. M. and Griffin, J. A. (1986) _Cell_ **44**, 507–515.

Sporn, M. B. and Roberts, A. B. (1988) _Nature_ **332**, 214–219.

Stead, R. H., Bienenstock, J. and Stanisz, A. M. (1987) _Immunol. Rev._ **100**, 333–360.

Stein, P., Dubois,P., Greenblatt, D. and Howard, M. (1986) _J. Immunol._ **136**, 2080–2089.

Suda, T., Okada, S., Suda, J., Miura, Y., Ito, M., Sudo, T., Hayashi, S.-I., Nishikawa, S.-I. and Nakauchi, H. (1989) _Blood_ **74**, 1936–1941.

Sudo, T., Ito, M., Ogawa, Y., Iizuka, M., Kodama, H., Kunisada, T., Hayashi, S.-I., Ogawa, M., Sakai, K., Nishikawa, S. and Nishikawa, S.-I. (1989) _J. Exp. Med._ **170**, 333–338.

Sung, S.-S. J., Jung, L. K. L, Walters, J. A., Jeffes III, E. W. B., Granger, G. A. and Fu, S. M. (1988) _J. Exp. Med._ **168**, 1539–1551.

Sung, S.-S. J., Jung, L. K. L., Walters, J. A., Jeffes I, E. W. B., Granger, G. A. and Fu, S. M. (1989) _J. Clin. Invest_ **84**, 236–243.

Suzuki, T. and Cooper, M. D. (1985) _J. Immunol._ **134**, 3111–3119.

Swain, S. L. and Dutton, R. W. (1982) _J. Exp. Med._ **156**, 1821–1834.

Swain, S. L., Howard, M., Kappler, J., Marrack, P., Watson, J., Booth, R., Wetzel, G. D. and Dutton, R. W. (1983) _J. Exp. Med._ **158**, 822–835.

Swain, S. L., McKenzie, D. T., Dutton, R. W., Tonkonogy, S. L. and English, M. (1988) _Immunol. Rev._ **102**, 77–105.

Swendeman, S. and Thorley-Lawson, D. A. (1987) _EMBO J._ **6**, 1637–1642.

Szakal, A. K. (1989) _Ann. Rev. Immunol._ **7**, 91–109.

Takatsu, K., Kikuchi, Y. H., Takahashi, N., Honjo, T., Matsumoto, M., Harada, N., Yamaguchi, N. and Tominaga, A. (1987) _Proc. Natl. Acad. Sci. USA_ **84**, 4234–4240.

Takeda, S., Gillis, S. and Palacios, R. (1989) _Proc. Natl. Acad. Sci. USA_ **86**, 1634–1638.

Tanaka, T., Saiki, O., Doi, S., Suemura, M., Negoro, S. and Kishimoto, S. (1988) _J. Clin. Invest._ **82**, 316–321.

Thorley-Lawson, D. A. and Mann, K. P. (1985) _J. Exp. Med._ **162**, 45–59.

Thorley-Lawson, D. A., Nadler, L. N., Bhan, A. K. and Schooley, R. T. (1985) _J. Immunol._ **134**, 3007–3012.

Thorley-Lawson, D. A., Swendeman, S. L. and Edson, C. M. (1986) _J. Immunol._ **136**, 1745–1751.

Tigges, M. A., Casey, L. S. and Koshland, M. E. (1989) _Science_ **243**, 781–786.

Tominaga, A., Mita, S., Kikuchi, Y., Hitoshi, Y. and Takatsu, K. (1989) _Growth Factors_ **1**, 135–146.

Tosato, G., Seamon, K. B., Goldman, N. D., Sehgal, P. B., May, L. T., Washington, G. C., Jones, K. D. and Pike, S. E. (1988) _Science_ **239**, 502–504.

Tsudo, M., Uchiyama, T. and Uchino, H. (1984) _J. Exp. Med._ **160**, 612–617.

Uchibayashi, N., Kikutani, H., Barsumian, E. L., Hauptmann, R., Schneider, F.-J., Schwendenwein, R., Sommergruber, W., Spevak,W., Maurer-Fogy, I., Suemura, M. and Kishimoto, T. (1989) *J. Immunol.* **142**, 3901–3908.

Uckun, F., Fauci, A. S., Heerema, N. A., Song, C. W., Mehta, S. R., Gajl-Peczalska, K., Chandan, M. and Ambrus, J. L. (1987) *Blood* **70**, 1020–1034.

Uckun, F. M. and Ledbetter, J. A. (1988) *Proc. Natl. Acad. Sci. USA* **85**, 8603–8607.

Umland, S. P., Go, N. F., Cupp, J. E. and Howard, M. (1989) *J. Immunol.* **142**, 1528–1535.

Vallé, A., Zuber, C. E., Defrance,T., Djossou, O., De Rie, M. and Banchereau, J. (1989) *Eur. J. Immunol.* **19**, 1463–1467.

Van Snick, J., Vink, A., Cayphas, S. and Uyttenhove, C. (1987) *J. Exp. Med.* **165**, 641–649.

Van Snick,J., Goethals, A., Renauld, J.-C., Van Roost, E., Uyttenhove, C., Rubira, M. R., Moritz, R. L. and Simpson, R. J. (1989) *J. Exp. Med.* **169**, 363–368.

Vandenabeele, P., Jayaram, B., Devos, R., Shaw, A. and Fiers, W. (1988) *Eur. J. Immunol.* **18**, 1027–1031.

Vazquez, A., Auffredou, M.-T., Gerard, J.-P., Delfraissy, J.-F. and Galanaud, P. (1987) *J. Immunol.* **139**, 2344–2348.

Vink, A., Coulie, P. G., Wauters, P., Nordan, R. P. and Van Snick, J. (1988) *Eur. J. Immunol.* **18**, 607–612.

Vitetta,E. S., Brooks, K., Chen, Y. W., Isakson, P., Jones, S., Layton, P., Mishira, G. C., Pure, E., Weiss, E., Ward, C., Yvan, D., Tucker, P., Uhr, J. W. and Krammer, P. H. (1984) *Immunol. Rev.* **78**, 137–157.

Wakasugi, H., Rimsky, L., Mahe, Y., Kamel, A. M., Fradelizi, D., Tursz, T. and Bertoglio, J. (1987) *Proc. Natl. Acad. Sci. USA* **84**, 804–808.

Wakefield, L. M., Smith, D. M., Flanders, K. C. and Sporn, M. B. (1988) *J. Biol. Chem.* **263**, 7646–7654.

Wakelam, M. J. O., Murphy, G. J., Hruby, V. J. and Houslay, M. D. (1986) *Nature* **323**, 68–71.

Waldmann, T. A. and Broder, S. (1982) *Adv. Immunol.* **32**, 1–55.

Walker, L., Guy, G., Brown, G., Rowe, M., Milner, A. E. and Gordon, J. (1986) *Immunol.* **58**, 583–589.

Warrington, R. J., Rutherford, W. J., Wong, S.-K., Cook, J. M. and Rector, E. S. (1989) *J. Immunol.* **143**, 2546–2552.

Weigent, D. A. and Blalock, J. E. (1987) *Immunol. Rev.* **100**, 79–108.

Welch, P. A., Namen, A. E., Goodwin, R. G., Armitage, R. and Cooper, M. D. (1989) *J. Immunol.* **143**, 3562–3567.

Wetzel, G. D. (1989) *Eur. J. Immunol.* **19**, 1701–1707.

Whitlock, C. A. and Witte, O. N. (1982) *Proc. Natl. Acad. Sci. USA* **79**, 3608–3612.

Williamson, B. D., Carswell, E. A., Rubin, B. Y., Prendergast, J. S. and Old, L. J. (1983) *Proc. Natl. Acad. Sci. USA* **80**, 5397–5401.

Wörmann, B., Mehta, S. R., Maizel, A. L. and LeBien, T. W. (1987) *Blood* **70**, 132–138.

Xia, X. and Choi, Y. S. (1988) *J. Biol. Resp. Modif.* **7**, 283–295.

Yamaoka, K. A., Claesson, H.-E. and Rosen, A. (1989) *J. Immunol.* **143**, 1996–2000.

Yang, Y.-C., Ricciardi, S., Ciarletta, A., Calvetti, J., Kelleher, K. and Clark, S. C. (1989) *Blood* **74**, 1880–1884.

Yee, C., Biondi, A., Wang, X. H., Iscove, N. N., de Sousa, J., Aarden, L. A.,

Wong, G. G., Clark, S. C., Messner, H. A. and Minden, M. D. (1989) *Blood* **74**, 798–804.

Yokota, A., Kikutani, H., Tanaka, T., Sato, R., Barsumian, E. L., Suermura, M. and Kishimoto, T. (1988) *Cell* **55**, 611–618.

Yoshizaki, K., Nakagawa, T., Fukunaga, K., Kaieda, T., Maruyama, S., Kishimoto, S., Yamamura, Y. and Kishimoto, T. (1983) *J. Immunol.* **130**, 1241–1252.

Yukawa, K., Kikutani, H., Owaki, H., Yamasaki, K., Yokota, A., Nakamura, H., Barsumian, E. L., Hardy, R. R., Suemura, M. and Kishimoto, T. (1987) *J. Immunol.* **138**, 2576–2580.

Zhang, X.-G., Bataille, R., Jourdan, M., Saeland, S., Banchereau, J. and Klein, B. (1990) Submitted.

Zola, H. and Nikoloutsopoulos, A. (1989) *Immunology* **67**, 231–236.

Zuber, C. E., Galizzi, J. P., Vallé, A., Harada, N., Howard, M. and Banchereau, J. (1990) *Eur. J. Immunol.* **20**, 551–555.

Zubler, R. H., Lowenthal, J. W., Erard, F., Hashimoto, N., Devos, R. and MacDonald, H. R. (1984) *J. Exp. Med.* **160**, 1170–1183.

Zubler, R. H., Werner-Favre, C., Wen, L., Sekita, K.-I. and Straub, C. (1987) *Immunol. Rev.* **99**, 281–299.

5
Cytokine regulation of B-cell differentiation

RICHARD J. ARMITAGE, KENNETH H. GRABSTEIN
AND MARK R. ALDERSON

Introduction

Over the last decade much attention has been focused on the rôle of T cells and T-cell derived soluble factors in B-cell differentiation and immunoglobulin (Ig) secretion. Following initial observations that antibody production was dependent on the interaction between T and B cells, it was found that supernatants from lymphocytes activated with polyclonal mitogens such as concanavalin A (Con A) or in a mixed lymphocyte reaction (MLR) contained much of the B-cell stimulatory activity previously ascribed to T cells (Dutton et al., 1971; Schimpl and Wecker, 1972). These T-cell derived mediators, termed T-cell replacing factors (TRF), were found to be active in a wide range of different assays for both T- and B-cell function. Initially, it was not clear how many different biological entities or cytokines were present in TRF. Subsequently, purification and, more recently, molecular cloning and production of recombinant factors has allowed the study of the distinct biological activities of these cytokines on various haemopoietic cell types.

The first T-cell derived cytokine to be cloned was interleukin 2 (IL-2), which was found in high concentrations in the supernatants of activated T cells. Although originally thought to specifically act on T cells, IL-2 was subsequently found to exert a multiplicity of actions on other cell types and, in particular, B cells. IL-2 not only provides a powerful proliferative signal to activated human B cells (Mingari et al., 1984) but also induces polyclonal Ig secretion from activated primary B cells and B-cell lines (Muraguchi et al., 1985). From early work on TRF, it became clear that IL-2 was not the only factor present which could exert an effect on B-cell function. Howard et al. (1982) described a cytokine termed B-cell growth factor, later called B-cell

CYTOKINES AND B LYMPHOCYTES
ISBN 0–12–155145–8

stimulatory factor 1 (BSF-1), which was distinct from IL-2 and had activity in B-cell proliferation. Vitetta *et al.* (1984) reported a factor that induced IgG1 secretion from lipopolysaccharide (LPS) induced B cells. The cloning of the cDNA for this activity (Noma *et al.*, 1986) demonstrated that it was identical to BSF-1 and led to its identification as IL-4. Interleukin 5 was first described by Swain and co-workers as B-cell growth factor II (BCGF-II) due to its ability to induce the *in vitro* proliferation of the BCL_1 *in vivo* cell line and to co-stimulate with dextran sulphate to cause normal murine B cells to proliferate (Swain *et al.*, 1983). Concurrent with the characterization of BCGF-II, Takatsu and colleagues reported on a TRF found in the supernatant of the B151-K12 T-cell hybridoma (Takatsu *et al.*, 1980a,b, 1985). It was shown that B151-TRF promotes IgM secretion by BCL_1 cells and induces hapten-specific IgG production *in vitro* by *in vivo* antigen-primed B cells. Molecular cloning of the B151-TRF gene proved that it also encoded BCGF-II activity, hence the designation IL-5 (Kinashi *et al.*, 1986).

Human IL-6 was first described by Hirano and colleagues (Hirano *et al.*, 1985), and its B-cell differentiation activity demonstrated by the ability to increase IgM secretion from an Epstein–Barr virus (EBV) transformed B-cell line. In contrast, murine IL-6 was first identified by its activity as a hybridoma and plasmacytoma growth factor (Nordan and Potter, 1986; Van Snick *et al.*, 1986). With the recent availability of recombinant material (Hirano *et al.*, 1986; Chiu *et al.*, 1988; Van Snick *et al.*, 1988), IL-6 has been shown to have differentiation activity on normal human and murine B cells, especially in combination with other cytokines.

In addition to these cytokines, the actions of which have been found to have important consequences for B-cell differentiation, several other recombinant proteins have been shown to modulate immunoglobulin secretion, including interferon (IFN) α, β and γ, interleukin 1, interleukin 3, tumour necrosis factor (TNF) α and β, and transforming growth factor (TGF) β.

In this chapter we will review the rôle cytokines play in proliferation and the production of immunoglobulin by murine and human B cells, with particular emphasis on the regulatory effects imparted on this process by combinations of cytokines. A summary of these effects of cytokines alone or in combination, discussed in this chapter, is contained in Tables 7 and 8.

Interleukin 2

Early studies on murine B-cell differentiation suggested that in high-density cultures of partially purified B cells, IL-2 may be acting via contaminating non-B cells (Howard and Paul, 1983). However, numerous reports indicate

Table 1 Effect of cytokines on the production of anti-SRBC plaque forming cells (PFC) in the TRF assay.[a]

	PFC per culture (S.D.)	
Addition to whole spleen	Exp. 1	Exp. 2
—	3,520 (453)	7,190 (144)
IL-2	10,040 (768)	16,733 (411)
IL-5	9,520 (534)	9,500 (279)
IL-6	8,560 (196)	—
IFN-γ	1,013 (75)	—
Addition to T-depleted spleen	Exp. 1	Exp. 2
—	553 (175)	1,033 (66)
IL-2	18,347 (868)	26,640 (320)
IL-5	3,870 (156)	5,460 (467)
IL-6	706 (54)	—
IFN-γ	127 (25)	—

[a]TRF assay: C57BL/6 spleen cells were depleted of T cells by treatment with a cocktail of antibodies and complement including anti-thymocyte serum (liver and marrow absorbed) and monoclonal antibodies against Thy 1 (T24) and CD4 (GK1.5). Treated or untreated spleen cells were cultured at 5×10^6 per culture for 5 days in the presence of SRBC and the indicated additive. PFC values were determined using a Jerne hemolytic plaque assay. Purified IL-2 and IFN-γ were each used at a final concentration of 10 ng ml^{-1}, IL-5 and IL-6 were used at 1/20 and 1/100 dilution of cos cell s/n, respectively.

that a proportion of B cells can express IL-2 receptors upon appropriate stimulation (Zubler *et al.*, 1984; Nakanishi *et al.*, 1984; Lowenthal *et al.*, 1985; Loughnan *et al.*, 1987; Harada *et al.*, 1987). Furthermore, Zubler *et al.* (1984) observed that with murine B cells activated with anti-Ig plus LPS, IL-2 could induce optimal proliferation. In addition, studies by Pike *et al.* (1984) demonstrated that a small, though significant, proportion of single hapten-specific B cells were induced to grow and differentiate by recombinant human IL-2 acting in the presence of a T-independent antigen.

IL-2 has also been shown to be important in the development of murine antibody forming cells. With the availability of recombinant IL-2, it can be shown that IL-2 is sufficient to stimulate primary *in vitro* anti-sheep red blood cell (SRBC) antibody responses in murine spleen cells from which T cells have been depleted, as originally described for TRF (Table 1). Leibson *et al.* (1982) demonstrated that optimal development of anti-SRBC plaque-forming cells (PFC) from purified B cells was stimulated by a combination of cytokines, specifically IL-1, IL-2 and IFN-γ. Similar results are given in Table 2. Despite this strong evidence for the direct action of IL-2 on murine

Table 2 Induction of anti-SRBC plaque forming cells (PFC) from purified murine B cells.[a]

Addition	PFC per culture (S.D.)
—	0
IL-1	90 (20)
IL-2	0
IFN-γ	0
IL-1 + IL-2	437 (45)
IL-2 + IFN-γ	508 (56)
IL-1 + IL-2 + IFN-γ	1,225 (72)
IL-5	240 (33)
IL-1 + IL-5	600 (57)
IL-2 + IL-5	637 (33)
IL-1 + IL-2 + IL-5	1,310 (233)
LPS	151 (21)
MLR S/n[b]	1,313 (154)
LPS + MLR s/n	6,633 (435)

[a] Murine splenic B cells were purified by a combination of T-cell depletion (as described in Table 1), passage over Sephadex G10 to remove adherent cells and positive selection using anti-IgM-coated pans. Purified B cells were cultured at 3×10^5 cells per culture for 4 days in 16 mm dishes in the presence of SRBC and the indicated additive. PFC values were determined using a Jerne hemolytic plaque assay and are expressed as PFC per culture. Purified IL-1 was used at a final concentration of 10 ng ml^{-1}, IL-2, IFN-γ and IL-5 were added as described in Table 1.
[b] Mixed lymphocyte reaction supernatant.

B cells, recent studies have claimed that the activity of IL-2 in B-cell cultures can be accounted for by its influence on contaminating T cells (Leanderson and Julius, 1986; Julius et al., 1987).

Interleukin 2 has been shown by several groups to be a potent differentiation factor for polyclonally activated human B cells (Waldmann et al., 1984; Muraguchi et al., 1985; Nakagawa et al., 1985; Jelinek et al., 1986), but only if added in the first 24 h of culture (Devos et al., 1985). In addition to its co-stimulatory action on mitogen-activated B cells, IL-2 has been reported to induce secretion of IgM, IgG and IgA from tonsil B lymphocytes and IgM from chronic lymphocytic leukaemia (CLL) B cells in the absence of in vitro activation, and this effect appears not to be related to the expression of the p55 subunit of the IL-2 receptor (Bich-Thuy and Fauci, 1985). Furthermore, high concentrations of IL-2 can induce p55-negative B cells activated with SAC to secrete Ig, and this response is not inhibited by addition of neutralizing anti-p55 antibody (Ralph *et al.*, 1984), suggesting IL-2 can induce differentiation solely through an alternative IL-2-binding surface protein, possibly the p75 subunit of the IL-2 receptor. Interleukin 2 has also been shown to be a potent TRF in specific antibody responses by human B cells (Callard *et al.*, 1986; Smith *et al.*, 1989). In this response, IL-2 acted directly on the B cells (Callard *et al.*, 1986), but only on low density (activated) and not high density B cells (Callard and Smith, 1988). Taken together, data from experiments examining the influence of IL-2 on B-cell function show this lymphokine to be a potent differentiation factor for *in vitro*, and perhaps *in vivo*, activated human B cells.

Interleukin 4

The effects of IL-4 on B cells are manifested by several different *in vitro* biological assays. Interleukin 4 stimulates the proliferation as well as the differentiation of B cells and induces increased surface expression of major histocompatibility complex (MHC) class II molecules (Noelle *et al.*, 1984) and CD23 (Kikutani *et al.*, 1986; Defrance *et al.*, 1987). Despite the fact that IL-4 is a strong growth factor for anti-IgM or antigen co-stimulated B cells, under these conditions IL-4 fails to stimulate significant IgM secretion (Howard *et al.*, 1982; Alderson *et al.*, 1987a).

Interleukin 4 has been shown to induce both IgG1 and IgE secretion by LPS-activated murine B cells cultured *in vitro* (Vitetta *et al.*, 1984; Sideras *et al.*, 1985; Coffman *et al.*, 1986; Snapper and Paul, 1987a). This effect of IL-4 is on cells that lack surface expression of IgG to cause IgG1 secretion (Snapper and Paul, 1987a). Snapper *et al.* (1988a) have reported that stimulation of murine B cells with LPS plus increasing concentrations of IL-4 resulted in bimodal production of IgG1, with peaks of antibody production seen with 100 and 10,000 U ml^{-1} of IL-4. In contrast, augmentation of IgE secretion was directly related to an increase in the concentration of IL-4 and was maximum at 10,000 U ml^{-1}.

Single resting B cells can be induced by IL-4 plus either LPS or antigen-specific T cells to generate IgG1 and IgE secreting clones *in vitro* (Pike *et al.*, 1987; Coffman *et al.*, 1988; Lebman and Coffman 1988a). In addition, it has been observed that IL-4 can induce transcription of germ-line γ1 and ε RNA in the presence of LPS (Rothman *et al.*, 1988; Berton *et al.*, 1989). These results suggest that IL-4 promotes Ig class-switching, rather than preferential expansion of previously switched cells.

Probably the best documented cytokine interaction on mouse B cells occurs between IL-4 and IFN-γ. Interleukin 4 is able to cause a 100- to 1,000-fold enhancement in the levels of IgG1 and IgE secreted by LPS-stimulated

Table 3 Interferon γ inhibits the effects of IL-4 and IL-5 on murine B cells cultured with a T-independent antigen.[a]

	Antigen + IL-4		Antigen + IL-5		
IFN-γ (units/ml)	proliferating clones (%)	IgM secreting clones (%)	proliferating clones (%)	IgM secreting clones (%)	pg IgM/clone
0	13.3	4.6	12.9	14.9	123
1	10.5	3.8	11.8	15.7	101
10	8.7	4.8	9.9	16.5	81
100	4.4	4.2	7.1	12.4	73
1000	3.3	4.2	3.8	13.0	62

[a] Fluorescein (FLU)-specific B cells obtained by fractionation on Petri dishes coated with FLU-gelatin were cultured at approximately 5 cells per 10 μl Terasaki well in the presence of the T-independent antigen FLU-polymerized flagellin and cytokines as indicated. After 5 days of culture, wells were assessed for the presence of proliferating B-cell clones by microscopy, and IgM-secreting clones by ELISA. rIL-4 and rIL-5 were added at final concentrations of 100 units per ml^{-1} and 0.3% (v/v), respectively. Values represent the mean of three experiments.

B-cells, and the addition of IFN-γ to such cultures can totally block the IL-4 effect (Coffman and Carty, 1986; Snapper and Paul, 1987b). Similarly, small quantities of IFN-γ can inhibit the ability of IL-4 to act in the anti-IgM co-stimulator assay (Mond *et al.*, 1985) and to cause the proliferation of hapten-specific B cells (Table 3; Stein *et al.*, 1986). Conversely, IFN-γ can enhance IgG2a secretion by LPS-activated B cells, an effect which is inhibited by IL-4 (Snapper and Paul, 1987b). Interleukin 4 has been reported to inhibit IgM secretion by murine B cells stimulated with IL-1 and/or IL-2 in the presence of antigen (Alderson *et al.*, 1987a). In addition, IL-4 has been shown to potently suppress IgM, IgG3 and IgG2b secretion by LPS-stimulated B cells (Jones *et al.*, 1983; Snapper and Paul, 1987b). These *in vitro* studies have been extended by Finkelman and co-workers to *in vivo* models of isotype regulation. Using antibodies against murine IL-4 or against the IL-4 recep-tor it was found that IL-4 is absolutely required for IgE secretion *in vivo*, whereas alternative, IL-4 independent, pathways for IgG1 production may exist (Finkelman *et al.*, 1990).

Interleukin 4 has also been shown to regulate IgE secretion from human blood mononuclear cells, and this response can be inhibited by either IFN-α or -γ (Pene *et al.*, 1988a; Sarfati *et al.*, 1988). However, highly purified peripheral blood (PB) B lymphocytes activated with IL-4 alone fail to differentiate to Ig secreting cells. Therefore, IL-4-induced IgE secretion is either an indirect effect on accessory cells or a direct effect on B cells requiring an additional signal. In this regard, in the presence of EBV, IL-4 induces highly purified PB B cells to produce IgM, IgG and IgA and, after several weeks in culture, to secrete considerable amounts of IgE (Thyphronitis *et al.*, 1989). Therefore, IL-4 does appear to directly affect Ig secretion from B cells. However, recent reports have suggested that IL-4 induced IgE production from human B cells is T-cell dependent (Pene *et al.*, 1988a; Del Prete *et al.*, 1988). Verchelli *et al.* (1989a) have published data which suggest a necessity for cognate interactions between the T-cell receptor–CD3 (TCR–CD3) complex on T cells and MHC class II molecules on B cells for the induction of IgE secretion. Monocytes, together with T-cell and monocyte-derived cytokines, also appear to be required in this interaction, with IL-6 playing an apparently obligatory rôle in IL-4 induced IgE secretion (Verchelli *et al.*, 1989b). This response is enhanced by addition of IL-6, although IL-4, -5, and -6 together fail to induce B cells to differentiate in the absence of accessory cells.

Addition of IFN-γ to EBV-activated B cells inhibits IL-4 induced production of IgE but not that of other isotypes, suggesting that both IL-4 and IFN-γ have direct effects on B-cell differentiation. In contrast, purified tonsil B cells stimulated with *Staphylococcus aureus* Cowan (SAC) are induced by IL-4 to secrete IgG and IgM but not IgE (Defrance *et al.*, 1988a) and, as with EBV-activated B cells, production of these isotypes is not inhibited by addition of IFN-γ.

Using a mouse thymoma (EL4) co-culture method originally described by Zubler *et al.* (1987), Lundgren and colleagues (1989) found IL-4 to induce PMA-activated human splenic B cells to secrete high levels of IgE and IgG4. Production of IgE was in this system augmented by the presence of IL-2. Limiting-dilution analysis suggested that the addition of PMA and IL-4 together caused an increase in the precursor frequency for IgE-secreting cells over that seen with PMA alone, indicating that IL-4 induced an isotype switch in human B cells similar to that reported for murine B lymphocytes.

It has recently been reported (Smeland *et al.*, 1989) that IL-4 selectively induces secretion of IL-6 from PB B cells and that this effect is enhanced in the presence of anti-IgM. This finding, together with the apparent necessity for IL-6 to be present for IL-4 mediated IgE production, suggests that in many experimental systems using highly purified B cells, endogenous IL-6 production may play a rôle in the production of IgE in IL-4-stimulated cultures. The question of whether endogenous IL-6 production plays a rôle in LPS plus IL-4-derived IgE secretion by murine B cells remains to be addressed, though it is notable that Kunimoto *et al.* (1989) recently detected substantial levels of IL-6 in the supernatant of LPS-stimulated splenic B cells. Clearly, this apparently indirect effect of IL-4 on IgE secretion may also exist in the murine system.

While IL-4 obviously plays an important rôle in IgE production by both human and murine B cells, no clear parallel has been found in the human to the distinct actions, already discussed, of IL-4 and IFN-γ on murine IgG secretion. Although IgG4 in the human and IgG1 in the mouse are specifically enhanced by IL-4, and these isotypes share an ability to fix complement, human IgG4, unlike murine IgG1, is a minor subclass in serum. Furthermore, while IFN-γ appears to inhibit IL-4 induced human IgE secretion in certain assays (Pene et al., 1988a; Delespesse et al., 1989) in a manner reminiscent to that seen in the mouse, it has not been shown to enhance production of any human IgG isotype in the way that IgG2a is enhanced with IFN-γ plus LPS-stimulated murine B cells (Snapper and Paul, 1987b).

Under certain conditions IL-4 appears to be able to exert an inhibitory effect on human antibody production. Secretion of IgG1, IgG2 and IgE by PB, spleen or lymph node B cells activated with SAC and IL-2 is depressed if IL-4 is added at the onset of culture (Jelinek and Lipsky, 1988; Splawski et al., 1989). If, however, cells are pre-activated with SAC and IL-2 for 48 h, subsequent addition of IL-4 gives slight enhancement of Ig production. In contrast, under the same culture conditions Ig secretion by LPS- and IL-2-activated B cells can not be inhibited by IL-4. It has been suggested that the IgE response described in this system derives from memory B cells that have already switched to IgE at the DNA level. Interestingly, the inhibitory effects of IL-4 can be partially reversed by IFN-α or IFN-γ. The necessity for IL-4 to be present for the duration of culture with SAC and IL-2 for its inhibitory effects to be seen may explain the lack of inhibition noted by others in this type of culture system (Defrance et al., 1988b).

Interleukin 5

As mentioned previously, IL-5 is a potent growth and differentiation factor for activated murine B cells. Interleukin 5 has been shown to be a potent inducer of proliferation and IgM secretion by antigen co-stimulated single hapten-specific B cells (Alderson et al., 1987b) or populations of purified splenic B cells (Table 2). It also stimulates polyclonal B-cell differentiation in the absence of antigen (Table 4). In the presence of LPS, IL-5 enhances IgA secretion, though it appears that the mode of action of IL-5 is to selectively promote the growth and differentiation of B cells already committed to IgA secretion, rather than inducing a switch to IgA secretion per se (Harriman et al., 1988). Several groups have now shown that IL-5 can

Table 4 Polyclonal plaque forming cell (PFC) production from purified murine B cells.[a]

Addition	± IL-4	PFC per culture (S.D.)
—	—	92 (13)
—	+	193 (11)
IL-1	—	200 (24)
IL-1	+	179 (10)
IL-2	—	114 (15)
IL-2	+	127 (6)
IL-5	—	561 (14)
IL-5	+	1,345 (36)
IL-6	—	72 (7)
IL-6	+	128 (5)
IL-7	—	49 (7)
IL-7	+	96 (8)
IFN-γ	—	30 (6)
IFN-γ	+	30 (6)

[a]Murine splenic B cells were purified as described in Table 1. Purified B cells were cultured at 6×10^4 cells per well in 96-well culture plates for 3 days. PFC values were determined by reverse plaque assay using Protein A-coupled SRBC and rabbit anti-mouse IgG, A and M anti-serum. IL-7 was used at a final concentration of 10 ng ml^{-1}, other additions were made as described in Tables 1 and 2.

induce high levels of IgA secretion by surface IgA positive, but not negative, splenic or Peyer's patch B cells (Beagley *et al.*, 1988; Harriman *et al.*, 1988; Lebman and Coffman, 1988b; Tonkonogy *et al.*, 1989). Recent studies by Coffman and colleagues (1989) have implicated TGF-β in the class switch to IgA by IgM positive B cells.

A combination of cytokines that has positive modulatory effects on Ig secretion is IL-4 and IL-5. A synergistic effect between IL-4 and IL-5 has been reported for the induction of IgM and IgG3 secretion by murine B cells cultured in the absence of any other intentional stimulus, and for IgG1, IgE and IgA secretion by LPS co-stimulated B cells (Tonkonogy *et al.*, 1989; Coffman *et al.*, 1988). Interleukin 4 plus IL-5 is also a significantly more potent combination than either cytokine acting alone, for the proliferation of normal B cells and for the proliferation and IgM secretion by antigen co-stimulated hapten-specific B cells (Figure 1) and the formation of polyclonal PFC in the absence of antigen (Table 4).

Recent studies have indicated that IL-5 can enhance the expression of the

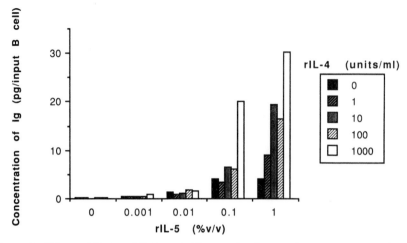

Figure 1 Effect of IL-4 and IL-5 on IgM secretion by murine antigen-specific B cells. Fluorescein (FLU)-specific B cells obtained by fractionation on Petri dishes coated with FLU-gelatin were cultured at 100 cells per 10 μl well in the presence of the T-independent antigen FLU-Ficoll and various concentrations of IL-4 and IL-5. After 5 days, supernatants from 12 replicate wells were pooled and IgM content determined by ELISA. Values represent the average amount of IgM secreted per input B cell.

p55 chain of the IL-2 receptor on normal resting murine B cells (Loughnan *et al.*, 1987; Harada *et al.*, 1987). In addition, these studies suggested that IL-5 pre-activated B cells could preferentially proliferate in response to exogenous IL-2 when compared to B cells pre-cultured with medium alone. Studies by Loughnan and Nossal (1989) have also suggested that IL-4 pre-cultured B cells may proliferate in response to high concentrations of IL-2, with the implication that IL-4 induces the high affinity p75 chain of the IL-2 receptor on murine B cells. In support of these observations, it was recently reported that optimal IgG1 secretion by anti-Ig treated B cells requires the cooperative action of IL-2, IL-4 and IL-5 (Purkerson *et al.*, 1988).

Recently, it was reported that in addition to the inhibitory effects of IFN-γ on IL-4-induced B-cell growth and differentiation, IFN-γ also inhibits the activity of IL-5. Interferon γ was shown to markedly suppress the IL-5 induced proliferation of BCL_1 cells (Lohoff *et al.*, 1989), an observation we have confirmed in our laboratory (Figure 2). Similarly, IFN-γ can inhibit antigen-specific B-cell proliferation and clonal IgM secretion, but not clone frequency, induced by IL-5 in the presence of T-independent antigen (Table 3).

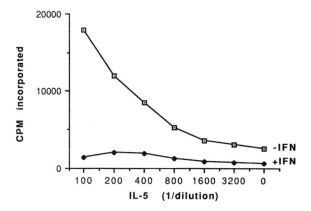

Figure 2 Interferon-γ inhibits IL-5-induced proliferation of BCL1 cells. BCL1 cells (5 × 10⁴ per well) were cultured with a titrating amount of IL-5 cos cell supernatant either in the presence or absence of a constant concentration of IFN-γ (1/200 dilution of cos cell supernatant). After 3 days, cells were pulsed with tritiated-thymidine for the final 6 h of culture. Results are expressed as mean incorporated CPM of triplicate cultures.

Similar to observations with murine B cells, IL-4-induced IgE secretion by human PB or tonsil B cells is enhanced by addition of IL-5 (Pene *et al.*, 1988b). Production of IgE under these conditions is inhibited by IFN-γ, suggesting that IL-5 acts by directly enhancing the action of IL-4 rather than exerting its effect through an alternative pathway. This synergy has a clear parallel with the interaction between IL-4 and IL-5 seen in IgE production in the murine system (Coffman *et al.*, 1988).

Despite the considerable literature concerning the biological activity of murine IL-5, the effects of human IL-5 on B-cell differentiation in the absence of other cytokines have not been well defined. Early studies by two groups using human IL-5 in the form of oocyte supernatant (Azuma *et al.*, 1986) and cos7 cell supernatant (Yokota *et al.*, 1987) reported IL-5 to be moderately effective at inducing IgM and IgA secretion from activated PB and splenic B cells. However, in a later extensive study involving four separate institutions, partially purified recombinant IL-5 was found to have no activity in a wide range of proliferation and differentiation assays using primary, leukaemic and transformed human B cells (Clutterbuck *et al.*, 1987). At the same time, this preparation of IL-5 was found to have potent activity as an eosinophil differentiation factor and to stimulate murine B cells.

Interleukin 6

Interleukin 6 has BCDF activity in both the human and murine systems. It has been shown to have relatively weak, though significant, effects on murine B-cell differentiation, when acting alone or in combination with antigen, anti-IgM antibodies of dextran sulphate (Takatsuki *et al.*, 1988; Vink *et al.*, 1988; Alderson and Pike, 1989). Kishimoto and colleagues (Suematsu *et al.*, 1989) recently reported on the generation of a mouse line carrying the human IL-6 transgene, and one of its characteristics was a 120- to 400-fold increase in serum IgG1 levels. Interleukin 6 has also been shown to enhance IgA secretion by surface IgA positive, but not IgA negative, murine Peyer's patch B cells (Beagley *et al.*, 1989).

Several reports have suggested that IL-6 has strong activity on murine B cells in the presence of other cytokines. Vink *et al.* (1988) showed that, in the presence of IL-1, IL-6 became a potent growth and differentiation factor for B cells either in the presence or absence of anti-Ig or dextran-sulphate. Similarly, the combination of IL-6 plus IL-1 induces far higher levels of IgM secretion by antigen co-stimulated B cells than either cytokine acting alone (Figure 3). Interleukin 6 was also shown to be a potent co-factor with IL-1 in IgM synthesis by Peyer's patch B cells (Kunimoto *et al.*, 1989).

Both IL-5 and IL-6 have been implicated in the induction of high rate IgA secretion by Peyer's patch B cells. Recently, it was reported that when

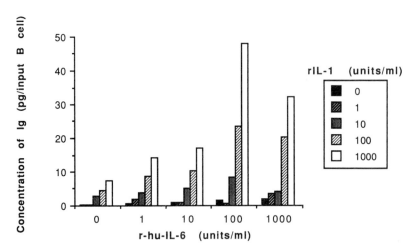

Figure 3 Effect of IL-1 and IL-6 on IgM secretion by murine antigen-specific B cells. FLU-specific B cells were cultured with FLU-Ficoll, as described for Figure 1, and various concentrations of IL-1 and/or IL-6. Values represent the average amount of IgM secreted per input B cell.

Peyer's patch B cells were stimulated by either cytokine alone, IgA secretion was only modestly enhanced, but was greatly increased by IL-5 and IL-6 in combination (Kunimoto *et al.*, 1989).

The BCDF activity of human IL-6 was first identified by its ability to induce Ig secretion from activated primary and EBV-transformed B cells (Hirano *et al.*, 1985, 1986). Human IL-6 has been shown to augment IgM, IgG and IgA production by PWM-stimulated PB mononuclear cells and is effective when added as late as day 4 of an 8-day culture (Muraguchi *et al.*, 1988), suggesting that IL-6, unlike IL-2, is a late acting differentiation factor. The presence of IL-6 has also been found to increase secretion of IgG and IgM by EBV-transformed (Rawle *et al.*, 1987; Muraguchi *et al.*, 1988) and leukaemic (Rawle *et al.*, 1987) B cells.

Although IL-6 clearly possesses BCDF activity in various different *in vitro* assay systems, it is not clear how dependent this activity is on the presence of other cytokines or accessory-cell populations. It has already been mentioned that IL-6 appears to play an obligatory rôle in IL-4-induced secretion of IgE (and, perhaps that of other isotypes) by PB B cells (Verchelli *et al.*, 1989b), and yet cytokines alone could not replace T cells and monocytes in this assay system, suggesting that cell contact in addition to their soluble factors is an essential requirement for IL-6 mediated Ig secretion. Highly purified blood or tonsil B cells activated with SAC will not differentiate to Ig secreting cells if IL-6 is the only exogenous cytokine added (Tadmori *et al.*, 1989; R. J. Armitage, personal observation). However, in the presence of SAC and low concentrations of IL-2, IL-6 is effective at inducing a level of Ig production above that seen with IL-2 alone, and this response can be further enhanced by the addition of IL-1β (Emilie *et al.*, 1988). There is no firm evidence therefore that human IL-6 can act as a differentiation factor for normal B cells in the absence of other cytokines or accessory cells. On the other hand, IL-6 seems to play a central rôle in IL-4-induced secretion of antibody, and IL-6 itself appears to be secreted from B cells in response to IL-4 (Smeland *et al.*, 1989). Thus, IL-6 may be involved in some of the reported effects of IL-4 and, perhaps, other cytokines in both human and murine systems.

Interferon γ and α

Leibson and co-workers (1982, 1984) originally described a factor which synergized with IL-1 and IL-2 in the *in vitro* PFC response to sheep erythrocytes, a factor they later showed to be IFN-γ (Table 2). Meanwhile, Sidman *et al.* (1984) reported that IFN-γ induced the maturation of resting murine B cells to a state of active immunoglobulin secretion. More recently,

IFN-γ has been shown to have a number of inhibitory influences on murine B-cell activation, especially responses induced by IL-4, as already described. Additionally, when LPS-activated B cells are treated with IFN-γ, they display enhanced IgG2a production (Snapper and Paul, 1987b; Snapper et al., 1988c).

We have already discussed several effects on human B-cell differentiation exerted by IFN-γ in the presence of other cytokines. Interferon γ augments Ig secretion when added to SAC-activated B cells together with IL-2 (Devos et al., 1985; Bich-Thuy and Fauci, 1986; Delfraissy et al., 1988) and inhibits IL-4 induced production of IgE, but not IgG or IgM (Defrance et al., 1988a; Pene et al., 1988a; Sarfati et al., 1988). In addition, IFN-γ has been shown to induce secretion of antibody from IL-2 stimulated CLL B cells (Ostlund et al., 1986; Karray et al., 1987). Although IFN-γ has been shown to induce proliferation of anti-IgM-activated human B cells, particularly in combination with IL-2 (Defrance et al., 1986; Romagnani et al., 1986), it has not been shown to have an effect on human B-cell differentiation in the absence of co-stimuli. In addition to IFN-γ, IFN-α and -β have also been found to be co-stimulatory for anti-IgM-activated human B cells (Table 5). The range of action of IFN-α on human B cells is still poorly understood. It has been reported to both suppress (Peters et al., 1986a) and enhance (Rodriguez et al., 1983) antibody production, with these contradictory effects apparently

Table 5 Interferon α, β and γ induce proliferation of anti-IgM-activated human B cells.[a]

	Counts per minute (S.D.)	
Addition	Exp. 1	Exp. 2
—	740 (59)	206 (2)
IFN-α	19,643 (1,229)	6,367 (963)
IFN-β	25,382 (3,072)	7,941 (1,681)
IFN-γ	3,453 (293)	4,425 (400)
IL-2	227 (100)	3,705 (157)
IL-2 + IFN-γ	6,527 (2,063)	14,167 (1,839)

[a] Human B cells were isolated from Ficoll-Hypaque (FH) purified tonsillar mononuclear cells by a combination of T-cell depletion by rosetting with AET-treated SRBC followed by further FH centrifugation, depletion of adherent cells by passage over Sephadex G10 and positive selection on rabbit anti-human IgM-coated pans. Purified B cells were cultured at 10^5 cells per well in 96-well plates for 3 days in the presence of F(ab')$_2$ goat anti-human IgM (1 μg ml^{-1}) and the indicated additive. Cultures were pulsed with tritiated-thymidine for the final 16 h of culture and data are expressed as incorporated counts per minute. Cytokine additions were all made at a final concentration of 10 ng ml^{-1}.

due to cytokine concentration. Thus, low concentrations of IFN-α enhance PWM- or SAC-driven Ig production, but high concentrations are suppressive (Peters *et al.*, 1986b). It appears from recent reports that IFN-α, like IFN-γ in both the human and the mouse, can suppress IL-4-induced IgE secretion (Delespesse *et al.*, 1989).

Purified human B cells specifically activated by trinitrophenol (TNP) can be induced to differentiate in the presence of IL-2, and this effect is enhanced by the addition of IFN-α (Delfraissy *et al.*, 1988). The effects of IFN-α in this system appear to be exerted at an earlier stage of the B-cell response than those of IL-2 and so differ from the synergistic activity reported for IFN-γ, which enhances the later stages of Ig secretion by IL-2-activated B cells (Nakagawa *et al.*, 1985; Bich-Thuy and Fauci, 1986).

Interleukin 1

Numerous reports have claimed a rôle for IL-1 in murine B-cell activation. For example, prior to the molecular cloning of IL-1, Leibson *et al.* (1982, 1984) showed that IL-1 was an important component in the PFC response to sheep erythrocytes, and Booth and Watson (1984) reported that IL-1 had activity in both the dextran-sulphate and anti-IgM co-stimulator assays for B-cell growth. However, with some of the earlier studies there was controversy over whether the effects seen on B cells were direct or via activation of contaminating T cells in the apparently purified B-cell populations (reviewed by Booth *et al.*, 1985). More recently, it was demonstrated that recombinant murine IL-1 could act in the presence of a T-independent antigen to promote the growth and differentiation of single hapten-specific B cells, though its activity was weak in comparison to other B-cell active cytokines such as IL-4 and IL-5 (Pike and Nossal, 1985; Pike *et al.*, 1987). The activity of recombinant IL-1 on mouse B cells has since been confirmed by Chiplunkar *et al.* (1986).

There is some evidence that IL-1 and IL-2 act synergistically to stimulate murine B cells in the PFC response to SRBC (Leibson *et al.*, 1982; Table 2). Similarly, Pike and Nossal (1985) reported that the combination of recombinant murine IL-1 and recombinant human IL-2 had more activity in the growth and differentiation of antigen co-stimulated single hapten-specific B cells than either factor acting alone.

Information concerning the action of IL-1 on human B cells has been limited and somewhat contradictory. The ability of IL-1 to enhance human Ig secretion has been demonstrated using partially purified B-cell preparations with pokeweed mitogen (PWM) as co-stimulus (Lipsky *et al.*, 1983). Addition of neutralizing anti-IL-1 antisera to B cells activated with

SAC and IL-2 suppressed the formation of antibody-secreting cells (Lipsky *et al.*, 1983); however, addition of IL-1 to such cultures did not consistently increase Ig production (Falkoff *et al.*, 1983, 1984). A difficulty in the interpretation of early studies results from the use of somewhat crude IL-1 preparations and partially purified B-cell populations. Recent reports using purified recombinant IL-1 show it to be capable of augmenting Ig secretion by highly purified blood B cells in the presence of SAC plus IL-2 (Jelinek and Lipsky, 1987) and by a B-lymphoblastoid cell line (Jandl *et al.*, 1988).

As mentioned previously, recombinant human IL-1β has been shown to act in synergy with IL-6 to increase Ig production by blood B cells stimulated with SAC plus IL-2 (Emilie *et al.*, 1988) and it is possible that the enhancing effects of IL-1 seen by others are, at least in part, mediated by a similar interaction between added IL-1 and endogenously produced IL-6.

Other cytokines

Several cytokines not normally considered to play a significant rôle in the humoral immune response have been shown to have an influence, either directly or indirectly, on B-cell differentiation. Recombinant human TNF-α has been shown to suppress IgG and IgM secretion from PWM-stimulated mononuclear cells (Kashiwa *et al.*, 1987). This may not be a direct effect targeted at B cells; it appears to be mediated via the inhibition of helper T-cell function. Addition of TNF-α as late as day 4 of culture reduces Ig production, suggesting that TNF-α affects a late stage of T-cell help for B-cell differentiation. The same study found TNF-α did not inhibit spontaneous Ig secretion by the CESS EBV-transformed B-cell line, although others have reported TNF-α to inhibit EBV-induced but not anti-IgM- or PWM-induced differentiation of purified B cells (Janssen and Kabelitz, 1985). In contrast, Jelinek and Lipsky (1987) have found TNF-α to significantly augment antibody production from highly purified blood B cells co-stimulated with SAC plus IL-2. The major effect of TNF in this assay is to enhance the responsiveness of SAC-activated B cells to IL-2. Similarly, Kehrl *et al.* (1987a) showed TNF-α to stimulate DNA synthesis and enhance Ig secretion by human B cells in the presence of SAC plus IL-2. This group also reported that recombinant lymphotoxin (TNF-β), acting alone, enhanced proliferation of activated human B cells and, acting with IL-2, augmented both proliferation and Ig secretion (Kehrl *et al.*, 1987b).

A recent report has demonstrated a synergistic action for IL-3 on Ig secretion by tonsil or blood B cells when co-stimulated with SAC plus IL-2 (Tadmori *et al.*, 1989). The late-acting B-cell differentiation activity seen with IL-3 is similar to that seen with IL-6 in that addition of IL-3 as late as

Table 6 Transforming growth factor β inhibits anti-SRBC (PFC) production in the TRF assay.[a]

Addition	PFC per culture (S.D.)
—	2,967 (96)
TGF-β	387 (68)
IL-1	9,800 (849)
IL-1 + TGF-β	2,827 (377)

[a]Murine spleen cells were cultured as in Table 1, in the presence of SRBC and the indicated additive. PFC levels were determined using a Jerne hemolytic plaque assay. TGF-β and IL-1 were each added at a final concentration of 10 ng ml^{-1}.

day 4 of culture is effective at augmenting antibody production. In the same study, a spontaneous B-cell line derived from peripheral blood lymphocytes secreted increased levels of Ig upon addition of IL-3. Others have shown IL-3 induced differentiation resulting in mature B cells from an IL-3 dependent precursor cell line which secretes IgG and IgM in co-culture with stromal or dendritic cells and T cells (Kinashi *et al.*, 1988).

Transforming growth factor (TGF) β has been implicated in murine IgA switching, since this cytokine, in the presence of LPS, can induce surface IgA negative B cells to synthesize mRNA that encodes α-chain, to express IgA on their surface and to secrete antibody of this isotype (Coffman *et al.*, 1989). In addition, TGF-β has been found to inhibit anti-SRBC PFC induction in the presence or absence of IL-1 (Table 6).

Discussion

The wide availability of highly purified recombinant lymphokines has paved the way for detailed analysis of the rôles of individual cytokines and combinations of cytokines in the B-cell activation pathway. How cytokines regulate the immune response *in vivo* is an area of considerable interest. *In vivo* murine studies have suggested that preferential production of cytokines by a particular TH subset may influence the mode of the immune response. Studies by Mosmann and Coffman have demonstrated the existence of two distinct types of CD4$^+$ long-term T-helper cell lines (termed TH1 and TH2) which are distinguished by their profiles of cytokine secretion. Each subset secretes cytokines unique to that cell type. For example, TH1 clones secrete IL-2 and IFN-γ but not IL-4 or IL-5, whereas TH2 clones produce IL-4 and IL-5 but neither IL-2 nor IFN-γ (Mosmann *et al.*, 1986; Mosmann and

Table 7 Summary of the effects of individual cytokines on immunoglobulin secretion.

Cytokine	Species[a]	Effect on Ig secretion
IL-1	H	Increased Ig from PWM-activated PBM Increased Ig from EBV-transformed lines
	M	Antigen specific Ig secretion
IL-2	H	Polyclonal Ig secretion from activated B cells Ig from leukaemic and tonsil B cells
	M	Increased anti-SRBC PFC formation Antigen-specific Ig secretion
IL-3	H	Increased Ig from B-cell line
IL-4	H	IgE from activated PBM and EBV-stimulated B cells IgG and IgM from SAC-activated B cells IgE and IgG4 from PMA-activated B cells
	M	IgG1 and IgE from LPS-stimulated B cells Inhibits IgM, IgG3, IgG2a, IgG2b from LPS-stimulated B cells
IL-5	H	IgM from SAC-activated PB and spleen cells IgA from non-stimulated and SAC-stimulated B cells
	M	IgM from BCL_1 Antigen specific IgM and IgG secretion IgA from LPS-stimulated B cells
IL-6	H	IgM, IgG and IgA from PWM-activated PBM Increased Ig from EBV-transformed lines and leukaemic B cells
	M	Increased IgG, IgM and IgA Increased IgG1 in transgenic mice
IFN-α	H	Modulation of Ig from PWM- or SAC-activated B cells
IFN-γ	M	Increased IgG2a from LPS-stimulated B cells
TFN-α	H	Decreased IgG and IgM from PWM- and EBV-activated PBM
TNF-β	M	IgA from LPS-stimulated B cells Inhibits PFC induction

[a] H = human; M = mouse.

Table 8 Synergistic or inhibitory effects of cytokines on immunoglobulin secretion.

Cytokine	Species[a]	Effect on Ig secretion
IL-1	H	↑ IL-2 induced Ig ± Il-6
	M	↑ Ig in presence of IL-2 ↑ Ig in presence of IL-6
IL-2	H	↑ IL-4 induced IgE
	M	↑ IL-4 induced IgG1 in presence of IL-5 ↑ Ig in presence of IL-1 and IFN-γ
IL-3	H	↑ IL-2 induced Ig
IL-4	H	↑ or ↓ IL-2 induced IgG1 and IgE
	M	↓ IFN-γ induced IgG2a ↑ IL-5 induced IgM, IgG3, IgA
IL-5	H	↑ IL-4 induced Ig ↑ IL-4 plus IL-6 induced Ig
	M	↑ IL-4 induced IgG1 and IgE ↑ IgG1 in the presence of IL-2 and IL-4 ↑ IgA in the presence of IL-6
IL-6	H	↑ IL-2 induced Ig ± IL-1 Required for IL-4 induced Ig
	M	↑ IgM in the presence of IL-1 ↑ IgA in the presence of IL-5
IFN-α	H	↑ IL-2 induced antigen-specific Ig ↓ IL-4 induced IgE
IFN-γ	H	↑ IL-2 induced Ig ↓ IL-4 induced IgE
	M	↓ IL-4 induced IgG1 and IgE ↓ IL-5 induced antigen-specific IgM
TNF-α	H	↑ IL-2 induced Ig

[a] H = human; M = mouse.

Coffman, 1989). In addition, both subsets share the ability to secrete a number of other cytokines including IL-3 and granulocyte–macrophage colony stimulating factor. It is becoming increasingly apparent that certain arms of the immune system predominate in the response to particular infectious agents. For example, IgG1 and IgE secretion are dominant in helminth infections where they are able to mediate antibody-dependent cytotoxicity by eosinophils (Ramalho-Pinto *et al.*, 1979; Capron *et al.*, 1981). The involvement of the TH2 products IL-4 and IL-5 in IgG1 and IgE secretion and eosinophil differentiation *in vitro* (Sanderson *et al.*, 1986; Yokota *et al.*, 1987) suggests preferential stimulation of TH2 cells in parasitized animals. On the other hand, TH1 products appear to be central to immune responses to *Brucella* and many viral infections. Responses to these pathogens are typically characterized by elevated IgG2a levels (Coutelier *et al.*, 1987) and delayed-type hypersensitivity (DTH), both of which are mediated by TH1 cells and TH1-derived cytokines (Cher and Mosmann, 1987; Snapper *et al.*, 1988c). Thus, it appears that different antigens preferentially activate different types of TH cells. The mechanism of differential induction of TH cells is purely speculative although it may be linked to the nature of the antigen (soluble or particulate), the route of administration and the type of antigen-presenting cell involved.

Despite the attractiveness of this model, recent studies have suggested that the TH1 and TH2 classifications may be too simplistic. Considerable numbers of murine T-cell clones and the majority of human T-cell clones produce both IL-4 and IFN-γ (Gajewski and Fitch, 1988; Kelso and Gough, 1988; Maggi *et al.*, 1988; Paliard *et al.*, 1988; Wong *et al.*, 1988). Although the existence of TH1 and TH2 cells remains to be demonstrated *in vivo*, it is clear that certain diseases have a predominantly "TH1-like" or "TH2-like" nature. For example, in the murine model for *Leishmaniasis*, resistance to infection by certain mouse strains appears to be associated with TH1 characteristics, whereas disease susceptibility resulting in death of the animal is linked to a characteristic TH2 type immune response (Scott *et al.*, 1988; Heinzel *et al.*, 1989).

Some of the predictions of the rôle that cytokines play in B-cell differentiation obtained from *in vitro* systems have been supported in animal models of disease. Finkelman and colleagues have found that the high levels of IgE detected during parasitic infections, or in mice immunized with goat anti-mouse δ (GaMδ) antibody, are strongly associated with the production of IL-4 *in vivo* (Finkelman *et al.*, 1990). Treatment of mice with neutralizing antibodies against IL-4 or against the IL-4 receptor (IL-4R) almost completely abrogated IL-4-induced IgE production. Interestingly, use of these antibodies had significantly less effect on IgG1 levels, suggesting that IgG1 production *in vivo* is in part IL-4 independent. Anti-IL-4R antibodies were found to be approximately five-fold more potent than anti-IL-4 at inhibiting GαMδ-mediated IgE secretion. Similar suppressive effects of antibodies against the murine IL-4R have been described for *in vitro* IgE production (Maliszewski *et al.*, 1990).

If the numerous *in vitro* studies reviewed in this chapter were to be criticized, the predominant feature would be the target B-cell populations used. In many cases, especially those involving human B cells, only partially purified B-cell populations were used for assessing cytokine activities. The possibility of a particular factor acting indirectly via non-B cells, which contaminate apparently purified B-cell populations, is ever present and has been demonstrated in a number of cases. For example, both IL-1 and TNF-α have been shown to induce IL-6 production by a number of cell types, including monocytes and fibroblasts (Van Damme *et al.*, 1987), and it is becoming increasingly apparent that biological effects originally attributed to IL-1 and TNF-α may, in fact, be mediated by IL-6. In addition, several recent reports have described the production of IL-1α and IL-1β (Pistoia *et al.*, 1986; Acres *et al.*, 1987), TNF (Sung *et al.*, 1988) and IL-6 (Horii *et al.*, 1988; Smeland *et al.*, 1989) by activated human B cells and B-cell lines. It is therefore possible that many of the effects on B-cell differentiation orig-inally ascribed to the actions of a single cytokine, are mediated through the secondary factors produced by the B cells themselves. Of particular interest is the recent observation that IL-4-stimulated human B cells produce IL-6 (Smeland *et al.*, 1989). This, together with the previous report that IL-4-induced IgE secretion is dependent on the presence of IL-6 (Vercelli *et al.*, 1989b), suggests that the specific effects attributed to IL-4 in Ig production need to be re-appraised. These recent findings highlight the need for highly purified target B-cell populations and low cell density cultures, in particular single-cell B-cell cultures, where the possibility of cytokine cascades is virtually eliminated. The availability of neutralizing antibodies against cytokines and their receptors will prove valuable in future attempts to define interactions complicated by the induction of endogenous cytokine production.

The discovery of soluble forms of IL-2R (Rubin *et al.*, 1985) and, more recently, IL-4R (Mosely *et al.*, 1989), IL-6R and IFN-γR (Novick *et al.*, 1989), raises the possibility that release of such cytokine receptors may provide a further mechanism by which cytokine involvement in the immune response can be regulated *in vivo*. Interleukin 1 and IL-4 induced prolifer-ation of anti-IgM-stimulated murine B cells can be inhibited by the presence of soluble IL-1R or IL-4R, respectively. In addition, soluble IL-4R has been found to effectively inhibit the IL-4-induced IgG1 and IgE secretion by LPS-stimulated B cells (Maliszewski *et al.*, 1990). The potential potency of soluble cytokine receptors, and the fact that there are naturally occurring forms, suggests a possible use for them as therapeutic agents, particularly when in the case of neutralizing antibodies the introduction of large amounts of foreign proteins is an inherent problem.

Examining the cytokine requirements for *in vivo* immune responses using animal models has already begun to reveal important differences from the predictions made from *in vitro* studies. For example, the essential requirement for IL-4 for IgG1 production *in vitro* by murine B cells appears to contrast the IL-4 independent production of IgG1 *in vivo*. Similarly, *in vitro* studies have failed to show a rôle for IL-6 in IgG1 production, yet IL-6 transgenic mice display highly elevated serum IgG1 levels. The increasing availability of antibodies against cytokines and cytokine receptors and soluble forms of receptors will undoubtedly provide some of the tools necessary for dissection of cytokine requirements *in vivo*.

Acknowledgements

We wish to thank Linda Troup for preparation of the manuscript.

References

Acres, R. B., Larsen, A., Gillis, S. and Conlon, P. J. (1987) *Mol. Immunol.* **24**, 479–485.
Alderson, M. R., Pike, B. L. and Nossal, G. J. V. (1987a) *Proc. Natl. Acad. Sci. USA* **84**, 1389–1393.
Alderson, M. R., Pike, B. L., Harada, N., Tominaga, A., Takatsu, K. and Nossal, G. J. V. (1987b) *J. Immunol.* **139**, 2656–2660.
Alderson, M. R. and Pike, B. L. (1989) *Int. Immunol.* **1**, 20–28.
Azuma, C., Tanabe, T., Konishi, M., Kinashi, T., Noma, T., Matsuda, F., Yaoita, Y., Takatsu, K., Hammarstrom, L., Smith, C. I. E., Severinson, E. and Honjo, T. (1986) *Nucleic Acid Res.* **14**, 9149–9158.
Beagley, K. W., Eldridge, J. H., Kiyono, H., Everson, M. P., Koopman, W. J., Honjo, T. and McGhee, J. R. (1988). *J. Immunol.* **141**, 2035–2042.
Beagley, K. W., Eldridge, J. H., Lee, F., Kiyono, H., Everson, M. P., Koopman, W. J., Hirano, T., Kishimoto, T. and McGhee, J. R. (1989) *J. Exp. Med.* **169**, 2133–2148.
Berton, M. T., Uhr, J. W. and Vitetta, E. S. (1989) *Proc. Natl. Acad. Sci. USA* **86**, 2829–2833.
Bich-Thuy, L. and Fauci, A. S. (1985) *Eur. J. Immunol.* **15**, 1075–1079.
Bich-Thuy, L. and Fauci, A. S. (1986) *J. Clin. Invest.* **77**, 1173–1179.
Booth, R. J. and Watson, J. D. (1984) *J. Immunol.* **133**, 1346–1349.
Booth, R. J., Prestidge, R. L. and Watson, J. D. (1985) *Lymphokines* **12**, 75–85.
Callard, R. E. and Smith, S. H. (1988) *Eur. J. Immunol.* **18**, 1635–1638.
Callard, R. E., Smith, S. H., Shields, J. G. and Levinsky, R. J. (1986) *Eur. J. Immunol.* **16**, 1037–1042.

Capron, M., Bazin, H., Joseph, M. and Capron, A. (1981) *J. Immunol.* **126**, 1764–1768.

Cher, D. J. and Mosmann, T. R. (1987) *J. Immunol.* **138**, 3688–3694.

Chiplunkar, S., Langhorne, J. and Kaufman, S. H. E. (1986) *J. Immunol.* **137**, 3748–3752.

Chiu, C.-P., Moulds, C., Coffman, R. L., Rennick, D. and Lee, F. (1988) *Proc. Natl. Acad. Sci. USA* **85**, 7099–7103

Clutterbuck, E., Shields, J. G., Gordon, J., Smith, S. J., Boyd, A., Callard, R. E., Campbell, H. D., Young, I. G. and Sanderson, C. J. (1987) *Eur. J. Immunol.* **17**, 1743–1750.

Coffman, R. L. and Carty, J. (1986) *J. Immunol.* **136**, 949–954.

Coffman, R. L., Ohara, J., Bond, M. W., Carty, J., Zlotnik, A. and Paul, W. E. (1986) *J. Immunol.* **136**, 4538–4541.

Coffman, R. L., Shrader, B., Carty, J., Mosmann, T. R. and Bond, M. W. (1987) *J. Immunol.* **139**, 3685–3590.

Coffman, R. L., Seymour, B. W. P., Lebman, D. A., Hiraki, D. D., Christiansen, J. A., Shrader, B., Cherwinski, H. M., Savelkoul, H. F. J., Finkelman, F. D., Bond, M. W. and Mosmann, T. R. (1988) *Immunol. Rev.* **102**, 5–28.

Coffman, R. L., Lebman, D. A. and Shrader, B. (1989) *J. Exp. Med.* **170**, 1039–1044.

Coutelier, J.-P., van der Logt, J. T. M., Heessen, F. W. A., Warnier, G. and Van Snick, J. (1987) *J. Exp. Med.* **165**, 64–69.

Defrance, T., Aubry, J. P., Vanbervliet, B. and Banchereau, J. (1986) *J. Immunol.* **137**, 3861–3867.

Defrance, T., Aubry, J. P., Rousset, F., Vanbervliet, B., Bonnefoy, J. Y., Arai, N., Takebe, Y., Yokota, T., Lee, F., Arai, K., DeVries, J. and Banchereau, J. (1987) *J. Exp. Med.* **165**, 1459–1467.

Defrance, T., Vanbervliet, B., Pene, J. and Banchereau, J. (1988a) *J. Immunol.* **141**, 2000–2005.

Defrance, T., Vanbervliet, B., Aubry, J.-P. and Banchereau, J. (1988b) *J. Exp. Med.* **168**, 1321–1337.

Delespesse, G., Sarfati, M. and Peleman, R. (1989) *J. Immunol.* **142**, 134–137.

Delfraissy, J. F., Wallow, C. and Galanaud, P. (1988) *Eur. J. Immunol.* **18**, 1379–1384.

Del Prete, G., Maggi, E., Parronchi, P., Chretien, I., Tiri, A., Macchia, D., Ricci, M., Banchereau, J., DeVries, J. and Romagnani, S. (1988) *J. Immunol.* **140**, 4193–4198.

Devos, R., Jayaram, B., Vandenabeele, P. and Fiers, W. (1985) *Immunol. Lett.* **11**, 101–105.

Dutton, R. W., Falkoff, R., Hirst, J. A., Hoffmann, M., Kappler, J. W., Kettman, J. R., Lesley, J. F. and Vann, D. (1971) *Prog. Immunol.* **1**, 355–373.

Emilie, D., Crevon, M.-C., Auffredou, M. T. and Galanaud, P. (1988) *Eur. J. Immunol.* **18**, 2043–2047.

Falkoff, R. J. M., Muraguchi, A., Hong, J.-X., Butler, J. L., Dinarello, C. and Fauci, A. S. (1983) *J. Immunol.* **131**, 801–805.

Falkoff, R. J. M., Butler, J. L., Dinarello, C. and Fauci, A. S. (1984) *J. Immunol.* **133**, 692–696.

Finkelman, F. D., Holmes, J., Katona, I. M., Urban, J. F., Beckman, M. P., Schooley, K. A., Coffman, R. L., Mosmann, T. R. and Paul, W. E. (1990) *Ann. Rev. Immunol.*, in press.

138   *R. J. Armitage, K. H. Grabstein and M. R. Alderson*

Gajewsкi, T. F. and Fitch, F. W. (1988) *J. Immunol.* **140**, 4245–4252.
Harada, N., Matsumoto, M., Koyama, N., Shimizu, A., Honjo, T., Tominaga, A. and Takatsu, K. (1987a) *Immunol. Lett.* **15**, 205–215.
Harriman, G. R., Kunimoto, D. Y., Elliot, J. F., Paetkau, V. and Strober, W. (1988) *J. Immunol.* **140**, 3033–3039.
Heinzel, F. P., Sadick, M. D., Holaday, B. J., Coffman, R. L. and Locksley, R. M. (1989) *J. Exp. Med.* **169**, 59–72.
Hirano, T., Taga, T., Nakano, N., Yasukawa, K., Kashiwamura, S., Shimizu, K., Kanakajima, K., Pyun, K. H. and Kishimoto, T. (1985) *Proc. Natl. Acad. Sci. USA* **82**, 5490–5494.
Hirano, T., Yasukawa, K., Harada, H., Taga, T., Watanabe, Y., Matsuda, T., Kashiwamura, S., Nakajima, K., Koyama, K., Iwamatsu, A., Tsunasawa, S., Sakiyama, F., Matsu, H., Takahara, Y., Taniguchi, T. and Kishimoto, T. (1986) *Nature (London)* **324**, 73–76.
Horii, Y., Muraguchi, A., Suematsu, S., Matsuda, T., Yoshizaki, K., Hirano, T. and Kishimoto, T. (1988) *J. Immunol.* **141**, 1529–1535.
Howard, M., Farrar, J., Hilfiker, M., Johnson, B., Takatsu, K., Hamaoka, T. and Paul, W. E. (1982) *J. Exp. Med.* **155**, 914–923.
Howard, M. and Paul, W. E. (1983) *Ann. Rev. Immunol.* **1**, 307–333.
Jandl, R. C., Flanagan, R. G. and Schur, P. H. (1988) *Clin. Immunol. Immunopathol.* **46**, 115–121.
Janssen, O. and Kabelitz, D. (1988) *J. Immunol.* **140**, 125–130.
Jelinek, D. F., Splawski, J. B. and Lipsky, P. E. (1986). *Eur. J. Immunol.* **16**, 925–932.
Jelinek, D. F. and Lipsky, P. E. (1987) *J. Immunol.* **139**, 2970–2976.
Jelinek, D. F. and Lipsky, P. E. (1988) *J. Immunol.* **141**, 164–173.
Jones, S., Chen, Y., Isakson, P., Layton, J., Pore, E., Word, C., Krammer, P. H., Tucker, P. and Vitetta, E. S. (1983) *J. Immunol.* **131**, 3049–3051.
Julius, M. H., Paige, C. J., Leanderson, T. and Cambier, J. C. (1987) *Scand. J. Immunol.* **25**, 195–202.
Karray, S., Vazquez, A., Merle-Beral, H., Olive, D., Debre, P. and Galanaud, P. (1987) *J. Immunol.* **138**, 3824–3828.
Kashiwa, H., Wright, S. C. and Bonavida, B. (1987) *J. Immunol.* **138**, 1383–1390.
Kehrl, J. H., Miller, A. and Fauci, A. S. (1987a) *J. Exp. Med.* **166**, 786–791.
Kehrl, J. H., Alvarez-Mon, M., Delsing, G. A. and Fauci, A. S. (1987b) *Science* **238**, 1144–1146.
Kelso, A. and Gough, N. M. (1988) *Proc. Natl. Acad. Sci. USA* **85**, 9189–9193.
Kinashi, T., Harada, N., Severinson, E., Tanabe, T., Sideras, P., Konishi, M., Azuma, C., Tominaga, A., Bergstedt-Lindqvist, S., Takahashi, M., Matsuda, F., Yaoita, Y., Takatsu, K. and Honjo, T. (1986) *Nature (London)* **324**, 70–73.
Kinashi, T., Inaba, K., Tsubata, T., Tashiro, K., Palacios, R. and Honjo, T. (1988) *Proc. Natl. Acad. Sci. USA* **85**, 4473–4477.
Kikutani, H., Inui, S., Sato, R., Barsumian, E. L., Owaki, H., Yamasaki, K., Kaisho, T., Uchibayashi, N., Hardy, R. R., Hirano, T., Tsunasawa, S., Sakiyama, F., Suemura, M. and Kishimoto, T. (1986) *Cell* **47**, 657–665.
Kunimoto, D. Y., Nordan, R. P. and Strober, W. (1989) *J. Immunol.* **143**, 2230–2235.
Leanderson, T. and Julius, M. H. (1986) *Eur. J. Immunol.* **16**, 182–187.
Lebman, D. A. and Coffman, R. L. (1988a) *J. Exp. Med.* **168**, 853–862.
Lebman, D. A. and Coffman, R. L. (1988b) *J. Immunol.* **141**, 2050–2056.

Leibson, H. J., Marrack, P. and Kappler, J. (1982) *J. Immunol.* **129**, 1398–1402.
Leibson, H. J., Gefter, M., Zlotnik, A., Marrack, P. and Kappler, J. W. (1984) *Nature* **309**, 799–801.
Lipsky, P. E., Thompson, P. A., Rosenwasser, L. J. and Dinarello, C. (1983) *J. Immunol.* **130**, 2708–2714.
Lohoff, M., Sommer, F. and Rollinghoff, M. (1989) *Eur. J. Immunol.* **19**, 1327–1329.
Loughnan, M. S., Takatsu, K., Harada, N. and Nossal, G. J. V. (1987) *Proc. Natl. Acad. Sci. USA* **84**, 5399–5403.
Loughnan, M. S. and Nossal, G. J. V. (1989) *Nature (London)* **340**, 76–79.
Lowenthal, J. W., Zubler, R. H., Nabholz, M. and MacDonald, H. R. (1985) *Nature* **315**, 669–672.
Lundgren, M., Persson, U., Larsson, P., Magnusson, C., Smith, C. I. E., Hammarstrom, L. and Severinson, E. (1989) *Eur. J. Immunol.* **19**, 1311–1315.
Maggi, E., Del Prete, G., Macchia, D., Parronchi, P., Tiri, A., Chretien, I., Ricci, M., Romagnani, S. (1988) *Eur. J. Immunol.* **18**, 1045–1050.
Maliszewski, C. R., Sato, T. A., Vanden Bos, T., Waugh, S., Dower, S. K., Slack, J., Beckmann, M. P. and Grabstein, K. H. (1990) *J. Immunol.* **144**, 3028–3033.
Mingari, M. C., Gerosa, F., Carra, G., Accolla, R. S., Moretta, A., Zubler, R. H., Waldmann, T. A. and Moretta, L. (1984) *Nature (London)* **312**, 641–643.
Mond, J. J., Finkelman, F. D., Sarma, C., Ohara, J. and Serrate, S. (1985) *J. Immunol.* **135**, 2513–2517.
Mosley, B., Beckmann, M. P., March, C. J., Idzerda, R. L., Gimpel, S. D., Vanden Bos, T., Friend, D., Alpert, A., Anderson, D., Jackson, J., Wignall, J. M., Smith, C., Gallis, B., Sims, J. E., Urdal, D., Widmer, M. B., Cosman, D. and Park, L. S. (1989) *Cell* **59**, 335–348.
Mosmann, T. R. and Coffman, R. L. (1989) *Ann. Rev. Immunol.* **7**, 145–173.
Mosmann, T. R., Cherwinski, H., Bond, M. W., Giedlin, M. A. and Coffman, R. L. (1986) *J. Immunol.* **136**, 2348–2357.
Muraguchi, A., Kehrl, J., Iongo, D. L., Volkman, D. J., Smith, K. A. and Fauci, A. S. (1985) *J. Exp. Med.* **161**, 181–197.
Muraguchi, A., Hirano, T., Tang, B., Matsuda, T., Horri, Y., Nakajima, K. and Kishimoto, T. (1988) *J. Exp. Med.* **167**, 332–334.
Nakagawa, T., Hirano, T., Nakagawa, N., Yoshizaki, K. and Kishimoto, T. (1985) *J. Immunol.* **134**, 959–966.
Nakanishi, K., Malek, T. R., Smith, K. A., Hamaoka, T., Shevach, E. M. and Paul, W. E. (1984) *J. Exp. Med.* **160**, 1605–1621.
Noelle, R., Krammer, P. H., Ohara, J., Uhr, J. W. and Vitetta, E. S. (1984) *Proc. Natl. Acad. Sci. USA* **81**, 6149–6153.
Noma, Y., Sideras, P., Natto, T., Bergstedt-Lindqvist, S., Azuma, C., Severinson, E., Tanabe, T., Kinashi, T., Matsuda, F., Yaoita, Y. and Honjo, T. (1986) *Nature (London)* **391**, 640–646.
Nordon, R. P. and Potter, M. (1986) *Science* **233**, 566–569.
Novick, D., Engelmann, H., Wallach, D. and Rubinstein, M. (1989) *J. Exp. Med.* **170**, 1409–1414.
Ostlund, L., Einhorn, S., Robert, K.-H., Juliusson, G. and Biberfeld, P. (1986) *Blood* **67**, 152–159.
Paliard, X., de Waal Malefijt, R., Yssel, H., Blanchard, D., Chretien, I., Abrams, J., de Vries, J. and Spits, H. (1988) *J. Immunol.* **141**, 849–855.
Pene, J., Rousset, F., Brierre, F., Chretien, I., Bonnefoy, J. Y., Spits, H., Yokota,

T., Arai, K., Banchereau, J. and deVries, J. (1988a) *Proc. Natl. Acad. Sci. USA* **85**, 6880–6884.

Pene, J., Rousset, F., Briere, F., Chretien, I., Wideman, J., Bonnefoy, J. Y. and deVries, J. F. (1988b) *Eur. J. Immunol.* **18**, 929–935.

Peters, M., Walling, D. M., Kelly, K., Davis, G. L., Waggoner, J. G. and Hoofnagle, J. H. (1986a) *J. Immunol.* **137**, 3147–3152.

Peters, M., Ambrus, J. L., Zheleznyak, A., Walling, D. and Hoofnagle, J. H. (1986b) *J. Immunol.* **137**, 3153–3157.

Pike, B. L., Raubitschek, A. and Nossal, G. J. V. (1984) *Proc. Natl. Acad. Sci. USA* **81**, 7917–7921.

Pike, B. L. and Nossal, G. J. V. (1985) *Proc. Natl. Acad. Sci. USA* **82**, 8153–8157.

Pike, B. L., Alderson, M. R. and Nossal, G. J. V. (1987) *Immunol. Rev.* **99**, 117–152.

Pistoia, V., Cozzolino, F., Rubarbtelli, A., Torcia, M., Roncella, S. and Ferrarini, M. (1986) *J. Immunol.* **136**, 1688–1692.

Purkerson, J. M., Newberg, J., Wise, G., Lynch, K. R. and Isakson, P. C. (1988) *J. Exp. Med.* **168**, 1175–1180.

Ralph, P., Jeong, G., Welte, K., Mertelsmann, R., Rabin, H., Henderson, L. E., Souza, L. M., Boone, T. C. and Robb, R. J. (1984) *J. Immunol.* **133**, 2442–2445.

Ramalho-Pinto, F. J., DeRossi, R. and Smithers, S. R. (1979) *Parasite Immunol.* **1**, 295–302.

Rawle, F. C., Armitage, R. J. and Beverley, P. C. L. (1987) *Trends in Leukemia VII* **31**, 123–125.

Rodriguez, M. A., Prinz, W. A., Sibbitt, W. L., Bankhurst, A. D. and Williams, R. C. (1983) *J. Immunol.* **130**, 1215–1219.

Romagnani, S., Givoizi, M. G., Biagiotti, R., Almerigogna, F., Mingari, C., Maggi, E., Liang, C. and Moretta, L. (1986) *J. Immunol.* **136**, 3513–3516.

Rothman, P., Lutzker, S., Cook, W., Coffman, R. and Alt, F. W. (1988) *J. Exp. Med.* **168**, 2385–2389.

Rubin, L. A., Kurman, C. C., Fritz, M. E., Biddison, W. E., Boutin, B., Yarchoan, R. and Nelson, D. L. (1985) *J. Immunol.* **135**, 3172–3177.

Sanderson, C. J., O'Garra, A., Warren, D. J. and Klaus, G. G. B. (1986) *Proc. Natl. Acad. Sci. USA* **83**, 437–440.

Sarfati, M. and Delespesse, G. (1988) *J. Immunol.* **141**, 2195–2199.

Schimpl, A. and Wecker, E. (1972) *Nature (New Biol.)* **237**, 15–17.

Scott, P., Natovitz, P., Coffman, R., Pearce, E. and Sher, A. (1988) *J. Exp. Med.* **168**, 1675–1684.

Sideras, P., Bergstedt-Lindqvist, S., MacDonald, H. R. and Severinson, E. (1985) *Eur. J. Immunol.* **15**, 586–593.

Sidman, C. L., Paige, C. J. and Schreider, M. H. (1984) *J. Immunol.* **132**, 209–222.

Smeland, E. B., Blomhoff, H. K., Funderud, S., Shalaby, M. R. and Espevik, T. (1989) *J. Exp. Med.* **170**, 1463–1468.

Smith, S. H., Shields, J. G. and Callard, R. E. (1989) *Eur. J. Immunol.* **19**, 2045–2049.

Snapper, C. M. and Paul, W. E. (1987a) *J. Immunol.* **139**, 10–17.

Snapper, C. M. and Paul, W. E. (1987b) *Science* **236**, 944–947.

Snapper, C. M., Finkelman, F. D. and Paul, W. E. (1988a) *J. Exp. Med.* **167**, 183–196.

Snapper, C. M., Finkelman, F. D. and Paul, W. E. (1988b) *Immunol. Rev.* **102**, 51–75.

Snapper, C. M., Peschel, C. and Paul, W. E. (1988c) *J. Immunol.* **140**, 2121–2127.
Splawski, J. B., Jelinek, D. F. and Lipsky, P. E. (1989) *J. Immunol.* **142**, 1569–1575.
Stein, P., Dubois, P., Greenblatt, D. and Howard, M. (1986) *J. Immunol.* **136**, 2080–2089.
Suematsu, S., Matsuda, T., Aozasa, K., Akira, S., Nakano, N., Ohno, S., Miyazaki, J., Yamamura, K., Hirano, T. and Kishimoto, T. (1989) *Proc. Natl. Acad. Sci. USA* **86**, 7547–7551.
Sung, S-S. J., Jung, L. K. L., Walters, J. A., Chen, W., Wang, C. Y. and Fu, S. M. (1988) *J. Exp. Med.* **168**, 1539–1551.
Swain, S. L., Howard, M., Kappler, J., Marrack, P., Watson, J., Booth, R., Wetzel, G. D. and Dutton, R. W. (1983) *J. Exp. Med.* **158**, 822–835.
Tadmori, W., Feingersh, D., Clark, S. C. and Choi, Y. S. (1989) *J. Immunol.* **142**, 1950–1955.
Takatsu, K., Tanaka, K., Tominaga, A., Kumahara, Y. and Hamaoka, T. (1980a) *J. Immunol.* **125**, 2646–2653.
Takatsu, K., Tominaga, A. and Hamaoka, T. (1980b) *J. Immunol.* **124**, 2414–2422.
Takatsu, K., Harada, N., Hara, Y., Takahama, Y., Yamada, G., Dobashi, K. and Hamaoka, T. (1985) *J. Immunol.* **134**, 382–389.
Takatsuki, F., Okano, T., Suzuki, C., Chieda, R., Takahara, Y., Hirano, T., Kishimoto, T., Hamuro, J. and Akiyama, Y. (1988) *J. Immunol.* **141**, 3072–3077.
Thyphronitis, G., Tsokos, G. C., June, C. H., Levine, A. D. and Finkelman, F. D. (1989) *Proc. Natl. Acad. Sci. USA* **86**, 5580–5584.
Tonkonogy, S. L., McKenzie, D. T. and Swain, S. L. (1989) *J. Immunol.* **142**, 4351–4360.
Van Damme, J., Opdenakker, G., Simpson, R. J., Rubira, M. R., Cayphas, S., Vink, A., Billiau, A. and Van Snick, J. (1987) *J. Exp. Med.* **165**, 914–919.
Van Snick, J., Cayphas, S., Vink, A., Uyttenhove, C., Coulie, P. G., Rubira, M. R. and Simpson, R. J. (1986) *Proc. Natl. Acad. Sci. USA* **83**, 9679–9683.
Van Snick, J., Cayphas, S., Szikora, J., Renauld, J., Van Roost, E., Boon, T. and Simpson, R. J. (1988) *Eur. J. Immunol.* **18**, 193–197.
Vercelli, D., Jabara, H. H., Arai, K.-I. and Geha, R. S. (1989a) *J. Exp. Med.* **169**, 1295–1307.
Vercelli, D., Jabara, H. H., Arai, K.-I., Yokota, T. and Geha, R. S. (1989b) *Eur. J. Immunol.* **19**, 1419–1424.
Vink, A., Coulie, P. G., Wauters, P., Nordan, R. P. and Van Snick, J. (1988) *Eur. J. Immunol.* **18**, 607–612.
Vitetta, E. S., Brooks, K., Chen, Y-W., Isakson, P., Jones, S., Layton, J., Mishra, G. C., Pure, E., Weiss, E., Word, C., Yuan, D., Tucker, P., Uhr, J. W. and Krammer, P. H. (1984) *Immunol. Rev.* **78**, 137–157.
Waldmann, T. A., Goldman, C. K., Robb, R. J., Depper, J. M., Leonard, W. J., Sharrow, S. O., Bongiovanni, K. F., Korsmeyer, S. J. and Greene, W. C. (1984) *J. Exp. Med.* **160**, 1450–1466.
Wong, R. L., Ruddle, N. H., Padula, S. J., Lingenheld, E. G., Gergman, C. M., Rugen, R. V., Epstein, D. I. and Clark, R. B. (1988) *J. Immunol.* **141**, 3329–3334.
Yokota, T., Coffman, R. L., Hagiwara, H., Rennick, D. M., Takebe, Y., Yokota, K., Gemmell, L., Shrader, B., Yang, G., Meyerson, P., Luh, J., Hoy, P., Pene, J., Briere, F., Spits, H., Banchereau, J., DeVries, J., Lee, F. D., Arai, N. and Arai, K.-I. (1987) *Proc. Natl. Acad. Sci. USA* **84**, 7388–7392.

Zubler, R. H., Lowenthal, J. W., Erard, F., Hashimoto, N., Devos, R. and MacDonald, H. R. (1984) *J. Exp. Med.* **160**, 1170–1183.
Zubler, R. H., Werner-Favre, C., Wen, L., Sekita, K.-I. and Straub, C. (1987) *Immunol. Rev.* **99**, 281–299.

6
Collaboration between T and B cells

VIRGINIA M. SANDERS AND ELLEN S. VITETTA

Introduction

Cellular collaboration is an important feature of the immune system and it involves the recognition of cell surface-associated molecules on one cell by specific receptors on another. Recognition of some cell surface molecules stabilizes cellular interactions, while recognition of others is involved in the transduction of regulatory signals. Cellular interactions regulate cell activation, differentiation, suppression, and lysis.

Two well-characterized cellular interactions are those occurring between cytolytic T lymphocytes (Tc) and their target cells and T helper (TH) lymphocytes and macrophages. The interaction between Tc and target cells leads to specific lysis while those between TH cells and macrophages induces secretion of cytokines, expression of cytokine receptors and proliferation of TH cells. Another cellular interaction occurs between TH cells and resting B lymphocytes; this induces TH cell activation and leads to B cell proliferation, differentiation and the production of specific antibodies of different isotypes.

In this chapter we discuss the physiological mechanisms by which a B cell is stimulated to differentiate into an antibody-secreting cell. Our working model describes three stages. Firstly, B cells expressing clonally-distributed antigen-specific immunoglobulin (Ig) receptors capture antigen, internalize it, process it and re-express antigenic fragments on their surface in association with major histocompatibility complex (MHC) class II molecules. Secondly, processed antigen plus class II molecules on the B cell are recognized by clonally-distributed receptors on T cells. This event, coupled with the recognition of a number of other accessory or adhesion molecules, induces close membrane interaction between the TH cell and the B cell, and the transduction of signals across the membrane of the B cell to induce a state of lymphokine responsiveness. It also induces the T cell to release lymphokines into the area of cell contact. Thirdly, lymphokines interact

CYTOKINES AND B LYMPHOCYTES
ISBN 0–12–155145–8

with their appropriate receptors on the B cell to initiate proliferation, differentiation and isotype switching. In this manner, only *specific* B cells become activated to secrete antibodies, the isotype of which is determined by the specific lymphokines secreted by the TH cell with which the B cell interacts.

Since our working model involves findings reported over the past 30 years, we first present a brief synopsis of these earlier findings. The reader is referred to reviews by Vitetta *et al.* (1989) and Jelinek and Lipsky (1987) for detailed discussions on the activation of murine and human B cells, respectively.

Historical perspective on the rôle of cellular collaboration in the generation of an antibody response

Cellular collaboration is mediated by thymus-derived and bone marrow-derived cells

Ovary and Benacerraf (1963) first suggested that the simultaneous recognition of both the "hapten" and "carrier" portions of a protein antigen were responsible for the production of anti-hapten antibody.

The first insight into which cells of the immune system were involved in the recognition of the carrier resulted from a report by Claman *et al.* (1966). Adoptive transfer of thymocytes and bone marrow cells, compared with either alone, was far more efficient in the subsequent production of antibody. Davies *et al.* (1967) and Mitchell and Miller extended these findings and determined that bone marrow-derived cells were responsible for antibody production (Miller and Mitchell, 1967; Mitchell and Miller, 1968). However, *both* bone marrow-derived and thymus-derived cells had to recognize antigen in order to obtain a maximal antibody response. These findings indicated that bone marrow cells contained the precursors for antibody-producing cells and that antigen-reactive cells from the thymus induced the differentiation of bone marrow-derived cells into antibody-producing cells.

Cellular collaboration is mediated by "antigen-bridging"

Rajewsky (1969) and Mitchison (1971) independently investigated the "carrier effect" as a mechanism involved in cellular cooperation. Using different *in vivo* approaches, both groups concluded that a good secondary response to the hapten occurred only if the animals were challenged with the hapten chemically *coupled* to a carrier protein with which the animal had been previously immunized. This implied that hapten-primed and carrier-primed cells were necessary for the response and that the two different cells interacted via a hapten-carrier bridge.

The results of these experiments suggested that the stimulating antigen was composed of at least two antigenic determinants, each of which was recognized by receptors on different cells. Therefore, both Rajewsky and Mitchison envisaged recognition of the hapten determinants by bone marrow-derived cells and the carrier determinants by thymus-derived cells.

Definitive evidence that thymus-derived lymphocytes were the cells responsible for the recognition of carrier determinants was first reported by Raff (1970). Using adoptive transfer of cells from carrier-primed or hapten-primed mice, treated before transfer with anti-theta (Thy-1) serum plus complement to selectively eliminate thymus-derived cells, they demonstrated that the carrier-specific helper cells were thymus-derived, while the hapten-specific cells were bone marrow-derived.

Mishell and Dutton (1967) introduced a method for *in vitro* induction of an antibody response. This approach facilitated the elucidation of the cellular requirements for an anti-sheep red blood cell (SRBC) antibody response. Utilizing *in vitro* techniques, three different groups determined that thymus-derived cells were critical for induction of antibody responses. Mosier *et al.* (1970) and Munro and Hunter (1970) showed that spleens from thymectomized mice were deficient in cells required for an *in vitro* response. This deficiency could be overcome by supplying thymus-derived cells. Schimpl and Wecker (1970) showed that the *in vitro* response to SRBC could be inhibited by treating spleen cell suspensions with anti-Thy-1 serum and complement prior to *in vitro* culture. These results supported and extended the hypothesis that an interaction between thymus-derived and bone marrow-derived cells was essential in the induction of an antibody response. Unfortunately, the "carrier effect" could not be studied *in vitro* utilizing SRBC since this was a large, complex antigen. In 1971, Cheers *et al.* (1971) produced the "carrier effect" *in vitro* by culturing spleen cell suspensions from mice immunized with less complex hapten-protein antigens, such as dinitrophenol keyhole limpet hemocyanin (DNP-KLH). Taken together, the results of these experiments supported the concept that separate cell populations were hapten- and carrier-specific.

Cellular collaboration is mediated by MHC-encoded molecules

Cooperation between T (thymus-derived) and B (bone marrow-derived) cells occurred only when the two types of cells were syngeneic. Kindred and Shreffler (1972) and Katz *et al.* (1973b) investigated the rôle of the MHC in the cooperative interaction between T and B cells. They concluded that the

MHC must play a rôle in cellular cooperation in the generation of an antibody response, since a potent antibody response was attained only when T and B cells were derived from histocompatible donors. Hence, the cooperative interaction between T and B cells was "genetically restricted", i.e. a strain-specific gene product had to be expressed and recognized by one or both of the interacting cells in order to generate an antibody response to hapten-protein conjugates. Subsequently, Katz and colleagues reported that the interaction between histocompatible T and B lymphocytes was controlled by genes encoded in the I region (Katz et al., 1975) of the MHC complex (Katz et al., 1973a). These findings were confirmed by Sprent (1978).

Thus, two major findings supported the hypothesis that the effective triggering of B cells occurred during T cell–B cell contact: (1) antigenic epitopes stimulating both T and B cells had to be present on the same antigenic molecule; and (2) the two cells had to be histocompatible.

Cellular collaboration is mediated by T cell recognition of processed antigen presented in the context of MHC molecules

The physical interaction between the antigen-specific T and B cells was challenged by evidence indicating that T cells became activated only after recognizing degraded fragments of native protein antigen (reviewed in Kourilsky and Claverie, 1989), while B cells recognized native protein. Therefore, a mechanism for obtaining degraded fragments of native antigen had to be defined. To this end, Mosier et al. (1968) demonstrated that macrophages were essential for the in vitro antibody response to the particulate antigen, SRBC, and Ziegler and Unanue (1981, 1982) showed that the macrophage was capable of internalizing native antigen, degrading it and recycling the degraded antigen to its surface, where it could be presented to T cells. Rosenthal and Shevach (1973) and Paul et al. (1977) showed that presentation of processed antigen by macrophages to T cells was restricted by the ability of the macrophage to form a cell surface-associated complex, consisting of MHC-encoded molecules and processed antigen. Thus, the specificity of the T cell was directed both to the degraded antigen and to the MHC-encoded molecule on the macrophage surface. Using electron microscopy and cell adherence techniques, it was demonstrated that macrophages physically interacted with T cells in an antigen-specific, MHC-restricted manner (Lipsky and Rosenthal, 1974; Nielsen et al., 1974). These interactions could be inhibited by antibodies to class II determinants and could not be inhibited by antibodies to native antigen. Following this interaction, macrophage-bound T cells proliferated. In view of the participation of the macrophage in T cell activation, interactions between T and B cells were re-evaluated. Two different mechanisms were proposed to explain T cell–B cell collaboration by a "bridging" of the two cells via a macrophage. Firstly, T cell–macrophage interaction could lead to the secretion of T cell-derived soluble factors which could then act on antigen-specific B cells. Such B cells were made responsive to these factors as a consequence of binding native antigen (Dutton *et al.*, 1971; Schimpl and Wecker, 1972). Secondly, cell collaboration could be mediated by a mechanism through which the T and B cells were focused on the macrophage surface by the simultaneous presentation of both *native* antigen to B cells and *degraded* antigen (in the context of MHC-encoded class II antigens) to T cells. This type of cell "focusing" brought the antigen-reactive T and B cells into close proximity so that soluble factors released from the T cell could act on the neighbouring B cell.

Benacerraf (1978) postulated another mechanism by which T–B cell collaboration occurred via "antigen bridging". This mechanism involved the processing of antigen by antigen-specific B cells, followed by the presentation of antigen fragments in the context of B cell-associated class II molecules to antigen-specific T cells. This proposal was difficult to test, however, since B cells specific for a given antigen were present in the normal spleen at a low frequency, as opposed to antigen-nonspecific macrophages which were numerous.

Benacerraf's proposal became testable when Chesnut and Grey (1981) developed a model system to evaluate the capacity of B cells to serve as antigen-presenting cells (APC). Rabbit anti-mouse Ig (RAMIg) was chosen for the antigen since this antibody would bind to the surface Ig (sIg) receptors on all B cells. T cells specific for processed rabbit Ig in the context of class II determinants were used as the indicator cells to determine if B cells could act as APC. Results showed that purified, macrophage-depleted B cells bound antigen (RAMIg) via their Ig receptors. These B cells internalized, processed and presented degraded fragments of antigen to T cells to stimulate a proliferative response.

Other investigators also overcame the difficulty of working with limited numbers of antigen-specific B cells. Lanzavecchia (1985) generated clones of human T cells and Epstein–Barr Virus (EBV) -transformed B cells specific for tetanus toxoid (TT) to study their interaction *in vitro* in the presence of antigen. His results showed that (1) native TT was recognized only by the B cells, (2) B cells internalized and degraded TT to present it to T cells, and (3) TT-specific B cells were at least 1,000 times more efficient than other APC in the presentation of TT to T cells, due to their ability to capture TT with their specific sIg receptors.

Another approach to study antigen-specific interactions between T and B cells was to enrich the B cells expressing sIg specific for a particular hapten, for example trinitrophenyl (TNP). Presentation of B cell-bound TNP-carrier to T cells by B cells was enhanced at least 1,000-fold compared with presentation by other cells (Rock *et al.*, 1984).

Taken together, these results showed that the "antigen bridging" model could be explained by a sequential recognition of native antigen by B cells and processed antigen by T cells. At high antigen concentrations, T cells interact with all APCs that can bind antigen non-specifically, while at low antigen concentrations, T cells interact only with antigen-specific B cells that preferentially capture the majority of the antigen via their sIg receptors. In this manner, only antigen-specific B cells are the recipients of "help" from antigen-specific T cells.

Mechanisms by which T cells provide help to B cells during cellular collaboration

The nature of T cell-derived "help" which resulted in the differentiation of B cells into antibody-secreting cells remained controversial. "Help" could be due solely to the soluble factors released into the intraction site between the T and B cells, or "help" could be due to both a transmembrane activating signal generated during the T–B cell interaction and signals from the soluble factors released into the immediate vicinity of the activated, responsive B cell.

If the first type of "help" were sufficient to drive B cell differentiation, then it might be possible to stimulate B cells via their sIg alone, to induce a state of lymphokine responsiveness. If, on the other hand, a T cell-induced transmembrane signal and lymphokines were both required for B cell activation, signalling of either B cell sIg or lymphokine receptors alone would not induce a B cell response. Initial experiments using high concentrations of anti-Ig antibodies demonstrated that the two signals could be separated. In contrast, later experiments, employing lower, more physiologically-relevant concentrations of anti-Ig, demonstrated the need for signals from sIg, T cells and lymphokines for B cell activation. Bretscher and Cohn (1968) proposed that one of the initial events in B cell activation was the interaction of sIg with antigen. They also proposed that additional signals from soluble factors would be involved in the differentiation of the activated B cell into an antibody-secreting cell. Thus, the only rôle of T–B cell interaction would be to induce the release of lymphokines from T cells into the vicinity of an antigen-activated B cell following the recognition of antigen fragments in association with class II molecules on the surface of these B cells. B cells would be made responsive to the lymphokines as a consequence of prior encounters with antigen. This was supported by the following findings:

(1) T cell-derived soluble factors by themselves were incapable of driving the growth and differentiation of resting murine or human B cells (Andersson *et al.*, 1980; Principato *et al.*, 1983).

(2) Perturbation of sIg alone was sufficient to induce a state of lymphokine responsiveness in resting B cells.

Sell and Gell (1965) were the first to show that anti-Ig alone activated B cells to proliferate, but not to differentiate. It was subsequently found that high concentrations of anti-Ig alone were able to activate B cells as determined by increased levels of RNA, cell enlargement, membrane depolarization, induction of the catabolism of phosphatidylinositol, increased expression of c-*myc* and c-*fos* mRNA, and increased DNA synthesis (reviewed in Cambier and Ransom, 1987; Cambier *et al.*, 1987). Parker *et al.* (1979) and Kishimoto and Ishizaka (1975) reported that T cell-derived soluble factors were essential for anti-Ig-stimulated B cells to differentiate into antibody-secreting cells.

It must be emphasized that the above experiments employed high concentrations of anti-Ig. In contrast, if low concentrations of anti-Ig were used, viable TH cells were essential to induce B cell differentiation (Tony and Parker, 1985). Soluble factors alone or in the presence of low concentrations of anti-Ig were not sufficient. In addition, the B cell response required linked recognition of antigen and was MHC-restricted. This suggested that the second type of T cell "help" (contact *and* factors) may be more physiologically relevant. Thus, the remainder of this chapter will focus on the rôle of both cell contact and soluble factors in the generation of an antibody response.

Current perspectives on the rôle of cellular collaboration in generation of an antibody response

Cell contact

The rôle of cell–cell contact in antigen-specific antibody responses. Among the first reports on the rôle of T cell–B cell contact in B cell activation were those by Melchers and colleagues (reviewed in Melchers and Andersson, 1984), who reported that blast transformation of small, resting B cells required antigen-specific, MHC-restricted interactions between B cells and TH cells. In contrast, the differentiation of B cell blasts into antibody-secreting cells required only antigen-nonspecific, MHC-unrestricted soluble factors. These factors were produced by TH cells which had interacted specifically with MHC-compatible adherent cells in the presence of specific antigen.

Using an enriched population of TNP-antigen-binding B cells (TNP-ABCs), Noelle *et al.* (1983) reported that only B cells that had specifically interacted with T cells became responsive to T cell-derived lymphokines and differentiated into antibody-secreting cells. The results of these experiments indicated for the first time that resting TNP-ABCs must be exposed to both antigen and activated by T cells via cell–cell contact, to induce responsiveness to lymphokines. However, it was still possible that lymphokines released at the contact site during the interaction, instead of the contact event itself, were responsible for the initial activation event. This possibility was addressed by Krusemeier and Snow (1988) who cultured TNP-ABCs with antigen-specific T cells that had been treated (prior to interaction) with cyclosporin A to inhibit the release of lymphokines from B cell-activated T lymphocytes. They found that although cyclosporin A-treated T lymphocytes were unable to release lymphokines, they could still physically interact with TNP-ABCs. TNP-ABCs which had interacted with cyclosporin A-treated T cells were able to differentiate into antibody-secreting cells only in the presence of exogenously-added T cell-derived lymphokines. Thus, cell–cell contact events could be distinguished from lymphokine-mediated events. Anti-class II antibodies partially blocked the development of lymphokine responsiveness by B cells cultured with cyclosporin A-treated T cells, suggesting that MHC-restricted interactions of TNP-ABCs with T cells render the TNP-ABCs responsive to lymphokines.

The above findings have been confirmed by a number of other investigators using different model systems (Ramussen *et al.*, 1988; Sekita *et al.*, 1988; Whalen *et al.*, 1988; Bartlett *et al.*, 1989). In addition, Noelle *et al.* (1989b) have recently shown that lymphokine-independent cell contact induced the B cell to progress into the G_1 phase of the cell cycle, whereas lymphokine-dependent events induced the B cell to proliferate.

The rôle of cell–cell contact in polyclonal responses. In contrast to MHC-restricted, antigen-specific activation of B cells, resting B cells can be induced to differentiate into antibody-secreting cells in a polyclonal fashion in the presence of histo-incompatible T cells. This phenomenon has been demonstrated by a number of recent experiments (Hirohata *et al.*, 1988; Julius and Rammensee, 1988; Julius *et al.*, 1988; Owens, 1988) showing that aggregation of T cell receptors (TcRs) by immobilized anti-CD3, antiTcR (F23.1) antibodies, or F23.1-conjugated B cells, can activate T cells to provide all the necessary signals to induce B cell differentiation in the absence of antigen or MHC compatibility, by a mechanism requiring direct cell–cell contact. The stimulated T cell can bind to B cells in a polyclonal, MHC-unrestricted manner, resulting in the acquisition by the B cell of a state of lymphokine responsiveness. The T cell then secretes lymphokines into the area of contact. Thus, aggregation of TcRs may induce the expression of a B cell-activating molecule which, upon contact with its receptor on B cells, induces a state of lymphokine responsiveness in the B cell. While the physiological relevance of this mode of cell activation is not clear, it is possible that it accounts for the bystander effect whereby massive activation of T cells in a lymph node induces activation of B cells of multiple specificities.

Characterization of the physical interaction between T and B lymphocytes. To characterize physical interactions at a cellular and biochemical level, two similar model systems were developed based on a modification of the system used to study the interaction between Tc cells and target cells (Berke *et al.*, 1975; Martz, 1975). Antigen-pulsed B lymphocytes and antigen-specific T lymphocytes were admixed and pelleted gently to increase the probability of their interaction. Cell pellets were resuspended and cell-conjugates were examined quantitatively and qualitatively.

Kupfer *et al.* (1986) showed that the formation of conjugates between class II-specific, antigen-nonspecific B hybridoma cells (LK35.2) and conalbumin-specific, class II-restricted cloned Tн cells (D10.G4.1) required antigen presentation by the B hybridoma cells and an MHC-restricted interaction between the two cells. In the presence of high concentrations of conalbumin, the LK35.2 cells were able to nonspecifically bind the antigen, process it and present it to the conalbumin-specific D10 cells. When LK35.2 cells and D10 cells were mixed, centrifuged and resuspended, tight-physical interactions or conjugates were formed and quantitated microscopically. Immunofluorescent staining showed that the formation of MHC-restricted conjugates induced reorientation of the microtubule organizing centre (MTOC) inside the Tн cell to face the site of T cell–B cell contact. In contrast, when conjugates formed in an antigen-nonspecific and MHC-nonrestricted manner, random orientation of the MTOC was observed.

Sanders *et al.* (1986) employed an antigen-specific system, utilizing a highly enriched population of B cells specific for the hapten TNP (TNP-ABCs) and T hybridoma cells specific for the carrier (KLH or ovalbumin, OVA). The T hybridoma cells recognized processed carrier in the context of class II molecules on the antigen-presenting TNP-ABCs. Because of the differences in size between the T hybridoma cells and the normal B cells, these cells could be visually distinguished and conjugates could be studied at the light and electron microscopic levels (Figure 1A). In this way, two types of interactions were described. One type involved the interdigitation of one or more microvilli from each cell type (i.e. loose interaction; Figure 1B), which occurred in the absence of antigen and, hence, was not considered immunologically specific. The second type of interaction, which was

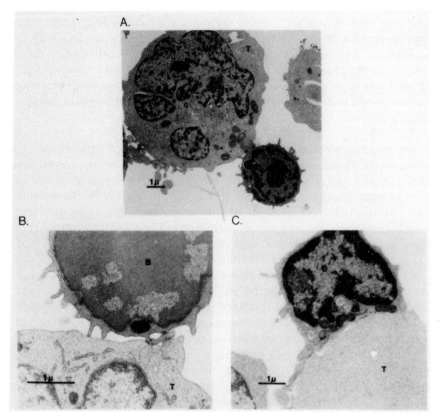

Figure 1 Transmission electron micrographs of T cell–B cell conjugates. (A) Lower magnification showing the morphologic difference between the two cells. The large cell is a T hybridoma cell, and the small cell is a TNP-ABC. (B) Interaction involving one or more microvilli. (C) Interaction involving a broad area of contact. The T and B cells are labelled; bars = 1 μm (Sanders *et al.*, 1986).

antigen-specific and MHC-restricted, increased as a function of time and involved an extensive area of close contact between the interacting cells (i.e. tight interaction; Figure 1C).

In both model systems, specific conjugates formed in both a time- and temperature-dependent manner and B cells required exposure to antigen for several hours before they were able to specifically conjugate to T cells. This suggested that antigen processing by the B cell was a rate-limiting step in the formation of specific T cell–B cell conjugates.

Tight physical interactions between normal T and B cells invariably involved one B cell and one T cell. The "monogamous" nature of the B cell–T cell interaction was experimentally tested using TNP-ABCs that could bind to either T_{H_1} [interleukin (IL) 2 producing and interferon (IFN) γ producing] or T_{H_2} (IL-4 and IL-5 producing) cells (Sanders *et al.*, 1988). (These two T_H cell types are described in more detail later in this chapter.) In competition studies, the number of cells of one type of T_H cell (e.g. T_{H_2}) was held constant in the presence of increasing numbers of the other type of T_H cell (e.g. T_{H_1}). Since the binding of one T_H cell type could be inhibited by increasing numbers of the other T_H cell type, it was concluded that the *same* antigen-specific B cell could bind to either a T_{H_1} or a T_{H_2} cell. In addition, it was observed that if one T_H cell had bound to a B cell, another T_H cell (of the same or different T_H cell type) was unable to do so at the same time. This does not rule out the possibility that, after the dissociation of the TNP-ABC from the T_H cell, the T_H cell can subsequently bind to another B cell.

The rôle of surface molecules on B cells in T–B cell contact. It is possible that the monogamy of B cells is due to membrane-associated molecules on the B cell which cluster at the interaction site and render them unavailable for interactions with other T_H cells. On the other hand, an initial interaction with one T_H cell may render the B cell incapable of interacting with another T_H cell, as a consequence of changes induced in the cell membrane. Whatever the mechanism involved, the monogamous nature of this inter-action suggests that a contact-mediated activating signal is delivered to the B cell by only one T cell.

Several B cell surface-associated molecules were examined for their ability to inhibit T–B cell conjugate formation and to localize at the site of cellular interaction. Cell surface molecules involved in the formation of conjugates between T and B cells include L3T4 (CD4), lymphocyte function-associated (LFA) 1α, Thy-1 and TcRs on the T cell, and class II molecules and LFA-1α on the B cell. This conclusion has been deduced from the observation that monoclonal antibodies (mAbs) directed against these molecules inhibit the formation of conjugates in a concentration-dependent manner (Sanders *et al.*, 1986, 1987b). Only two of these B cell-associated molecules (MHC class II and LFA-1) will be discussed in this chapter. For a more detailed discussion of other T cell and B cell surface molecules involved in cognate interactions, the reader is referred to recent reviews by Kupfer and Singer (1989) and Vitetta *et al.* (1989).

The rôle of MHC class II molecules. It has been shown that antigenic fragments of thymus-dependent (TD) antigens processed by APCs associate with class II molecules and are recognized by MHC-restricted, antigen-specific T_H cells. Hence, the production of antibody in response to a TD antigen is restricted by the expression of class II molecules on B cells (Sprent, 1978). The experiments of LoCascio *et al.* (1984) not only demon-strated the necessity for class II compatibility between B cells and T cells activated by TD antigens, but also implicated class II molecules as transmembrane signalling molecules. However, the state of activation of the B cell can determine its requirement for a class II-restricted T–B cell inter- action in the induction of an antibody response (Andersson *et al.*, 1980; Julius *et al.*, 1982; Ratcliffe and Julius, 1982). Resting B lymphocytes require a class II-restricted interaction, whereas activated B cells require only the lymphokines produced by T cells (previously activated by another APC in a class II-restricted manner). In contrast, recent observations have challenged the absolute requirement for the involvement of class II mol- ecules in the activation of resting B cells (Julius and Rammensee, 1988; Julius *et al.*, 1988; Owens, 1988; Riedel *et al.*, 1988).

A number of approaches have been used to show that class II molecules are involved in the events associated with the initial physical interaction between antigen-specific T and B cells. Kupfer *et al.* (1986, 1987a) have shown that specific reorientation of the MTOC in T cells occurs when class II-compatible, as opposed to class II-incompatible, B cells conjugate with T cells. Likewise, Sanders *et al.* (1986, 1987b) reported that anti-class II antibodies inhibit the formation of antigen-specific tight interactions be- tween T and B cells. In addition, pre-treatment of TNP-ABCs with IL-4, increased by two-fold both the density of class II molecules on the TNP- ABC and the number of antigen-pulsed TNP-ABC capable of conjugating to T cells (Sanders *et al.*, 1987a). The same two-fold increase in the number of IL-4 pre-treated TNP-ABCs differentiating into antibody-secreting cells was observed in bulk and limiting dilution cultures (Sanders *et al.*, 1987a; Vitetta *et al.*, 1987). Thus, these studies directly confirmed earlier obser- vations (Henry *et al.*, 1977; Bottomly *et al.*, 1983; Bekkhoucha *et al.*, 1984) that both the expression and the density of class II molecules on the B cell surface determines the number of successful T–B cell interactions leading to the activation of the B cells.

The rôle of class II molecules as signal transducing molecules in B cells has remained controversial (reviewed in Cambier and Ransom, 1987). The major approach that has been used to address this issue has been to utilize anti-class II antibodies to stimulate B cells. Although some monoclonal anti- class II antibodies can stimulate resting B cells in a T-independent manner, treatment of mitogen-stimulated B cells can result in either inhibition or stimulation of antibody secretion. Anti-class II antibodies also inhibit both anti-Ig induced B cell proliferation and the differentiation induced by antigen and T cells. In one instance, however, anti-class II antibodies synergized with anti-μ antibodies to enhance B cell proliferation (Balayut and Subbarao, 1988). In addition, Cambier and Lehman (1989) have reported that resting B cells primed with anti-Ig and IL-4 proliferate in response to immobilized anti-class II antibodies and differentiate, under these conditions, in the presence of additional lymphokines.

Cambier and colleagues (Cambier *et al.*, 1987; Chen *et al.*, 1987) have also shown that anti-class II antibodies can stimulate the translocation of protein kinase C (PKC) from the cytoplasmic pool to a nuclear membrane-associated pool, providing biochemical evidence that class II molecules have a signalling function. This observation may also explain the inhibitory effects of anti-class II antibodies on mitogen-induced B cell responses, since a class II-induced translocation of PKC to the nuclear membrane would deplete cytoplasmic stores of PKC which are usually translocated to the plasma membrane pool after mitogen stimulation (Chen *et al.*, 1986).

The rôle of MHC class II molecules in determining the monogamy of B cells was examined and it was found that:

(1) Class II molecules remain relatively uniformly distributed on the B cell surface after conjugation as determined by immunofluorescence staining of T–B cell conjugates (Sanders and Vitetta, unpublished observations).

(2) TNP-ABCs conjugated to antigen-specific Tн cells could not conjugate at the same time to alloreactive Tн cells (which recognize only class II molecules as opposed to class II/peptide complexes) (Sanders *et al.*, 1988).

The first finding suggests that class II molecules are not clustered to any large extent at the interaction site. However, it is possible that only a small fraction of the class II molecules are associated with the antigen fragment recognized by the specific TcR, and that it is this small fraction of the total class II molecules that clusters to the interaction site. This small change in the density of class II molecules at the contact site may not be detectable by immunofluorescence, but it may be sufficient for generation of a signal to the B cell.

However, clustering of a small proportion of the class II molecules to the site of cell interaction would not account for the monogamy of B cells since it would be unlikely that two different Tн cell types would recognize an identical class II/peptide complex, thus preventing the binding of more than one Tн cell type by steric hindrance. If class II molecules are involved in determining the occurrence of a monogamous interaction, they are not the only surface molecules involved. This view is supported by the second finding since one would expect alloreactive T cells, which recognize only class II molecules, to conjugate to a B cell already conjugated to a Tн cell whose TcRs did not bind to the majority of class II molecules. Thus, either another B cell surface molecule was totally involved in both Tн and alloreactive interactions or a permanent cellular change had been induced by the binding of the first T cell to prohibit the binding of another T cell.

In summary, class II molecules on B cells are involved in the MHC-restricted physical interactions between antigen-specific T and B cells but are not solely responsible for determining the monogamous nature of the B cell. These molecules may also be involved in the transduction of activating signals to the B cell. Modulation of the density of class II molecules on the B cell influences both the number of B cells capable of conjugating to T cells and, consequently, those B cells which differentiate into antibody-secreting cells. However, studies showing that resting B cells can be induced to differentiate in an MHC-independent manner by activated T cells demonstrate the lack of an absolute requirement of class II molecules in signalling B cells.

The rôle of LFA-1. Involvement of LFA-1 in cell adhesion has been demonstrated primarily in the interaction between Tc cells and target cells (reviewed in Springer *et al.*, 1987). Recently, LFA-1 has been implicated in interactions between T and B cells (Sanders *et al.*, 1986). T-dependent B cell proliferation and/or antibody responses can be inhibited by anti-LFA-1 antibodies (reviewed in Springer *et al.*, 1987; Vitetta *et al.*, 1989), and it has been postulated that this is due to an effect of LFA-1 on cellular interactions. The importance of LFA-1 as an adhesion molecule may be related to the avidity of the interaction between the antigen/class II molecule and the TcR. Golde *et al.* (1986) demonstrated that LFA-1 is involved in the interaction between T cells and APC only if the avidity of the TcR for processed antigen/class II molecules on the APC is low. Along the same lines, when TNP-ABCs from unprimed mice were used in the T–B cell conjugate assay, pre-treatment of either the T cells or TNP-ABCs with anti-LFA-1α antibody inhibited the formation of conjugates (Sanders *et al.*, 1986). In contrast, when TNP-ABCs from primed mice were used, pre-treatment of the T cells, but not the TNP-ABC, with anti-LFA-1α antibodies inhibited the formation of conjugates (Sanders *et al.*, 1987b). This finding has been confirmed in EBV-transformed human B cells from normal or LAD (LFA-1-deficient) individuals. Mazerolles *et al.* (1988) reported that there was no rôle for LFA-1 on these EBV-activated B cells in T–B cell conjugation. They found that LFA-1-negative B cells conjugated with LFA-1-positive T cells at a level equivalent to that of LFA-1-positive B cells. This contrasts to the obligatory rôle of LFA-1 on the T cells in T–B cell conjugation in both humans and mice.

A possible signalling function for LFA-1 on B cells was first reported by Mishra *et al.* (1986). In this study, a mAb recognizing LFA-1α (G-48) mimicked many of the actions of IL-4 on B cells. G-48 induced increased levels of expression of class II antigen on resting B cells, augmented the proliferation of anti-δ-stimulated B cells, and in insolubilized form, induced IgG1 secretion in lipopolysaccharide (LPS) activated B cells. This mAb enhanced, rather than inhibited, conjugate formation (Sanders and Vitetta, unpublished observations). Of 12 anti-LFA-1α antibodies tested, G-48 was unique in its stimulatory functions (Lee and Vitetta, unpublished observations). These data suggest a possible signalling function associated with antibodies directed against this particular epitope of LFA-1α.

van Noesel *et al.* (1988) presented a model system in which aggregation of T cells from normal individuals was not necessary for the proliferation induced by immbolized anti-CD3, thus facilitating dissection of the adhesion and signalling functions of the LFA-1 molecule. Addition of anti-LFA-1α antibodies to normal T cells stimulated with anti-CD3 enhanced T cell proliferation, IL-2 release and IL-2 receptor expression, while addition of anti-LFA-1β antibodies inhibited these responses. Wacholtz *et al.* (1989) have extended this finding to demonstrate that during the interaction of T cells with APCs, LFA-1α and β molecules amplify activation signals delivered to the T cell via stimulation of CD3 molecules.

Immunofluorescence localization studies show that LFA-1 on the B cell clusters to the T–B cell interaction site during the first 45 min of contact (Sanders and Vitetta, unpublished observations). If conjugates are observed after this time, very few B cells in the T–B cell conjugates show localization of LFA-1, but instead, LFA-1 molecules were uniformly distributed on the surface of the B cell. Localization of LFA-1 was shown using antibodies directed against two different epitopes on LFA-1α. As noted above, antibodies directed against one epitope (M17/4.2) inhibited conjugate formation, while antibodies directed against another epitope (G-48) had no inhibitory effect but enhanced conjugate formation. Since both antibodies identified LFA-1 at the T–B interaction site, but produced different effects on conjugate formation and B cell activity, one might speculate that certain epitopes on LFA-1 serve an adhesion function while other epitopes may be involved in a transmembrane signalling function.

The β chain of LFA-1 on B cells was also found to localize to the T–B interaction site during the first 45 min of contact. However, anti-LFA-1β antibodies (M18/4.2) have no effect on the ability of cells to conjugate (Sanders *et al.*, 1986), suggesting that the β chain of LFA-1 may not be involved in adhesion. However, since only one anti-murine β chain antibody has been available for testing, it is possible that the adhesive function of the β chain is associated with another epitope. Since at least one study has shown a signalling function associated with LFA-1β (Mazerolles *et al.*, 1988), one could postulate that this molecule may serve a signalling function during T–B cell contact.

The rôle of LFA-1 molecules on memory B cells is still unclear. Anti-LFA-1 antibodies have no effect on the ability of antibody pre-treated TNP-specific memory cells (TNP-MABC) to conjugate with T cells (Sanders *et al.*, 1987b). However, immunofluorescence studies show a time-dependent localization of LFA-1 on TNP-MABC to either the conjugation site or to a site directly opposite the conjugation site (Sanders and Vitetta, unpublished observations). The mechanisms underlying different patterns of localization of LFA-1 on memory B cells remain unclear.

As discussed above, the B cell which is involved in a tight interaction with a T cell appears to be monogamous in its interaction with that T cell. If LFA-1 molecules are essential for conjugation and signalling, the clustering of all the LFA-1 molecules to the site of contact may explain the monogamous nature of the B cell and the mechanism of its activation. The clustering of LFA-1 may also be important for signalling purposes, since a critical threshold of a signal may have to be generated in order for B cell activation to occur. Thus far, we have failed to identify any other surface molecule on B cells (Ig, B220, J11D, FcεR, or class I MHC) which clusters at the site of T–B contact.

Since LFA-1 molecules redistribute evenly on the B cell surface after their initial clustering, it appears that accessibility of LFA-1 molecules is not the only mechanism controlling B cell monogamy. Obviously, the B cell has changed biochemically or physiologically as a consequence of the initial clustering so that it cannot receive another activation signal. These changes might include a change in the structure of the LFA-1 molecule or a change in membrane fluidity, induced by the initial LFA-1 clustering, which would prohibit other interactions.

In summary, LFA-1 participates in T–B cell interactions. The degree of participation of LFA-1 in these interactions may be influenced by the avidity of the TcR for antigen/class II, and by the ability of B cells to process antigen and express high densities of class II molecules. LFA-1 may also be involved in the transduction of activating signals to the B cell.

The rôle of T cells

Types of TH cells involved in contact-dependent antibody responses. To understand the rôle of soluble factors in antibody responses resulting from T–B cell interactions, it is important to define the types of TH cells which are involved. Studies by Marrack and Kappler (1975) and Janeway (1975), suggested that heterogeneity exists among TH cells that provide help to B cells. This heterogeneity was characterized functionally by the type of help provided to B cells. One type of TH cell was MHC-restricted, carrier-specific and augmented antibody responses via cognate interactions with B cells. The other TH cell type helped B cells by providing "non-specific soluble factors" which activated B cells polyclonally.

Recently, Mosmann *et al.* (1986) have characterized two types of functionally distinct TH cell clones according to the lymphokines which they secrete. Cells of one type, TH_1, secrete IL-2, IFN-γ, lymphotoxin (LT)/tumor necrosis factor (TNF) and IL-3. The other type of TH cell, TH_2, secretes

IL-4, IL-5, IL-6 and IL-3. Bottomly and colleagues (reviewed in Bottomly, 1988) have proposed a similar classification which divides TH cells into "inflammatory" and "helper" subtypes. These two types are equivalent to TH_1 and TH_2 cells, respectively. More recently, a number of reports have described TH clones which secrete lymphokines usually produced by only one or the other type of TH clone. Thus, all TH clones do not fall into the TH_1 or TH_2 category. In humans, the distinction between TH_1 and TH_2 cells is not clear. This is a controversial area and the reader is referred to chapter 7 in this book for a thorough discussion of this topic, and to a recent review by Mosmann and Coffman (1989). Also, it is not known at this time whether the functional distinction observed for *in vitro* generated clones will apply to normal T cells *in vivo*.

Mosmann *et al.* (1986) originally determined that TH_1 and TH_2 cells could provide help to LPS-activated B cells for antibody responses, although TH_2 cells were better helper cells than TH_1 cells. Killar *et al.* (1987) reported three functional subtypes of TH cells based on their ability to induce an *in vitro* anti-hapten antibody response by small, resting splenic B cells. TH clones that did not produce IL-4 failed to provide help for antigen-specific B cells. In contrast, Stevens *et al.* (1988) found that TH_1 cells could induce TNP-ABCs to secrete IgM and IgG2a, while TH_2 cells could induce secretion of IgM and IgG1.

DeKruyff *et al.* (1989) found that the ability of TH cells to induce antibody synthesis by TNP-primed or unprimed splenic B cells could not be predicted solely by the lymphokines which they secreted. TH_1 and TH_2 cells were heterogeneous in their ability to induce antibody synthesis. Those TH_2 cells that provided help for hapten-specific antibody responses produced significantly greater quantities of IL-5 than TH_2 cells that did not provide help.

There is considerable discrepancy with regard to the ability of TH_1 cells to provide help to B cells. Two possible reasons for this discrepancy are that:

(1) IFN-γ (secreted by activated TH_1 cells) often provides negative signals to B cells (reviewed in Jurado *et al.*, 1989). Thus, TH_1 cells secreting large amounts of IFN-γ may prevent B cell help.

(2) B cells which respond to TH_1 clones may represent distinct subsets (e.g. memory vs. virgin B cells) or cells at different stages of activation. For example, Killar *et al.* (1987) used small, resting splenic B cells, Stevens *et al.* (1988) used small, resting TNP-ABCs, DeKruyff *et al.* (1989) used TNP-primed and unprimed splenic B cells, and Mosmann *et al.* (1986) used LPS-activated B cells.

A number of studies have now suggested that the ability of TH cells to help B cells is, in fact, dependent on the activation state of the B cells. Bottomly and colleagues (Kim *et al.*, 1985; Killar *et al.*, 1987; Rasmussen *et al.*, 1988) have reported that both types of clones (TH_1/inflammatory and TH_2/helper) are capable of mediating polyclonal B cell responses, whereas only TH_2/helper clones are able to mediate antigen-specific responses. Moreover, they have reported that antigen-specific responses are elicited from small B cells as a consequence of T–B cell contact and lymphokines, whereas polyclonal responses are elicited from large B cells in the presence of lymphokines alone. Taken together, the above studies suggest that TH cells with a TH_2 lymphokine secretion pattern, possibly because of their ability to secrete IL-4 and IL-5, are responsible for the major portion of the helper activity mediated by TH cells.

The rôle of soluble factors in specific antibody responses. The lymphokines secreted by TH_1 and TH_2 cells have potent effects on B cell activation, proliferation and differentiation. In the following section, we discuss the activities of IL-2, IL-4, IL-5, IL-6 and IFN-γ. We also describe the rôle of these lymphokines in T–B cell interactions and the rôle of T–B cell interaction in the function of these lymphokines. Directed secretion of lymphokines from the T cell to the B cell may be important during this interaction. An important intracellular event that follows specific T–B cell interactions is reorientation of the MTOC in the T cell to face the site of contact with the B cell (Kupfer *et al.*, 1986, 1987a). This event is reminiscent of the reorientation of the MTOC and Golgi apparatus in Tc cells interacting with target cells (Geiger *et al.*, 1982). This change in the MTOC may direct the release of lymphokines into the intercellular space between the conjugating cells such that small amounts of lymphokines can effectively stimulate the interacting B cells because of their close proximity. Hence, local transfer of lymphokines might not affect neighbouring cells. Two additional findings have supported this idea of directed lymphokine release during T–B cell interaction; (1) crosslinking of TcRs with anti-receptor antibodies activates T cells and results in the directed release of lymphokines to the site of clustered TcRs (Poo *et al.*, 1988), and (2) TcRs localize to the area of T–B contact (Kupfer *et al.*, 1987b), suggesting that directed secretion of lymphokines into the area of contact would occur, and result in B cell activation.

Interleukin 4. IL-4 can modulate the B cell response at many points in its activation/differentiation pathway. Its ability to do so may be programmed into the B cell when it is still in G_0. IL-4 acts on resting B cells, subsequently cultured with LPS, to induce the secretion of IgG1 and IgE and to decrease the secretion of IgG3 (reviewed in Coffman *et al.*, 1988; Snapper *et al.*, 1988a; Mosmann and Coffman, 1989), indicating that IL-4 is an "early"-acting factor that can program "later events". Layton *et al.* (1984), Bergstedt-Linqvist *et al.* (1988), and Coffman *et al.* (1988) have reported that IL-4 can programme uncommitted B lymphocytes to switch to IgG1 and

IgE production. Although it is not yet clear if B cells stimulated during cognate T–B cell interaction behave similarly to LPS-activated B cells, it is plausible that IL-4 secreted during cognate T–B cell interaction programmes the interacting B cell, and perhaps other B cells, to subsequently secrete IgG1 or IgE.

IL-4, in combination with LPS, induces B cells to secrete IgG1 (Isakson *et al.*, 1982). The enhanced secretion of IgG1 is accompanied by an IL-4-mediated increase in the transcription of $\gamma 1$ genes (Yuan *et al.*, 1985), and an increase in the precursor frequency of IgG1-secreting cells (Layton *et al.*, 1984), suggesting that IL-4 induces sIgM$^+$ sIgD$^+$ B cells to undergo a heavy chain class switch from IgM to IgG1. The mechanism by which IL-4 regulates IgG1 isotype switching is unknown, but recent studies on the molecular basis of isotype switching may provide some clues. Radbruch *et al.* (1986) and Kepron *et al.* (1989) have shown that isotype switching in normal B cells involves the deletion and rearrangement of specific C_H genes on both chromosomes. Hence, isotype switching may be regulated at the level of accessibility of the switch regions to a common switch recombinase (reviewed in Alt *et al.*, 1986). Stavnezer and colleagues (1986, 1988) have demonstrated that the specificity of class switching correlates with hypo-methylation and transcriptional activation of the corresponding germline C_H gene prior to switching. IL-4 induces transcription of the germline $\gamma 1$ constant region locus in normal B cells (Stavnezer *et al.*, 1988; Berton *et al.*, 1989) and induces DNase I hypersensitive sites in the S$\gamma 1$ region before switch recombination occurs (Berton *et al.*, in press). This induction is dependent on the dose of IL-4 and is markedly inhibited by IFN-γ. These studies demonstrate that IL-4 may initiate isotype switching very early by making these switching sites more accessible to a switch recombinase. The challenge now is to identify the regulatory proteins involved in this process.

The mechanism by which IL-4 works during T–B cell collaboration remains unclear. After cognate interaction between a T$_{H2}$ cell and a B cell, secreted IL-4 could act in combination with signals provided by the physical interaction itself to activate the B cell and induce its proliferation. DuBois *et al.* (1987) have reported that a cloned T cell line that does not secrete IL-4 can induce the proliferation of B cells only if exogenous IL-4 is provided. Rasmussen *et al.* (1988) have proposed that, in addition to cell–cell contact, IL-4 is essential for the induction of IL-5 responsiveness in a small, resting B cell. Noelle and McCann (1989) reported that IL-4 treated B cells respond more effectively to T$_H$-derived contact-mediated signals. These findings suggest that IL-4 may be involved in amplification and/or progression of the contact-mediated signal.

IL-4 induces an increase in the expression of class II molecules on small, resting B cells (Noelle *et al.*, 1984; Roehm *et al.*, 1984). T cells that have been activated previously by other APCs are secreting IL-4 into the milieu of resting B cells. This IL-4 could induce class II expression and prepare these B cells to interact more efficiently with T cells. This hypothesis has been tested and results show that treatment of small TNP-ABCs with IL-4 enhances the ability of such cells to physically interact with TH cells, an effect mediated by increased expression of class II molecules (Sanders *et al.*, 1987a). These B cells also generate more antibody-producing cells.

A recent study by Stevens *et al.* (1988) has placed some of the observations concerning lymphokine-mediated isotype switching into the context of T–B cell interactions involving subsets of TH_1 vs. TH_2 cells. Using two KLH-specific T cell clones of the TH_1 or TH_2 types, it was reported that the interaction between a TNP-ABC and a TH_2 cell (that secretes IL-4 and IL-5), resulted in the production of IgG1, whereas interaction between a TNP-ABC and a TH_1 cell (that secretes IL-2 and IFN-γ), resulted in the production of IgG2a. The addition of exogenous IL-4 to TNP-ABC and TH_1 cells resulted in the production of IgG1, instead of IgG2a. Conversely, B lymphocytes incubated with TH_2 cells and exogenous IFN-γ failed to produce IgG2a but also failed to produce IgG1. Since an individual TNP-ABC is capable of interacting with either a TH_1 or a TH_2 cell (Sanders *et al.*, 1988), we postulate that the interaction between a B cell and a T cell (TH_1 or TH_2) induces a state of responsiveness to many, but perhaps not all, lymphokines. These results suggest that the class of Ig secreted by a B cell is dependent upon the type of T cell with which it interacts and the lympho-kines that the activated T cell subsequently secretes. The monogamous nature of a T–B cell interaction may serve to prevent the B cell from receiving multiple, often conflicting, signals.

TH_2, but not TH_1, cells induce IgE responses (reviewed in Coffman *et al.*, 1988). This activity can be inhibited by anti-IL-4 antibodies, demonstrating that IL-4 is required for IgE production. Although IL-4 programmes the secretion of both IgG1 and IgE, Snapper *et al.* (1988b) have suggested that production of the two isotypes is differently regulated, since a 100-fold higher IL-4 concentration is required to induce a polyclonal IgE response. Vercelli *et al.* (1989b) have shown that physiological concentrations of IL-4 induce purified human B cells to synthesize IgE only after a cognate interaction with T cells. Optimal cytokine combinations alone were unable to induce IgE synthesis in human B cells. In addition to the requirements for both T–B cell contact and IL-4 for human B cell IgE synthesis, Vercelli *et al.* (1989a) have also found that endogenously produced IL-6 is essential for the IL-4 dependent induction of IgE synthesis. This requirement for IL-6 is interesting in light of a recent finding showing that IL-4 induces the production of IL-6 from resting human B cells. This implies that IL-6 may also serve an autocrine function in B cell responses (Smeland *et al.*, 1989).

These results suggest that at least three signals are required for induction of human IgE synthesis. One signal is provided by cell–cell contact and the other signals are delivered by IL-4 and IL-6. Lebman and Coffman (1988) used clonal cultures of sIgM-expressing B cells stimulated with T_{H2} cells specific for RAMIg to determine whether IL-4 (released by the T_{H2} cell) induced isotype switching or facilitated the maturation of pre-committed precursor cells. In the absence of anti-IL-4 antibodies, there was an increase in the proportion of clones secreting IgE and in the amount of IgE secreted per clone. This confirms the results from mitogen studies showing that IL-4 induces $C\varepsilon$ transcripts in B lymphoid cells (Rothman *et al.*, 1988) and suggests that this switching can be induced by lymphokines released during T_{H2}–B cell interaction.

Interleukin 5. In contrast to IL-4, IL-5 appears to act primarily on activated B cells (Swain, 1985) to enhance their proliferation and differentiation into IgM-secreting cells. Thus, in the context of a cognate T–B cell interaction, IL-5 should act on B cells previously stimulated by antigen, IL-4 and T_H cells, to enhance these activated B cells to proliferate and secrete IgM.

The molecular mechanism by which cells are stimulated to become IgM-secreting cells has recently been elucidated. Matsui *et al.* (1989) have reported that, in a neoplastic B cell clone, IL-5 induces an increase in the secretory form of μH chain mRNA expression and a modest increase in J chain mRNA expression. The J chain is critical for the formation of pentameric IgM. The level of J chain expression is greatly enhanced by IL-2 (Blackman *et al.*, 1986) and, thus, in IL-5-stimulated cells, IL-2 was found to further enhance IgM secretion (Matsui *et al.*, 1989). Thus, if B cells are simultaneously or sequentially stimulated with these lymphokines, IgM-secreting cells are generated.

IL-5 has been reported to have enhancing effects on IgA secretion by LPS-stimulated B cells. This effect of IL-5 on IgA secretion has been reported to occur only in B cells previously committed to IgA expression (Beagley *et al.*, 1988; Harriman *et al.*, 1988; Schoenbeck *et al.*, 1989). These results suggest that IL-5 does not function as a switch factor, but instead increases the clone size or enhances the level or rate of secretion of IgA from committed B cells.

The fact that IL-4 acts primarily on resting B cells, whereas IL-5 acts primarily on activated B cells, suggests that the presence of both lymphokines would result in enhanced proliferation and differentiation of B cells activated by T cells and antigen. Rasmussen *et al.* (1988) have reported that T–B cell contact is critical for the induction of a state of IL-5 responsiveness in small, resting B cells. Loughnan *et al.* (1987) and Harada *et al.* (1987) have observed that recombinant (r)IL-5 can induce the expression of IL-2 receptors and responsiveness to IL-2 in B cells. It could be postulated that the biological significance of the induction of both functional IL-5Rs (by TH₂-B cell contact) and functional IL-2Rs (by IL-5 secreted by T_{H2} cells) is that such cells would then acquire responsiveness to IL-2, a lymphokine secreted by T_{H1} cells. Thus, as discussed above, the small amount of mRNA synthesis for J chain induced by IL-5 will be amplified by IL-2 upon interaction with the IL-2Rs induced by IL-5. This would provide a means of regulating Ig production by both subsets of TH cells, and it suggests that the temporal order of lymphokine activities on B cells might be IL-4 → IL-5 → IL-2 and, finally, → IL-6 (which has been shown to induce the growth and secretion of Ig by plasma cells; Hirano et al., 1986; Muraguchi et al., 1988).

Interleukin 2. The rôle played by IL-2 in B cell proliferation and differentiation is less clear. Early studies suggested that IL-2, in combination with other factors, acted synergistically to induce a primary anti-SRBC response *in vitro.* These helper factors were later identified as IFN-γ and IL-1 (Liebson *et al.*, 1982). In contrast, other studies suggested that B cells lacked IL-2Rs and could not respond to IL-2. More recently it has become clear that although resting B cells express very few, if any, IL-2Rs, at least some activated B cells express functional IL-2Rs (Waldmann *et al.*, 1984). Zubler *et al.* (1984) reported that B cells stimulated with a mixture of LPS and anti-Ig expressed IL-2Rs and responded to IL-2, while B cells stimulated with LPS alone did not. In human B cells, IL-2 synergized with IL-4 and PMA for the production of IgE antibody (Lundgren *et al.*, 1989). IL-2 has been shown to induce the transcription of the *J chain* gene in murine BCL-1 lymphoma cells, thus inducing assembly of the IgM pentamer and enhancing IgM secretion (Blackman *et al.*, 1986; Brooks *et al.*, 1983).

Whether T–B cell interaction can induce responsiveness of the B cell to IL-2 remains to be determined. One study (Isakov and Morrow, 1989) has attempted to address this issue by employing the splenic fragment culture technique, which measures the antibody response on a clonal level. Irradiated, carrier-primed mice were injected with naive splenic B cells. Splenic fragments from the recipients were cultured *in vitro* with a hapten (DNP) carrier antigen in the absence or presence of IL-2. The frequency of DNP-responsive B cells was increased by IL-2, as was the amount of Ig secreted per clone, and IL-2 facilitated isotype switching. These effects of IL-2 may have resulted from enhanced IL-2R expression on B cells induced by their antigen-specific interaction with T cells.

Although most of the biological effects of IL-2 are thought to be induced via IL-2 receptors of high affinity (p75 plus p55 subunits), it has been reported that receptors of intermediate affinity (i.e. p75) can transmit signals after binding IL-2 (Saiki *et al.*, 1988; Tanaka *et al.*, 1988). Resting B cells may express only intermediate affinity IL-2Rs, and these cells may proliferate and/or differentiate in response to high concentrations of IL-2. When B cells are activated by certain stimuli, the expression of p55 might be induced on cells already expressing p75, which would result in the formation of high affinity IL-2Rs. Such cells would be expected to respond to IL-2 at much lower concentrations. As previously described, IL-5 enhances IL-2R expression (Harada *et al.*, 1987; Loughmann *et al.*, 1987). Hence, IL-5 probably induces the expression of p55 on B cells that already express p75, thus leading to the expression of high affinity IL-2Rs. This suggests that B cells would have to first encounter IL-5 (secreted by a TH₂ cell) before they could respond to IL-2 (secreted by a TH₁ cell). TH₁ cells would then amplify responses to IL-5. On the other hand, at least some TH₁ clones can activate B cells via cognate interaction in the apparent absence of TH₂ cells. Whether T–B cell interaction can substitute for IL-5 in rendering B cells responsive to IL-2, or whether some TH₁ clones *do* secrete both IL-5 and IL-2, remains to be determined.

Interferon γ. IFN-γ, a lymphokine secreted by activated TH₁ cells and several other cell types, has numerous rôles in the immune response. IFN-γ has both anti-viral and anti-proliferative activities and regulates the activities of cells involved in both humoral and cellular responses (Trinchieri and Perusia, 1985). IFN-γ synergizes with IL-2 and IL-1 in the generation of anti-SRBC antibody responses (Liebson *et al.*, 1982), and promotes Ig secretion by resting or activated murine and human B cells (Liebson *et al.*, 1982, 1984; Sidman *et al.*, 1984). Paradoxically, IFN-γ also has potent *inhibitory* effects on B cell activation, proliferation and differentiation (reviewed in Jurado *et al.*, 1989). IFN-γ inhibits the IL-4-mediated expression of class II antigens and CD23 molecules (FcεR) on resting B cells. IFN-γ also has inhibitory effects on the proliferation of B cells stimulated by anti-Ig and IL-4 and affects B cell differentiation by inhibiting the IL-4-mediated isotype switch to IgG1 and IgE. At the same time, IFN-γ promotes the secretion of IgG2a (Finkelman *et al.*, 1986, 1988; Snapper *et al.*, 1988c; Stevens *et al.*, 1988) in B cells cultured with LPS or antigen plus TH₁ cells. IFN-γ-containing supernatants from TH₁ cells (or inflammatory T cell clones) have a suppressive effect on the Ig production of TH₂-stimulated B cells (Bottomly, 1988; Coffman *et al.*, 1988). Stevens *et al.* (1988) have recently reported that TH₁, but not TH₂, cells induce IgG2a secretion by antigen-specific B cells after antigen stimulation and that this activity can be partially inhibited by antibodies against IFN-γ. Interestingly, IgM secretion was not affected by IFN-γ. *In vivo*, IFN-γ inhibits the secretion of IgG1 and IgE in mice treated with anti-IgD antibodies (Finkelman *et al.*, 1988). IFN-γ also enhances IgG2a secretion in mice immunized with *Brucella abortus* (Finkelman *et al.*, 1988). These results suggest that IFN-γ can regulate B cell function by acting both as a B cell differentiation factor (especially for the synthesis of IgG2a) and as a non-competitive antagonist of early IL-4-mediated effects on B cells. Hence, the isotype(s) of Ig ultimately secreted after stimulation by a particular antigen will probably be determined by the relative numbers of activated TH_1 vs. TH_2 cells and the levels of IL-4 and IFN-γ secreted. Antigens that induce predominantly IgG2a responses might preferentially activate TH_1 cells and antigens that induce IgG1 and/or IgE might activate TH_2 cells.

The molecular mechanisms underlying the antagonistic effects of IFN-γ on the IL-4-induced activities on B cells are not clear. However, binding studies have demonstrated that IFN-γ does not compete for IL-4 in binding to IL-4Rs (Ohara and Paul, 1987; Nakajima *et al.*, 1987; Park *et al.*, 1987; Lowenthal *et al.*, 1988), indicating that these two lymphokines do not compete for the same cell surface receptor. Berton *et al.* (1989) have recently reported that the induction of germline transcripts by IL-4 is inhibited by IFN-γ.

Interleukin 6. In the human, IL-6 is a late-acting factor that promotes Ig secretion by activated B lymphocytes and lymphoblastoid cell lines (Hirano *et al.*, 1986; Muraguchi *et al.*, 1988). In activated, normal B cells, IL-6 induces Ig secretion without proliferation. In contrast, IL-6 is a potent proliferative factor for lymphoblasts (Muraguchi *et al.*, 1988). These results suggest that IL-6 acts on B cells after IL-4, IL-5 and IL-2 to promote Ig secretion. For a comprehensive discussion on the biology of IL-6, the reader is referred to a recent review by Kishimoto (1989).

Conclusions

A T cell and a B cell must physically interact to initiate the complex processes of progression, activation, proliferation, differentiation and isotype switching. This interaction is antigen-specific and is restricted by the MHC class II determinants expressed on the B cell surface. We have presented several hypotheses concerning the sequence of events leading to the production of antibody by antigen-specific B cells. These events are summarized in Figure 2 and include antigen uptake by B cells, processing and presentation to a T cell and induction of a close physical interaction between T and B cells. This interaction stimulates lymphokine secretion by the T cell and lymphokine responsiveness by the B cell. The two ends of this spectrum—antigen processing and lymphokine secretion and responsiveness—are more clearly understood than the intermediate events involving cell–cell interaction *per se*. The events which occur during this interaction remain to be further explored.

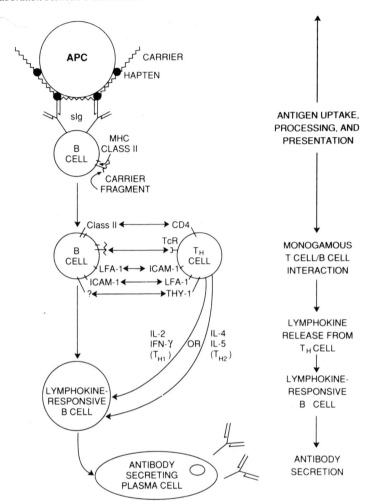

Figure 2 Cellular events leading to the production of antigen-specific antibody. High affinity sIg receptors on B cells either capture free antigen or are presented antigen by another APC such as a dendritic cell. The B cells process antigen and recycle antigenic fragments (or denatured antigen) to their surface in association with MHC class II molecules. A single B cell presents the antigenic fragment/class II complex to a T cell-associated TcR. This T cell can be either a TH1 or a TH2 cell. Other cell surface molecules involved in this monogamous interaction include B cell-associated LFA-1 and ICAM-1, and T cell-associated L3T4 (CD4), LFA-1, ICAM-1 and Thy-1. The T cell releases lymphokines directly onto the B cell, which has been made lymphokine-responsive as a consequence of the cell–cell interaction. The B cell then differentiates into an antibody-secreting cell whose isotype is determined by the type of lymphokines released.

Acknowledgements

We are indebted to Drs Mark Till, Rafael Fernandez-Botran, Michael Berton and Ms. Alexis Bossie for helpful comments concerning this manuscript. We thank Ms. M-M. Liu for excellent technical assistance, and Ms. G. A. Cheek and Ms. N. Stephens for their excellent secretarial assistance. This work is supported by NIH Grants AI-11851, AI-12789 and AI-07824.

References

Alt, F. W., Blackwell, T. K., DePinho, R. A., Reth, M. G. and Yancopoulos, G. D. (1986) *Immunol. Rev.* **89**, 5–30.

Andersson, J., Schreier, M. H. and Melchers, F. (1980) *Proc. Natl. Acad. Sci. USA* **77**, 1612–1616.

Baluyut, A. R. and Subbarao, B. (1988) *J. Mol. Cell. Immunol.* **4**, 45–57.

Bartlett, W. C., Michael, A., McCann, J., Yuan, D., Claassen, E. and Noelle, R. J. (1989) *J. Immunol.* **143**, 1745–1754.

Beagley, K. W., Eldridge, J. H., Kiyono, H., Everson, M. P., Koopman, W. J., Honjo, T. and McGhee, J. R. (1988) *J. Immunol.* **141**, 2035–2042.

Bekkhoucha, F., Naquet, P., Pierres, A., Marchetto, S. and Pierres, M. (1984) *Eur. J. Immunol.* **14**, 807–814.

Benacerraf, B. (1978) *J. Immunol.* **120**, 1809–1812.

Bergstedt-Lindqvist, S., Moon, H.-B., Persson, U., Moller, G., Heusser, C. and Severinson, E. (1988) *Eur. J. Immunol.* **18**, 1073—1077.

Berke, G., Gabison, D. and Feldman, M. (1975) *Eur. J. Immunol.* **5**, 813–818.

Berton, M. T., Uhr, J. W. and Vitetta, E. S. (1989) *Proc. Natl. Acad. Sci. USA.* **86**, 2829–2833.

Blackman, M. A., Tigger, M. A., Minnie, M. E. and Koshland, M. E. (1986) *Cell* **47**, 609–617.

Bottomly, K. (1988) *Immunol. Today* **9**, 268.

Bottomly, K., Jones, B., Kaye, J. and Jones, F. D. (1983) *J. Exp. Med.* **158**, 265–279.

Bretscher, P. A. and Cohn, M. (1968) *Nature* **220**, 444–448.

Brooks, K., Yuan, D., Uhr, J. W., Krammer, P. H. and Vitetta, E. S. (1983) *Nature* **302**, 825–826.

Cambier, J. C. and Lehmann, K. R. (1989) *J. Exp. Med.* **170**, 877–886.

Cambier, J. C. and Ransom, J. T. (1987) *Ann. Rev. Immunol.* **5**, 175–199.

Cambier, J. C., Justement, L. B., Newell, M. K., Chen, Z. Z., Harris, L. K., Sandoval, V. M., Klemsz, M. J. and Ransom, J. T. (1987) *Immunol. Rev.* **95**, 37–57.

Cheers, C., Breitner, J. C. S., Little, M. and Miller, J. F. A. P. (1971) *Nature* **232**, 248–250.

Chen, Z. Z., Coggeshall, K. M. and Cambier, J. C. (1986) *J. Immunol.* **136**, 2300–2304.

Chen, Z. Z., McGuire, J. C., Leach, K. L. and Cambier, J. C. (1987) *J. Immunol.* **138**, 2345–2352.

Chesnut, R. W. and Grey, H. M. (1981) *J. Immunol.* **126**, 1075–1079.

Claman, H. N., Chaperon, E. A. and Triplett, R. F. (1966) *Proc. Soc. Exp. Biol. Med.* **122**, 1167–1171.

Coffman, R. L., Seymour, B. W., Lebman, D. A., Hiraki, D. D., Christiansen, J. A., Shrader, B., Cherwinski, H. M., Savelkoul, H. F., Finkelman, F. D., Bond, M. W. *et al.* (1988) *Immunol. Rev.* **102**, 5–28.

Davies, A. J. S., Leuchars, E., Wallis, V., Marchant, R. and Elliott, E. V. (1967) *Transplantation* **5**, 222–231.

DeKruyff, R. H., Ju, S.-T., Hunt, A. J., Mosmann, T. R. and Umetsu, D. T. (1989) *J. Immunol.* **142**, 2575–2582.

DuBois, P., Stein, P., Ennist, D., Greenblatt, D., Mosmann, T. and Howard, M. (1987) *J. Immunol.* **139**, 1927–1934.

Dutton, R. W., Falkoff, R., Hirst, J. A., Hoffman, M., Kappler, J. W., Kottman, J. R., Lesley, J. F. and Vann, D. (1971) *Prog. Immunol.* **1**, 355.

Finkelman, F. D., Ohara, J., Goroff, D. K., Smith, J., Villacreses, N., Mond, J. J. and Paul, W. E. (1986) *J. Immunol.* **137**, 2878–2885.

Finkelman, F. D., Katona, I. M., Mosmann, T. R. and Coffman, R. L. (1988) *J. Immunol.* **140**, 1022–1027.

Geiger, B., Rosen, D. and Berke, G. (1982) *J. Cell Biol.* **95**, 137–143.

Golde, W. T., Gay, D., Kappler, J. and Marrack, P. (1986) *Cell. Immunol.* **103**, 73–83.

Harada, N., Matsumoto, M., Koyama, N., Shimizu, A., Honjo, T., Tominaga, A. and Takatsu, K. (1987) *Immunol. Lett.* **15**, 205–215.

Harriman, G. R., Kunimoto, D. Y., Elliott, J. F., Paetkau, V. and Strober, W. (1988) *J. Immunol.* **140**, 3033–3039.

Henry, C., Chan, E. L. and Kodlin, D. (1977) *J. Immunol.* **119**, 744–748.

Hirano, T., Yasukawa, K., Harada, H., Taga, T., Watanabe, Y., Matsuda, T., Kashiwamura, S., Nakajima, K., Koyama, K., Iwamatsu, A., Tsunasawa, S., Sakiyama, F., Matsiu, H., Takahara, Y., Taniguchi, T. and Kishimoto, T. (1986) *Nature* **324**, 73–76.

Hirohata, S., Jelinek, D. F. and Lipsky, P. E. (1988) *J. Immunol.* **140**, 3736–3744.

Isakov, N. and Morrow, P. R. (1989) *Cell. Immunol.* **120**, 366–374.

Isakson, P. C., Pure, E., Vitetta, E. S. and Krammer, P. H. (1982) *J. Exp. Med.* **155**, 734–748.

Janeway, C. A., Jr. (1975) *J. Immunol.* **114**, 1394.

Jelinek, D. F. and Lipsky, P. E. (1987) *Adv. Immunol.* **40**, 1–59.

Julius, M. H. and Rammensee, H. G. (1988) *Eur. J. Immunol.* **18**, 375–379.

Julius, M. H., Chiller, J. M. and Sidman, C. L. (1982) *Eur. J. Immunol.* **12**, 627–633.

Julius, M. H., Rammensee, H. G., Ratcliffe, M. J., Lamers, M. C., Langhorne, J. and Kohler, G. (1988) *Eur. J. Immunol.* **18**, 381–386.

Jurado, A., Carballido, J., Griffel, H., Hochkeppel, H. K. and Wetzel, G. D. (1989) In *Experientia*, pp. 521–526. Birkhauser Verlag, Basel, Switzerland.

Katz, D. H., Hamaoka, T., Dorf, M. E. and Benacerraf, B. (1973a) *Proc. Natl. Acad. Sci. USA* **70**, 2624–2628.

Katz, D. H., Hamaoka, T. and Benacerraf, B. (1973b) *J. Exp. Med.* **137**, 1405–1418.

Katz, D. H., Graves, M., Dorf, M. E., DiMuzio, H. and Benacerraf, B. (1975) *J. Exp. Med.* **141**, 263–268.

Kepron, M. R., Chen, Y-W., Uhr, J. W. and Vitetta, E. S. (1989) *J. Immunol.* **143**, 334–339.

Killar, L., MacDonald, G., West, J., Woods, A. and Bottomly, K. (1987) *J. Immunol.* **138**, 1674–1679.

Kim, J., Woods, A., Becker-Dunn, E. and Bottomly, K. (1985) *J. Exp. Med.* **162**, 188–201.

Kindred, B. and Shreffler, D. C. (1972) *J. Immunol.* **109**, 940–943.

Kishimoto, T. (1989) *Blood* **74**, 1–10.

Kishimoto, T. and Ishizaka, K. (1975) *J. Immunol.* **114**, 585–591.

Kourilsky, P. and Claverie, J-M. (1989) *Adv. Immunol.* **45**, 107–193.

Krusemeier, M. and Snow, E. C. (1988) *J. Immunol.* **140**, 367–375.

Kupfer, A. and Singer, S. J. (1989) *Ann. Rev. Immunol.* **7**, 309–337.

Kupfer, A., Swain, S. L., Janeway, C. A., Jr. and Singer, S. J. (1986) *Proc. Natl. Acad. Sci. USA* **83**, 6080–6083.

Kupfer, A., Swain, S. L. and Singer, S. J. (1987a) *J. Exp. Med.* **165**, 1565–1580.

Kupfer, A., Singer, S. J., Janeway, C. A., Jr. and Swain, S. L. (1987b) *Proc. Natl. Acad. Sci. USA* **84**, 5888–5892.

Lanzavecchia, A. (1985) *Nature* **314**, 537–539.

Layton, J. E., Vitetta, E. S., Uhr, J. W. and Krammer, P. H. (1984) *J. Exp. Med.* **160**, 1850–1863.

Lebman, D. A. and Coffman, R. L. (1988) *J. Exp. Med.* **168**, 853–862.

Liebson, H. J., Marrack, P. and Kappler, J. (1982) *J. Immunol.* **129**, 1398–1402.

Liebson, H. J., Gefter, M., Zlotnik, A., Marrack, P. and Kappler, J. W. (1984) *Nature* **309**, 799.

Lipsky, P. E. and Rosenthal, A. S. (1974) *J. Exp. Med.* **141**, 138–154.

LoCascio, N. J., Haughton, G., Arnold, L. W. and Corley, R. B. (1984) *Proc. Natl. Acad. Sci. USA* **81**, 2466–2469.

Loughnan, M. S., Takatsu, K., Harada, N. and Nossal, G. J. (1987) *Proc. Natl. Acad. Sci. USA* **84**, 5399–5403.

Lowenthal, J. W., Castle, B. E., Christiansen, J., Schreurs, J., Rennick, D., Arai, N., Hoy, Y., Takebe, Y. and Howard, M. (1988) *J. Immunol.* **140**, 456–464.

Lundgren, M., Persson, U., Larsson, P., Magnusson, C., Smith, C. I. E., Hammarstrom, L. and Severinson, E. (1989) *Eur. J. Immunol.* **19**, 1311–1315.

Marrack, P. and Kappler, J. W. (1975) *J. Immunol.* **114**, 1116.

Martz, E. (1975) *J. Immunol.* **115**, 261–267.

Matsui, K., Nakanishi, K., Cohen, D. I., Hada, T., Furuyama, J.-I., Hamaoka, T. and Higashino, K. (1989) *J. Immunol.* **142**, 2918–2923.

Mazerolles, F., Lumbroso, C., Lecomte, O., Le Deist, F. and Fischer, A. (1988) *Eur. J. Immunol.* **18**, 1229–1234.

Melchers, F. and Andersson, J. (1984) *Cell* **37**, 713–720.

Miller, J. F. A. P. and Mitchell, G. F. (1967) *Nature* **216**, 659–663.

Mishell, R. I. and Dutton, R. W. (1967) *J. Exp. Med.* **126**, 423–442.

Mishra, G. C., Berton, M. T., Oliver, K. G., Krammer, P. H., Uhr, J. W. and Vitetta, E. S. (1986) *J. Immunol.* **137**, 1590–1598.

Mitchell, G. F. and Miller, J. F. A. P. (1968) *J. Exp. Med.* **128**, 821–837.

Mitchison, N. A. (1971) *Eur. J. Immunol.* **1**, 18–27.

Mosier, D. E. and Coppelson, L. W. (1968) *Proc. Natl. Acad. Sci. USA* **61**, 542.

Mosier, D. E., Fitch, F. W., Rowley, D. A. and Davies, A. J. (1970) *Nature* **225**, 276–277.

Mosmann, T. R. and Coffman, R. L. (1989) *Adv. Immunol.* **46**, 111–147.

Mosmann, T. R., Cherwinski, H., Bond, M. W., Giedlin, M. A. and Coffman, R. L. (1986) *J. Immunol.* **136**, 2348–2357.

Munro, A. and Hunter, P. (1970) *Nature* **225**, 277–278.

Muraguchi, A., Hirano, T., Tang, B., Matsuda, T., Horii, Y., Nakajima, K. and Kishimoto, T. (1988) *J. Exp. Med.* **167**, 332–344.

Nakajima, K., Hirano, T., Koyama, K. and Kishimoto, T. (1987) *J. Immunol.* **139**, 774–779.

Noelle, R. J. and McCann, J. (1989). *J. Mol. Cell. Immunol.* **4**, 161–175.

Noelle, R. J., Snow, E. C., Uhr, J. W. and Vitetta, E. S. (1983) *Proc. Natl. Acad. Sci. USA* **80**, 6628–6631.

Noelle, R., Krammer, P. H., Ohara, J., Uhr, J. W. and Vitetta, E. S. (1984) *Proc. Natl. Acad. Sci. USA* **81**, 6149–6153.

Noelle, R. J., McCann, J., Marshall, L. and Bartlett, W. C. (1989b) *J. Immunol.* **143**, 1807–1814.

Ohara, J. and Paul, W. E. (1987) *Nature* **325**, 537–540.

Ovary, Z. and Benacerraf, B. (1963) *Proc. Soc. Exp. Biol. Med.* **114**, 72–76.

Owens, T. (1988) *Eur. J. Immunol.* **18**, 395–401.

Park, L. S., Friend, D., Grabstein, K. and Urdal, D. L. (1987) *Proc. Natl. Acad. Sci. USA* **84**, 1669–1673.

Parker, D. C., Fothergill, J. J. and Wadsworth, D. C. (1979) *J. Immunol.* **123**, 931–941.

Poo, W. J., Conrad, L. and Janeway, C. A., Jr. (1988) *Nature* **332**, 378.

Principato, M. A., Thompson, G. S. and Friedman, S. M. (1983) *J. Exp. Med.* **158**, 1444–1458.

Radbruch, A., Muller, W. and Rajewsky, K. (1986) *Proc. Natl. Acad. Sci. USA* **83**, 3954–3957.

Raff, M. C. (1970) *Nature* **226**, 1257.

Rajewsky, K., Schirrmacher, V., Nase, S. and Jerne, N. K. (1969) *J. Exp. Med.* **129**, 1131–1143.

Rasmussen, R., Takatsu, K., Harada, N., Takahashi, T. and Bottomly, K. (1988) *J. Immunol.* **140**, 705–712.

Ratcliffe, M. J. and Julius, M. H. (1982) *Eur. J. Immunol.* **12**, 634–641.

Riedel, C., Owens, T. and Nossal, G. J. (1988) *Eur. J. Immunol.* **18**, 403–408.

Rock, K. L., Benacerraf, B. and Abbas, A. K. (1984) *J. Exp. Med.* **160**, 1102–1113.

Roehm, N. W., Liebson, H. J., Zlotnik, A., Kappler, J., Marrack, P. and Cambier, J. C. (1984) *J. Exp. Med.* **160**, 679–694.

Rosenthal, A. S. and Shevach, E. M. (1973) *J. Exp. Med.* **138**, 1194–1212.

Rothman, P., Lutzker, S., Cook, W., Coffman, R. and Alt, F. W. (1988) *J. Exp. Med.* **168**, 2385–2389.

Saiki, O., Tanaka, T., Doi, S. and Kishimoto, S. (1988) *J. Immunol.* **140**, 853–858.

Sanders, V. M., Snyder, J. M., Uhr, J. W. and Vitetta, E. S. (1986) *J. Immunol.* **137**, 2395–2404.

Sanders, V. M., Fernandez Botran, R., Uhr, J. W. and Vitetta, E. S. (1987a) *J. Immunol.* **139**, 2349–2354.

Sanders, V. M., Uhr, J. W. and Vitetta, E. S. (1987b) *Cell. Immunol.* **104**, 419–425.

Sanders, V. M., Fernandez-Botran, R., Coffman, R. L., Mosmann, T. R. and Vitetta, E. S. (1988) *Proc. Natl. Acad. Sci. USA* **85**, 7724–7728.

Schimpl, A. and Wecker, E. (1972) *Nature* **237**, 15.

Schoenbeck, S., McKenzie, D. T. and Kagnoff, M. F. (1989) *Eur. J. Immunol.* **19**, 965–969.

Sekita, K., Straub, C., Hoessli, D. and Zubler, R. H. (1988) *Eur. J. Immunol.* **18**, 1405–1410.

Sell, S. and Gell, P. G. H. (1965) *J. Exp. Med.* **122**, 423.
Sidman, C. L., Marshall, J. D., Schultz, L. D., Gray, P. W. and Johnson, H. M. (1984) *Nature* **309**, 801.
Smeland, E. B., Blomhoff, H. K., Funderud, S., Shalaby, M. R. and Espevik, T. (1989) *J. Exp. Med.* **170**, 1463–1468.
Snapper, C. M., Finkelman, F. D. and Paul, W. E. (1988a) *Immunol. Rev.* **102**, 51–75.
Snapper, C. M., Finkelman, F. D. and Paul, W. E. (1988b) *J. Exp. Med.* **167**, 183–196.
Snapper, C. M., Peschell, C. and Paul, W. E. (1988c) *J. Immunol.* **140**, 2121–2127.
Sprent, J. (1978) *J. Exp. Med.* **147**, 1142–1158.
Springer, T., Dustin, M. L., Kishimoto, T. K. and Marlin, S. D. (1987) *Ann. Rev. Immunol.* **5**, 223–252.
Stavnezer-Nordgren, J. and Sirlin, S. (1986) *EMBO J.* **5**, 95–102.
Stavnezer, J., Radcliffe, G., Lin, Y.-C., Nietupski, J., Berggren, L., Sitia, R. and Severinson, E. (1988) *Proc. Natl. Acad. Sci. USA* **85**, 7704–7708.
Stevens, T. L., Bossie, A., Sanders, V. M., Fernandez-Botran, R., Coffman, R. L., Mosmann, T. R. and Vitetta, E. S. (1988) *Nature* **334**, 255–258.
Swain, S. L. (1985) *J. Immunol.* **134**, 3934–3943.
Tanaka, T., Saiki, O., Doi, S., Negoro, S. and Kishimoto, S. (1988) *J. Immunol.* **140**, 470–473.
Tony, H. P. and Parker, D. C. (1985) *J. Exp. Med.* **161**, 223–241.
Trinchieri, G. and Perusia, B. (1985) *Immunol. Today* **6**, 131.
van Noesel, C., Miedema, F., Brouwer, M., de Rie, M. A., Aarden, L. A. and Van Lier, R. A. W. (1988) *Nature* **333**, 850–852.
Vercelli, D., Jabara, H. H., Arai, K., Yokota, T. and Geha, R. S. (1989a) *Eur. J. Immunol.* **19**, 1419–1424.
Vercelli, D., Habara, H. H., Arai, K.-I. and Geha, R. S. (1989b) *J. Exp. Med.* **169**, 1295–1307.
Vitetta, E. S., Bossie, A., Fernandez Botran, R., Myers, C. D., Oliver, K. G., Sanders, V. M. and Stevens, T. L. (1987) *Immunol. Rev.* **99**, 193–239.
Vitetta, E. S., Fernandez-Botran, R., Myers, C. D. and Sanders, V. M. (1989) *Adv. Immunol.* **45**, 1–105.
Wacholtz, M. C., Patel, S. S. and Lipsky, P. E. (1989) *J. Exp. Med.* **170**, 431–448.
Waldmann, T. A., Goldman, C. L., Robb, R. J., Depper, J. M., Leonard, W. J., Sharrow, S. O., Bongiovanni, K. F., Korsmeyer, S. J. and Greene, W. C. (1984) *J. Exp. Med.* **160**, 1450.
Whalen, B. J., Tony, H-P. and Parker, D. C. (1988) *J. Immunol.* **141**, 2230–2239.
Yuan, D., Weiss, E. A., Layton, J. E., Krammer, P. H. and Vitetta, E. S. (1985) *J. Immunol.* **135**, 1465–1469.
Ziegler, K. and Unanue, E. R. (1981) *J. Immunol.* **127**, 1869–1875.
Ziegler, H. K. and Unanue, E. R. (1982) *Proc. Natl. Acad. Sci. USA* **79**, 175–178.
Zubler, R. H., Lowenthal, J. W., Erard, F., Hashimoto, N., Devos, R. and MacDonald, H. R. (1984) *J. Exp. Med.* **160**, 1170.

7
Immunoglobulin isotype regulation

JUDY M. TEALE AND D. MARK ESTES

Introduction

It has been known for many years that T helper cells (Tн cells) are required for optimal isotype switching and the production of multiple antibody classes during an antigen specific response (Taylor and Wortis, 1968; Torrigiani, 1972; Teale, 1983; Teale and Abraham, 1987). In recent years, the study of antibody class regulation has become an exciting research area, since the molecular mechanisms associated with isotype regulation by T lymphocytes are rapidly being elucidated. Of particular importance is the accumulating evidence for the rôle of cytokines produced by activated T cells in signalling B cells to synthesize specific antibody classes. Much of this chapter will be devoted to reviewing what is known about the rôle of cytokines in antibody class regulation.

It is important from the start, to point out some of the complexities inherent in the studies described. Most obvious is the fact that there are multiple cytokines and often multiple target cells for each cytokine. In addition, in many cases, several cell types can produce a given cytokine. Since many of the bioassays used to analyse the influence of particular lymphokines on isotype expression involve more than one cell type—i.e. B cell, T cell and macrophage—it is possible that the effects observed are not direct effects on the B cell itself. The addition of an exogenous lymphokine could potentially induce production of yet another cytokine which could then exert its influence on the B cell. This becomes especially significant in the light of the fact that we have not yet identified all of the relevant lymphokines. Moreover, many studies have indicated the importance of lymphokine concentration as well as the kinetics of addition of lymphokines. These problems are compounded by the knowledge that combinations of lymphokines can synergize with one another in inducing antibody synthesis. For example, the combination of interleukin 4 (IL-4) and IL-5 results in greater production of several isotypes (Coffman *et al.*, 1988; Lebman and

CYTOKINES AND B LYMPHOCYTES
ISBN 0–12–155145–8

Coffman, 1988a,b; Swain et al., 1988ab; Tonkonogy et al., 1989). In addition, interferon γ (IFN-γ) is known to inhibit the ability of IL-4 to enhance IgG1 and IgE synthesis (Coffman et al., 1986; Coffman and Carty, 1986).

Another level of complexity is that certain lymphokines can differentially affect a given B cell depending upon its maturational state (Roehm et al., 1984; Noelle et al., 1984; Callard and Smith, 1988). Thus, IL-4 can affect resting B cells by inducing class II histocompatibility molecules (Ia) expression, but it can also affect activated B cells by inducing the specific expression of IgG1 or IgE (Isakson et al., 1982; Coffman et al., 1986a; Snapper et al., 1988b). Importantly, lymphokines exogenously added to cultures have often led to different effects on isotype expression depending upon whether small, resting B cells or activated B cell blasts were used. For example, the synergy of IL-4 and IL-5 in enhancing the production of all isotypes is only observed when large, presumably activated, cells are used (Tonkonogy et al., 1989). In addition, the activation requirements of resting and previously activated cells appear to be different with the resting cells requiring cognate interactions with the T cell (Krusemeier and Snow, 1988; Stevens et al., 1988; DeKruyff et al., 1989; Noelle et al., 1989; Tonkonogy et al., 1989). Thus, in defining the exact mechanisms associated with isotype regulation by cytokines, it is critical that the maturational state of the B cell is known. This was not the case in many of the earlier experiments.

Another potential problem in several of the studies to date that have examined the rôle of cytokines in isotype regulation is the use of the mitogen lipopolysaccharide (LPS) as the B cell stimulant rather than an antigen-specific, T cell driven response. Presumably, LPS will result in different signals to the B cell which could enhance the effect of certain cytokines and obscure the effects of others in a non-physiological manner.

Finally, there is increasing evidence for T cell heterogeneity among CD4[+] TH cells that results in activated T cells producing distinct lymphokine profiles. Given the rôle of certain cytokines in the induction of specific isotypes, the particular TH cells activated during an immune response could profoundly influence the isotypes produced.

Distinct subsets of T helper cells

A case for distinct subsets of TH cells was established when a large number of mouse TH cell clones were analysed for lymphokine production (Kim et al., 1985; Mosmann et al., 1986; Cherwinski et al., 1987; Bottomly et al., 1988). TH$_1$ (T inflammatory) type T cell clones were found to produce IL-2, IFN-γ, and lymphotoxin, whereas TH$_2$ type T cell clones produce IL-4, IL-5 and

IL-6 (reviewed in Mosmann and Coffman, 1989). Both types of T cells synthesize granulocyte and macrophage colony stimulating factor (GM-CSF), tumour necrosis factor (TNF), IL-3 and preproenkephalin (Mosmann and Coffman, 1989). Subsequent studies have indicated distinct functional capabilities. T_{H1} cells appear to be more important for cell mediated immunity and are involved in the induction of both delayed type hypersensitivity and cytotoxic T cell response (Bottomly *et al.*, 1988; Mosmann and Coffman, 1989). Although T_{H1} cells have been shown to be effective in providing help to secondary antigen-specific responses with primed B cells, their ability to provide help to unprimed B cells has led to mixed results (Giedlin *et al.*, 1986; Killar *et al.*, 1987). T_{H2} cells, on the other hand, are very effective at providing help for B cell antibody responses (Tony and Parker, 1985; Kim *et al.*, 1985; Stevens *et al.*, 1988; Boom *et al.*, 1988; Coffman *et al.*, 1988).

It is still not clear how these different subsets of cells defined by *in vitro* propagated T cell clones relate to normal T cells *in vivo*. It is possible that the findings of distinct function described above relate to the maturational state of the T helper cell as opposed to truly different subsets (Swain *et al.*, 1988b; Powers *et al.*, 1988; Gajewski *et al.*, 1989). Moreover, more recent experiments suggest that the classification of T cells into just two subsets based on lymphokine production is an oversimplification. Thus, some clones do not fall into the T_{H1}–T_{H2} lymphokine pattern and produce both IL-4 and IFN-γ (Gajewski *et al.*, 1988; Bass *et al.*, 1989; Abraham and Teale, unpublished observations); lymphokines normally used to distinguish between T_{H1} (IFN-γ producing) and T_{H2} (IL-4 producing) subsets. In addition, the polymorphic cell surface glycoprotein-1 (Pgp-1$^-$) subset of CD4$^+$ T cells secretes substantial amounts of IL-2 but little or no IFN-γ (Budd *et al.*, 1987). Additional evidence for heterogeneity was observed when lymphokine profiles of mouse helper T cell clones were tested early (2–4 weeks) instead of late (months) after establishment in culture (Mosmann and Coffman, 1989), and evidence for distinct lymphokine patterns produced by T cell precursors has emerged (Swain *et al.*, 1988a,b; Gajewski *et al.*, 1989). Such heterogeneity may help to explain the results obtained with human T cell clones in which the two distinct patterns of lymphokine profiles originally found in mouse T_{H1} and T_{H2} clones were not apparent (Maggi *et al.*, 1988; Paliard *et al.*, 1988). Resolution of these issues may require definition of both lineage- and activation-specific markers. Although markers such as the leukocyte common antigen in humans and mice, and the OX22 marker in the rat appear to distinguish between functional T cell subsets (Arthur and Mason, 1986; Rudd *et al.*, 1987), it is not clear whether these markers represent lineage- or activation-specific markers.

Nevertheless, despite the basis for different lymphokine profiles of individual T cells, the phenomenon of selected lymphokine production appears to be biologically relevant. Thus, it seems clear from a number of infection models that distinct lymphokine patterns are induced (Scott *et al.*, 1988: Heinzel *et al.*, 1989: Estes and Teale, unpublished observations). The most convincing experiments have compared the lymphokines produced as a result of infection in both susceptible and resistant strains of mice. For example, when *Leishmania major* infects the susceptible strain, BALB/c, IL-4 was induced and an antibody response was apparent. In contrast, the non-susceptible strain C57BL/6, which resolved the infection, produced IFN-γ with evidence for cell mediated immunity (Heinzel *et al.*, 1989). Apparently, for defence against this particular organism, cell-mediated immunity is more important. Thus, the specific lymphokines produced as a result of infection can affect the outcome of the infectious disease process.

Distinct T helper cell subsets and isotype regulation

Mouse T cell clones that were classified as either T_{H_1} or T_{H_2} were also shown to differ in their ability to stimulate the various isotypes (Coffman *et al.*, 1988; Stevens *et al.*, 1988). The most convincing differences were observed with the isotypes IgE and IgG2a which appear to be specifically induced by the lymphokines IL-4 and IFN-γ, respectively (Coffman *et al.*, 1986; Snapper *et al.*, 1988a,b). In one study, the use of a panel of several T_{H_1} and T_{H_2} clones revealed that the vast majority of IL-4 producing T_{H_2} clones were capable of inducing IgE responses in contrast to none of the T_{H_1} clones lacking detectable IL-4 (Coffman *et al.*, 1988). On the other hand, T_{H_1} clones were able to induce substantially more IgG2a relative to the T_{H_2} clones. In another study using isolated trinitrophenyl-specific B cells, a T_{H_1} clone was shown to induce IgG2a whereas the T_{H_2} clone induced IgG1 (Stevens *et al.*, 1988). Both types of T_H clones were shown to induce IgM and IgG3. In this system, the regulation of isotype expression appeared to occur in at least two stages involving activation via cognate interaction between the T and B cell, and the interaction of T cell-derived lymphokines with the B cell (Stevens *et al.*, 1988). The major conclusion from these experiments is that the particular lymphokines produced by individual T cells affect the production of specific antibody classes.

As pointed out above, however, the designation of T_{H_1} and T_{H_2} is probably an oversimplification and not useful for an analysis of human systems. Therefore, the next section concentrates more on current knowledge of individual cytokines and their potential rôle in isotype regulation.

Cytokines and isotype regulation

IL-4

IL-4, first described in 1982, was originally isolated from crude supernatants of the EL-4 thymoma and characterized as the specific factor that supported the growth of anti-Ig stimulated blasts (Howard *et al.*, 1982). Derived primarily from T cells, its activities have been demonstrated to affect a wide range of cell types, including most cells of haemopoietic lineage (reviewed in Ohara and Paul, 1987). Among its activities on B cells, IL-4 enhances the expression of class II major histocompatibility antigens (Noelle *et al.*, 1984; Roehm *et al.*, 1984), stimulates IgG1 and IgE production by LPS blasts (Isakson *et al.*, 1982; Coffman *et al.*, 1986a,b), is necessary for generation and maintenance of IgE responses *in vivo* (Finkelman *et al.*, 1988a,b,c), and stimulates Thy-1 expression on normal B cells (Snapper *et al.*, 1988a,b,c). It also increases expression of CD23 (DeFrance *et al.*, 1987) and surface IgM (Shields *et al.*, 1989) on human B cells.

In terms of cytokines specifically inducing particular isotypes, the evidence is perhaps strongest for IL-4 and IgE synthesis. Initial studies tested the effect of exogenous IL-4 on mitogen-stimulated B cells. Culture of murine spleen cells with LPS results in activated B cells which then secrete largely IgM, IgG3 and IgG2b (Anderson *et al.*, 1979; Yuan and Vitetta, 1983). In contrast, spleen cells cultured with LPS and IL-4, selectively produce IgG1 and IgE, while expression of IgG3 and IgG2b are substantially suppressed (reviewed in Ohara and Paul, 1987). Importantly, the addition of anti-IL-4 profoundly inhibits IgE synthesis (Coffman *et al.*, 1986; Snapper *et al.*, 1988b; Mosmann and Coffman, 1989). Comparable systems for activating human B cells and studying the direct effects of human IL-4 have not been fully delineated as LPS is not a potent activator of human B cells. In a recent study, Thyphronitis *et al.* (1989) showed that IL-4 increases IgE secretion by highly purified human B cells stimulated with Epstein–Barr virus (EBV). Similarly, Lundgren *et al.* (1989) utilized IL-4, phorbol 12-myristate 13-acetate (PMA) and a mouse thymoma cell line in co-culture with human B cells, resulting in increased amounts of IgE and IgG4 production assayed by limiting dilution analysis. Although IgG4 and IgE appear to be co-regulated in humans (Hammarstrom *et al.*, 1987), IgG4 cannot be said to be analogous to murine IgG1. In fact, the IgG subclasses in humans and mice have apparently evolved independently and they are therefore unlikely to be subject to the same immunoregulatory mechanisms (Callard and Turner, 1990).

In both human and murine systems it is clear that IL-4 plays an obligatory rôle in IgE synthesis. Thus, in a variety of *in vitro* systems, it has been shown that either the absence of IL-4 or its inhibition by anti-IL-4 results essentially in no IgE response (Vitetta *et al.*, 1985; Coffman *et al.*, 1986; Snapper and Paul, 1987; Maggi *et al.*, 1988; Pene *et al.*, 1988; Vercelli *et al.*, 1989a,b; del Prete *et al.*, 1988). This conclusion was confirmed in an *in vivo* model in which the IgE response normally found in animals infected with *Nippostrongylus brasiliensis* could be virtually eliminated by the administration of anti-IL-4 (Finkelman *et al.*, 1988a). In mice, IL-4 appears to affect IgE production by increasing the frequency of B cells that switch to IgE as well as by increasing the clonal burst size (Lebman and Coffman, 1988b; Savelkoul *et al.*, 1988) but the mechanism in humans is not known. The examination of single B cell clones stimulated with T_{H2} cells strongly suggested that IL-4 was inducing IgM-bearing cells and their clonal progeny to subsequently switch to IgE synthesis (Lebman and Coffman, 1988b).

Although from both murine and human systems it seems clear that IL-4 is an absolute requirement for IgE production, there is evidence from studies with human B cells that IL-4 is not the sole lymphokine required. Thus, a recent study indicated that IgE production could be inhibited by both anti-IL-4 and anti-IL-6, suggesting a requirement for IL-6 (Vercelli *et al.*, 1989a,b). In addition, IgE production was optimally enhanced by the presence of IL-5. Another study used cyclosporin A treated, allogeneic T cell clones to stimulate B cells and then examine the effects of lymphokines (DeKruyff *et al.*, 1989). The cyclosporin A treatment results in the inability of T cells to secrete their own lymphokines (Krusemeir and Snow, 1988). In this system, an apparent requirement for low molecular weight B cell growth factor (LMW BCGF) was observed (DeKruyff *et al.*, 1989). It is unclear, at present, whether IgE is regulated in a fundamentally different manner in mice and humans, or whether further details of IgE regulation remain to be elucidated.

The precise molecular mechanisms by which IL-4 specifically induces IgE synthesis remain unresolved. However, recent studies suggest that IL-4 prepares the B cell for Ig rearrangement and isotype switching (see below).

IL-4 is also known to upregulate IgG1 production. Previous studies clearly showed that LPS-activated B cells in the presence of IL-4 switch to the production of IgG1 (Isakson *et al.*, 1982; Coffman *et al.*, 1986; Lee *et al.*, 1986; Noma *et al.*, 1986) as well as IgE. Moreover, a limiting dilution analysis indicated that IL-4 was inducing IgM-bearing cells to switch to IgG1 (Layton *et al.*, 1984). However, despite its strong IgG1 enhancing effects in mitogen-driven systems, its rôle in the specific regulation of IgG1 synthesis remains uncertain. Thus, a number of T_{H1} clones that do not produce IL-4 induce substantial IgG1 production (Coffman *et al.*, 1988). In addition, anti-IL-4 results in little or no inhibition of IgG1 responses either *in vitro* (Boom *et al.*, 1988; Coffman *et al.*, 1988) or *in vivo* (Finkelman *et al.*, 1986). Such studies indicate IL-4 independent mechanisms for IgG1 production. Additionally, studies of anti-Ig derived murine B cell blasts indicate that IL-4 alone cannot support proliferation and differentiation of B cells (Purkerson *et al.*, 1988). In order to obtain optimal stimulation and IgG1 production, further addition of IL-2 and IL-5 was required (Purkerson *et al.*, 1988).

Interestingly, it has been reported that IL-4 can affect resting B cells and presumably influence their commitment to IgG1 production upon subsequent activation (Snapper *et al.*, 1988b). This leads to the prediction that increased IL-4 levels *in vivo* would influence the potential of the resident, primary B cell pool. Infection of mice with *Mesocestoides corti* results in an antibody response restricted to IgM and IgG1 (Chapman *et al.*, 1979; Abraham and Teale, 1987a,b). Although increased IL-4 appears to be associated with the infection, the resting B cells were unaltered in their potential to produce multiple isotypes in response to hapten-carrier conjugates (Desai, Abraham and Teale, unpublished findings). Thus, no evidence was found for prior commitment to IgG1 synthesis. One of the major unresolved areas in isotype regulation by cytokines is when, during B cell activation and clonal proliferation, cytokines induce isotype-specific signals.

IL-4 induction of both IgE and IgG1 synthesis is inhibited by relatively low concentrations of IFN-γ (Coffman and Carty, 1986; Finkelman *et al.*, 1988b). The differences in the production of IL-4 and IFN-γ between T_{H_1} and T_{H_2} subsets of T cells can explain their differences in the ability to induce an IgE response. Additional evidence for this is the capacity to obtain an IgE response using T_{H_1} cells if IL-4 and anti-IFN-γ are added to the cultures (Coffman *et al.*, 1988).

IL-4 has also been shown to inhibit the enhanced expression of the IgG FcRII on LPS-activated B cells (Snapper *et al.*, 1989). Although the function of FcRII on B cells remains unclear, crosslinkage of surface Ig and FcRII with rabbit IgG specific for mouse Ig inhibits many B cell functions including activation and differentiation (Sidman *et al.*, 1986; Philips *et al.*, 1984; Bijsterbosch *et al.*, 1985). IL-4 has also been shown to regulate the expression of the low affinity receptor for IgE on lymphocytes (Conrad *et al.*, 1987; DeFrance *et al.*, 1987; Hudak *et al.*, 1987), adding yet another parameter through which IL-4 can potentially regulate IgE responses.

IFN-γ

IFN-γ, derived primarily from T lymphocytes, serves as a potent regulator of B cell development and differentiation in addition to its other numerous biological activities. IFN-γ has been shown to upregulate expression of secretory component necessary for IgM and IgA binding and transport, in addition to upregulation of IgG(Fc) receptors on polymorphonuclear cells (PMN) (Pace *et al.*, 1983; Sollid *et al.*, 1987).

IFN-γ appears to regulate both *in vitro* and *in vivo* antibody responses. Utilizing LPS-activated B cells *in vitro*, it was demonstrated that IFN-γ stimulates IgG2a secretion (Snapper *et al.*, 1988a). Marked increases in IgG2a production have also been demonstrated for resting B cells before LPS stimulation, suggesting that IFN-γ acts directly on B cells. Importantly, IFN-γ, as well as stimulating IgG2a synthesis, has been shown to inhibit IgG1, IgG2b, IgG3, and IgE secretion (Snapper *et al.*, 1988a,c). Such findings indicate that IFN-γ may play an inhibitory rôle in antibody production.

The importance of IFN-γ in IgG2a synthesis has also been shown in several *in vivo* models. Previous studies indicated that the administration of anti-IgD results in relatively large increases in serum levels of both IgG1 and IgE (Finkelman *et al.*, 1987; Mountz *et al.*, 1987). In mice treated with a goat antibody to mouse IgD, administration of IFN-γ inhibited production of IgG1 and IgE, and stimulated production of IgG2a (Finkelman *et al.*, 1988a, 1988b). In another model, monoclonal antibodies specific for IFN-γ were shown to block IgG2a responses elicited by the bacterium *Brucella abortus*, an organism which elicits primarily an IgG2a response in mice (Finkelman *et al.*, 1988a,b).

Infectious disease models indicate the physiological importance of the IgG2a response and the presumed rôle for IFN-γ. For example, it has been shown that infection with a large number of both DNA and RNA viruses elicits predominantly an IgG2a response (Coutelier *et al.*, 1987). Because interferons are produced as a result of viral infections, it was postulated that IFN-γ was responsible for the preferential expression of IgG2a antibodies. It has been suggested that IFN-γ is involved in humoral immune responses to a variety of pathogens that predominantly elicit IgG2a responses (Duran and Metcalf, 1987; Winter *et al.*, 1989). The advantages of an IgG2a response to microbial pathogens are evident when the effector functions of the various isotypes are compared. IgG2a can fix complement. In addition, antibodies of the IgG2a subclass bind with high avidity to Fc receptors on both macrophages and natural killer (NK) cells and more effectively mediate antibody-dependent cellular cytotoxicity reactions relative to other isotypes (Matthews *et al.*, 1981; Herlyn and Koprowski, 1982; Johnson *et al.*, 1985; Unkeless *et al.*, 1988). These effector mechanisms should be effective in combating intracellular infections.

Studies of mouse T_{H_1} clones are particularly relevant to understanding the functional consequences of IFN-γ production because detectable levels of

IFN-γ are not produced by T$_{H2}$ clones (Mosmann and Coffman, 1989). As indicated previously, T$_{H1}$ clones induce substantial quantities of IgG2a relative to amounts produced by T$_{H2}$ clones, and they have also been shown to suppress T$_{H2}$-induced *in vitro* responses (Mosmann and Coffman, 1989). In addition, differential selection of T$_{H1}$ clones in the presence of IFN-γ *in vitro* implies that preferential expansion of this subset may also occur *in vivo*, selectively altering the isotype distribution indirectly through regulation of T cell responses (Gajewski *et al.*, 1989; Mosmann and Coffman, 1989).

IL-5

IL-5, first isolated in the early 1970s as a potent activator of eosinophils (Sanderson *et al.*, 1988) also induces Ig synthesis and proliferation of B cells. This was first demonstrated by co-stimulation of mouse BCL-1 cells with dextran sulphate (Schimpl and Wecker, 1975; Swain *et al.*, 1982). IL-5 appears to have the capability to act directly on B cells, as an IL-5 receptor has been identified on murine BCL1-B20 cells (Takatsu *et al.*, 1988).

IL-5 induces differentiation and Ig secretion in murine splenic B cells (Takatsu *et al.*, 1980; Harada *et al.*, 1985; Kinashi *et al.*, 1986; Moller, 1988). In studies utilizing LPS-activated splenic B cells in the presence of IL-5, several investigators demonstrated increased production of IgA. Thus early evidence indicated that IL-5 may act as a possible IgA switch factor (Coffman *et al.*, 1987; Bond *et al.*, 1987; Murray *et al.*, 1987; Yokota *et al.*, 1987). However, several subsequent studies have demonstrated that IL-5 increased the IgA response by acting on surface IgA$^+$ B cells that are presumably already committed to IgA synthesis. Therefore, IL-5 appears to serve more as a terminal differentiation factor than as an isotype switch factor (Beagley *et al.*, 1988, 1989; Schoenbeck *et al.*, 1989).

In LPS-stimulated B cell cultures or cultures utilizing percoll-fractionated B cell blasts, IL-4 and IL-5 synergize to enhance the IgG1 response (Tonkonogy *et al.*, 1989; Estes and Teale, unpublished results). In studies of LPS-stimulated anti-Ig blasts, a requirement was demonstrated for both IL-5 and IL-2 for optimal IgG1 expression (Purkerson *et al.*, 1988). As previously shown for IgA secretion, IL-5 may act as a differentiation factor for IgG1-committed cells.

IL-5 can also influence IgM expression. Stimulation of LPS or anti-Ig blasts in the presence of IL-4 resulted in reduced IgM secretion. IL-4 dependent reduction in IgM expression was shown to be substantially overcome by the addition of IL-5 (Tonkonogy *et al.*, 1989; Purkerson *et al.*, 1988; Estes and Teale, unpublished results).

In contrast to the activities of IL-5 in the murine system, the effects of IL-5 on human B cell differentiation and proliferation are unresolved at present. Studies using human B cells have been unable to reproduce IL-5-induced effects on antibody production as observed in the murine system. Although at least one study indicated an effect of recombinant human IL-5 on B cell antibody production (Yokota *et al.*, 1987), it is possible that the predominant effect of IL-5 in humans is its rôle in eosinophil development (Clutterbuck *et al.*, 1987; Sanderson *et al.*, 1988).

While the precise mechanism of IL-5 action on B cells is poorly understood, IL-5 stimulation of a BCL-1 subline resulted in increased synthesis of u_s mRNA and modest increases in J chain mRNA (Matsui *et al.*, 1989). IL-5, together with IL-2 also appeared to augment J chain mRNA synthesis (Matsui *et al.*, 1989). In addition, B cells cultured with LPS plus IL-5 showed increased steady-state levels of mRNA for the secreted form of $\gamma1$ and α (Takatsu *et al.*, 1988). Such activities help to explain increases in IgM, IgA, and IgG1 secretion. They are also consistent with the notion that IL-5 is important as a B cell terminal differentiation factor.

IL-1

IL-1 is a highly pleiotropic cytokine. It is produced primarily by macrophages and monocytes and was first identified in 1972 (Gery *et al.*, 1972). Many different cell types have been shown to produce IL-1 or IL-1 like activities; including B cell lines and B lymphoblasts (Pistoia *et al.*, 1986; Rimsky *et al.*, 1986; Valentine *et al.*, 1986; Acres *et al.*, 1987; Hawrylowicz *et al.*, 1989). Expression of IL-1 or IL-1 like activities by B cells is especially relevant to their function as antigen-presenting cells (APCs) since IL-1 may be a necessary stimulus for effective activation of T cells.

Among the effects of IL-1 on immune function is the ability to co-stimulate B cell differentiation and proliferation, primarily in the presence of IL-6 (Vink *et al.*, 1988). IL-1 may also act indirectly on B cells through its ability to promote IL-2 and IL-2R transcriptional activity in certain populations of T cells, possibly by induction or enhancement of factors and receptors necessary for T cell activation (Garman *et al.*, 1987; Hagiwara *et al.*, 1987; Lowenthal *et al.*, 1988).

With regard to isotype expression, IL-1 may favour the proliferation of the helper/inducer T cell subpopulation (T_{H_2}), since T cell clones capable of providing antigen-specific B cell help can respond to the autocrine growth factor IL-4 only in the presence of IL-1 (Greenbaum *et al.*, 1988). Favouring the expansion T_{H_2} cells instead of T_{H_1} cells would presumably promote IgG1, IgE and IgA synthesis while minimizing IgG2a synthesis. IL-1 also acts synergistically both in enhancing IgM production in the presence of IL-6 and enhancing IgA production in the presence of IL-5 (Kunimoto *et al.*, 1989).

IL-2

Although IL-2 was originally described as a potent activator of T cells, subsequent studies have demonstrated that it plays a prominent rôle in B cell proliferation and differentiation. Although many of the effects of IL-2 are indirectly manifested through stimulation of other T cell-derived cytokines, the potential exists for direct stimulation of B cells as the presence of IL-2R like molecules have been demonstrated on both B cell lines and normal activated B cells (Malek *et al.*, 1983; Mingari *et al.*, 1984; Osawa and Diamanstein, 1984; Tsudo *et al.*, 1984; Zubler *et al.*, 1984). Additionally, B cells shown to be positive for IL-2R expression not only proliferate in the presence of exogenous IL-2 but also synthesize and secrete antibody (Teranishi *et al.*, 1983; Nakanishi *et al.*, 1984; Jelinek *et al.*, 1986). In accord with its rôle as a B cell differentiation factor, IL-2 induces J-chain transcription and synthesis in the BCL-1 B cell line and thus facilitates assembly of the pentameric form of IgM. The J chain has been shown to be the limiting factor for high rate synthesis of IgM (Blackman *et al.*, 1986; Matsui *et al.*, 1989).

The rôle of IL-2 in isotype expression is currently unresolved although several studies suggest that IL-2 is an essential cofactor for B cell differentiation and directed isotype switching. In studies of anti-Ig treated B cell blasts, it was demonstrated that while IL-4 was solely capable of suppressing IgM expression, other lymphokines, including IL-2, were necessary for secretion of IgG1 (Purkerson *et al.*, 1988). Additionally, in studies of IgE synthesis in humans, optimal expression of IgE in resting B cells occurred in the presence of T cells, IL-4, LMW-BCGF and IL-2 (DeKruyff *et al.*, 1989). However, IL-2 as the lone soluble factor is not sufficient to generate *in vitro* IgE responses under cognate conditions. Activated or low density B cells are capable of producing IgE in the presence of soluble IL-4 and IL-2, in the absence of T cells. Utilizing activated cells, IL-2 is also a potent B cell differentiation factor for IgG synthesis (DeKruyff *et al.*, 1989; Lundgren *et al.*, 1989; Splawski *et al.*, 1989). In addition, IL-2 has been shown to be a necessary cofactor for Ig synthesis by *Staphylococcus aureus* stimulated B cells, with little or no bias in specific isotype expression (Splawski *et al.*, 1989).

In addition to indirect effects of IL-2 addition, a recent study indicates that IL-2 may regulate isotype production, possibly through non-T cells, by production of IFN-γ and IL-4 (Amigorena *et al.*, 1989). Utilizing LPS-stimulated spleen cells derived from nude mice, IL-2 induced IgG2a secretion was blocked by both monoclonal and polyclonal antibodies to IFN-γ. In the case of the monoclonal antibody, blockade resulted in increased IgG1 production. Increased IgG1 production was countered by the addition of an anti-IL-4 monoclonal antibody. These results infer that IL-2 may regulate isotype production through an undefined T cell-independent mechanism involving both IFN-γ and IL-4.

IL-6

As is apparent for other lymphokines, IL-6 has a wide variety of effects on immune responsiveness, although largely in concert with other soluble mediators. Many of the biological activities formerly ascribed to IL-1 have now been shown to be due to IL-6 or at least due to synergy with IL-6. Among its many activities, IL-6 has the ability to promote the growth and differentiation of B cells (Hirano et al., 1986; Van Snick et al., 1986; Shields et al., 1987). IL-6 has been shown to enhance the production of IgM by activated murine splenic B cells, particularly when IL-1 is present (Kunimoto et al., 1989). It also supports both Ig synthesis by human tonsillar B cells stimulated with pokeweed mitogen (PWM) and growth and Ig secretion of a human B-lymphoblastoid cell line (reviewed in Kishimoto and Hirano, 1988). In concert with IL-5, murine IL-6 has been shown to be a potent cofactor in IgA synthesis by T cell-depleted Peyer's patch (PP) B cells (Beagley et al., 1989; Kunimoto et al., 1989).

IL-6 has been proposed to act as a relatively late acting lymphokine whose main function is directing terminal B cell differentiation. Purified IL-6 has been shown to increase Ig secretion without bias to particular isotypes (Muraguchi et al., 1988). However, introduction of a human IL-6 transgene into C57BL/6 mice resulted in high concentrations of human IL-6 accompanied by a 120- to 400-fold increase in polyclonal IgG1 expression in sera of all transgenic mice surveyed (Suematsu et al., 1989). In IL-6 transgenic mice, a large proportion of IgM-expressing plasma cells present in lymph nodes appear to undergo a rapid class switch to IgG1, suggesting that novel mechanisms for substantial IgG1 production may exist.

Recent studies indicate that IL-6 upregulates the synthesis of immunoglobulin mRNAs, preferentially increasing mRNAs encoding the secretory form of immunoglobulin relative to the membrane form (Raynal et al., 1989). This effect appears to be mediated either at the level of post-transcriptional processing and/or by affecting message stability.

IL-6 is also likely to function in a synergistic manner with IL-4 and affect isotype expression. In humans, as in mice, it is clear that IL-4 plays an essential rôle in the regulation of IgE production. In humans, rIL-4 has been shown to induce IgE synthesis by normal peripheral blood mononuclear cells (PBMC) (Del Prete *et al.*, 1988; Jabara *et al.*, 1988; Pene *et al.*, 1988; Sarfati and Delepese, 1988). Interestingly, in a recent study (Vercelli *et al.*, 1989a,b) of IL-4 driven IgE production by PBMC, IgE production was strongly inhibited by an anti-IL-6 monoclonal antibody, indicating a potential rôle for this cytokine in human IgE production. Isotype switching to IgE may be initiated by IL-4, as IL-4 is required for induction of responsiveness to IL-6 by increasing IL-6R expression on B cells. IL-4 has also been shown recently to induce IL-6 secretion by human B cells and it is possible that some IL-4 effects are indirectly mediated (Smeland *et al.*, 1989).

Regulation of IgG1 and IgE synthesis in mice, and potentially IgG4 and IgE synthesis in humans, may be due to a subset of T$_H$ cells that differentially secrete cytokines important for isotype expression. Defined patterns of lymphokine secretion have not been clearly demonstrated among human T cells. However, expression of IgG1 and IgE may be regulated by a specific T cell subset in the mouse, as T$_{H2}$ but not T$_{H1}$ cells have been shown to secrete both IL-6 and IL-4 (Mosmann and Coffman, 1989).

Transforming growth factor-beta (TGF-β)

TGF-β was originally described by its ability to induce abnormal growth patterns of non-malignant fibroblasts (Sporn *et al.*, 1986). TGF-β is produced by a variety of cell types including activated B cells (Kehrl *et al.*, 1986a), T cells (Kehrl *et al.*, 1986b) and macrophages (Assoian, 1987). Additionally, TGF-β has largely a suppressive effect on lymphoid cells and has been shown to inhibit the production of many immunoglobulin isotypes in LPS-stimulated B cell cultures (IgM, IgG1, IgG2a and IgG3) while not affecting others (IgG2b) (Coffman *et al.*, 1989; Sonoda *et al.*, 1989). Consequently TGF-β, like IFN-γ, may play an important rôle in negatively regulating antibody synthesis.

The predominance of IgA in mucosal secretions and various lymphoid tissues has led to a number of investigations of the cytokines present in these tissues as well as those which preferentially enhance IgA production *in vitro*. A number of factors have been shown to enhance IgA secretion including IL-5, IL-4, IL-2 and TGF-β. However, TGF-β, unlike the other factors known to affect IgA production, appears to specifically induce surface IgA$^-$ cells to switch to IgA production (Coffman *et al.*, 1989; Sonoda *et al.*, 1989). Therefore, TGF-β appears to be an IgA switch factor as opposed to a terminal differentiation factor such as IL-5. Importantly, TGF-β increases IgA production approximately 10-fold in LPS-stimulated cultures, whereas other cytokines (IL-5, IL-2 and IL-4) elicit less than 10-fold increases (Coffman *et al.*, 1989). Increased production of IgA by TGF-β is further enhanced by IL-2 and to some extent by IL-5. Whether TGF-β is preferentially expressed in mucosal tissues needs to be explored.

Cytokines and the induction of germline transcripts

Details of the isotype switch process are still uncertain. It has been postulated that antibody class switch recombination can be controlled either by isotype specific recombinases (Davis *et al.*, 1980) or by relaxing chromatin structure of the immunoglobulin switch regions providing accessibility for switch recombinases (Stavnezer-Nordgren and Sirlin, 1986; Lutzker *et al.*, 1988). Support for this latter model was provided by studies of B cell lines in which a preferential switch to certain isotypes occurs upon activation. Switching to these particular isotypes was shown to be preceded by transcription of the unrearranged constant region locus coding for the isotypes, including the 5′ switch region (Stavnezer-Nordgen and Sirlin, 1986; Lutzker and Alt, 1988).

Although much remains to be learned about lymphokines and how they might specifically regulate isotype expression, recent molecular studies of germline transcripts provide some interesting clues (Stavnezer-Nordgren and Sirlin, 1986; Lutzker *et al.*, 1988; Rothman *et al.*, 1988; Esser and Radbruch, 1989). Thus, it has been shown with both B cell lines and splenic B cells that the addition of IL-4 induces germline transcription of both the $C_{\gamma 1}$ and C_{ε} constant region loci (Rothman *et al.*, 1988; Esser and Radbruch, 1989). Moreover, this occurs within hours of the addition of IL-4 (Esser and Radbruch, 1989). It was postulated that IL-4 induces IgE and IgG1 expression by inducing accessibility of the associated switch regions, thus promoting the isotype switch to these constant region loci. Importantly, this phenomenon does not appear to be limited to IL-4 since it has been reported that TGF-β, which appears to induce IgA synthesis, results in the transcription of the unrearranged C_{α} locus prior to the appearance of detectable surface (s) IgA$^+$ cells or secreted IgA (Coffman *et al.*, 1989). Together, these data support the idea that cytokines induce isotype switching not by altering the specificity of the recombination but rather by changing the accessibility of specific C_H loci.

Concluding remarks

Significant progress has been made in defining how antibody classes are produced and regulated. Upon B cell activation, either as a result of mitogen- or antigen-dependent T–B cell interactions, a number of cytokines have been shown to affect the expression of particular isotypes. As discussed above, it appears that in some cases the cytokine is directly inducing the isotype switch. The strongest case can be made for IL-4 and its induction of IgE synthesis (reviewed in Mosmann and Coffman, 1989). Thus, IL-4 is an obligatory cytokine for IgE production, and apparently promotes the isotype switch in surface IgM-bearing B cells previously uncommitted to the production of IgE. Moreover, IL-4 induces germline transcripts of the C_ε constant region gene complex within hours of B cell activation, providing potential molecular mechanisms for promotion of the isotype switch to IgE (see above).

However, there is still much to be learned about the process. It seems clear that there will not be a single, unique lymphokine that controls each of the antibody classes. Even in the more defined analyses of murine IgE regulation, IL-4 promotes the synthesis of both IgE and IgG1 and results in germline transcripts of $C_{\gamma 1}$ and C_ε. Moreover, for synthesis of IgE in the human, there appear to be other obligatory signals apart from IL-4. Another unexplained observation is that IL-4 does not induce all activated B cells to switch to IgE.

A complete understanding of how the other isotypes are regulated requires even further refinement. For example, although production of IFN-γ by T_{H1} cells has clearly been shown to promote IgG2a synthesis, the addition of anti-IFN-γ does not substantially alter the IgG2a response (Stevens *et al.*, 1988). Moreover, the addition of IFN-γ to T_{H2}-stimulated cultures fails to significantly enhance the IgG2a response. If there is an obligatory signal for IgG2a synthesis, it remains to be established. The regulation of IgG1 is also uncertain. Although early reports indicated the importance of IL-4 in specifically inducing IgG1 production in LPS blasts, it is likely that there are IL-4 independent mechanisms for IgG1 induction, since anti-IL-4 causes little or no inhibition of IgG1 *in vitro* or *in vivo* (see above). This is of particular significance because studies suggest that IL-4 promotes IgG1 by inducing the isotype switch in previously uncommitted surface IgM bearing cells rather than acting as a terminal differentiation factor (Layton *et al.*, 1984). The regulatory mechanisms of IgA synthesis also continues to unfold. In this case, IL-5 has been shown to act as a terminal differentiation factor and induce IgA secretion in cells already committed to IgA. In contrast, TGF-β appears to induce the isotype switch to IgA (see above). Thus, the bulk of the evidence points to a multifaceted regulation of individual isotypes that will require detailed studies for full understanding.

In more general terms, it is interesting that many of the cytokines that affect isotype regulation are produced by a variety of cells and influence a number of target cells apart from the B cell. Under these circumstances, it would be somewhat surprising that each of them would convey an isotype-specific signal. It seems more likely that each cytokine or combination of cytokines would induce a particular activation pathway that favours the production of one or more antibody classes.

The purification and characterization of cytokines that affect isotype expression have resulted in significant new advances in determining mechanisms of antibody class regulation. The road is now paved for defining cytokine-induced second messengers and the cellular processes associated with the isotype switch. Significant areas of research will include determining when, during B cell activation, lymphokines act and elucidating the precise mechanisms involved.

References

Abraham, K. and Teale, J. (1987) *J. Immunol.* **138**, 1699–1704.
Abraham, K. and Teale, J. (1987) *J. Immunol.* **139**, 2530–2537.
Acres, R. B., Larsen, A., Gillis, S. and Conlon, P. (1987) *Mol. Immunol.* **24**, 479–485.
Amigorena, S., Teillaud, J. and Fridman, W. (1989) In *Abstracts of the 7th International Congress of Immunology (Berlin)*, p. 23. Gustav Fischer, New York.
Anderson, J., Coutinho, A. and Melchers, F. (1979) *J. Exp. Med.* **147**, 1744–1754.
Arthur, R. and Mason, D. (1986) *J. Exp. Med.* **163**, 1147–1186.
Assoian, R., Fleurdlys, B., Stevenson, H., Miller, P., Madtes, D., Raines, E., Ross, R. and Sporn, M. (1987) *Proc. Natl. Acad. Sci. USA* **84**, 6020–6024.
Bass, H., Mosmann, T. and Stober, S. (1989) *J. Exp. Med.* **170**, 1495–1511.
Beagley, K. W., Eldridge, J. H., Kiyono, H., Everson, M. P., Koopman, W. J., Honjo, T. and McGhee, J. R. (1988) *J. Immunol.* **141**, 2035–2042.
Beagley, K. W., Eldridge, J. H., Lee, F., Kiyono, H., Everson, M. P., Koopman, W., Hirano, T., Kishimoto, T. and McGhee, J. R. (1989a) *J. Exp. Med.* **169**, 2133–2148.
Bergstedt-Lindquist, S., Sideras, P., MacDonald, H. R. and Severinson, E. (1984) *Immunol. Rev.* **78**, 25–50.
Bijsterbosch, M. and Klaus, G. (1985) *J. Exp. Med.* **162**, 1825–1836.
Blackman, M. A., Tigges, M. A., Minie, M. E. and Koshland, M. E. (1986) *Cell* **47**, 609–617.
Bond, M., Sharder, B., Mosmann, T. and Coffman, R. (1987) *J. Immunol.* **139**, 3685–3691.
Boom, W. H., Liano, D. and Abbas, A. I. (1988) *J. Exp. Med.* **167**, 1352–1363.
Bottomly, K. (1988) *Immunol. Today* **9**, 268–274.
Budd, R., Cerottini, S. and MacDonald, H. (1987) *J. Immunol.* **138**, 3583–3587.
Callard, R. and Smith, S. (1988) *Eur. J. Immunol.* **18**, 1635–1638.
Callard, R. E. and Turner, M. W. (1990) *Immunol. Today* **11**, 200–203.
Chapman, C., Knopf, P., Hicks, J. and Mitchell, G. (1979) *Aust. J. Exp. Med. Sci.* **57**, 369–387.

Cherwinski, H. C., Schumacher, J. H., Brown, K. D. and Mosmann, T. R. (1987) *J. Exp. Med.* **166**, 1229–1244.

Clutterbuck, E., Shields, J., Gordon, J., Smith, S., Boyd, A., Callard, R., Campbell, H., Young, I. and Sanderson, C. (1987) *Eur. J. Immunol.* **17**, 1743–1750.

Coffman, R. L. and Carty, J. (1986) *J. Immunol.* **136**, 949–954.

Coffman, R., Ohara, J., Bond, M., Carty, J., Zlotnik, A. and Paul, W. (1986a) *J. Immunol.* **136**, 4538–4541.

Coffman, R., Shrader, B., Carty, J., Mosman, T. and Bond, M. (1987) *J. Immunol.* **139**, 3685–3690.

Coffman, R., Seymour, B., Lebman, D., Hiraki, D., Christiansen, J., Shrader, B., Cherwinski, H., Savelkoul, H., Finkelman, F., Bond, M. and Mosmann, T. (1988) *Immunol. Rev.* **102**, 5–28.

Coffman, R., Lebman, D. and Shrader, B. (1989) *J. Exp. Med.* **170**, 1039–1044.

Conrad, D., Waldschmidt, T., Lee, W., Rao, M., Keegan, A., Noelle, R., Lynch, R. and Kehry, M. (1987) *J. Immunol.* **139**, 2290–2296.

Coutelier, J., van der Logt, J., Heesen, F., Warnier, G. and Van Snick, J. (1987) *J. Exp. Med.* **165**, 164–167.

Davis, M., Kim, S. and Hood, L. (1980) *Science* **209**, 1360–1365.

DeFrance, T., Aubry, J. P., Rousset, F., Vandervliet, B., Bonnefoy, Y.-V., Arai, N., Takebe, Y., Yokota, T., Lee, F., Arai, K., deVries, J. and Banchereau, J. (1987) *J. Exp. Med.* **165**, 1459–1467.

Del Prete, G., Maggi, E., Parronchi, P., Chr'etien, I., Tiri, A., Macchia, D., Ricci, M., Banchereau, J., DeVries, J. and Romagnini, J. (1988) *J. Immunol.* **140**, 4193–4198.

Duran, L. and Metcalf, E. (1987) *J. Exp. Med.* **165**, 340–358.

DeKruyff, R. H., Turner, T., Abrams, J. S., Palladino, M. A. and Umetsu, D. T. (1989) *J. Exp. Med.* **170**, 1477–1493.

Esser, C. and Rabruch, A. (1989) *EMBO J.* **8**, 483–488.

Finkelman, F., Snapper, C., Mountz, J. and Katona, I. (1987) *J. Immunol.* **138**, 2826–2830.

Finkelman, F., Katona, I., Urban, J., Holmes, J., Ohara, J., Tung, A., Sample, J. and Paul, W. (1988a) *J. Immunol.* **141**, 2335–2341.

Finkelman, F., Katona, I., Mosmann, T. and Coffman, R. (1988b) *J. Immunol.* **140**, 1022–1027.

Gajewski, T., Joyce, J. and Fitch, F. (1989) *J. Immunol.* **143**, 15–22.

Garman, R., Jacobs, K., Clark, S. and Raulet, D. (1987) *Proc. Natl. Acad. Sci. USA* **84**, 7629–7633.

Gery, I. and Waksman, B. (1972) *J. Exp. Med.* **136**, 143–148.

Giedlin, M. A., Longenecker, B. M. and Mosmann, T. R. (1986) *Cell. Immunol.* **97**, 357–370.

Greenbaum, L. A., Horowitz, J. B., Woods, A., Pasqualine, T., Reich, E. and Bottomly, K. (1988) *J. Immunol.* **140**, 1555–1560.

Hagiwara, H., Huang, H., Arai, N., Herzenberg, L., Arai, K. and Zlotnik, A. (1987) *J. Immunol.* **138**, 2514–2519.

Hammarstrom, L. and Smith, C. I. E. (1987) *Allergy* **42**, 529–534.

Harada, N., Kikuchi, Y., Tominaga, A., Takaki, S. and Takatsu, K. (1985) *J. Immunol.* **134**, 3944–3951.

Harriman, G., Kunimoto, D., Elliot, J., Paetkau, V. and Strober, W. (1988) *J. Immunol.* **140**, 3033–3039.

Hawrylowicz, C., Duncan, L., Fuhlbrigge, R. and Unanue, E. (1989) *J. Immunol.* **142**, 3361–3368.

Heinzel, F., Sadick, M., Holaday, B., Coffman, R. and Lockslay R. (1989) *J. Exp. Med.* **169**, 59–72.

Herlyn, D. and Koprowski, H. (1982) *Proc. Natl. Acad. Sci. USA* **79**, 4761–4765.

Hirano, T., Yasukawa, K., Harada, H., Taga, T., Watanabe, Y., Matsuda, T., Kashiwamura, S., Nakajima, K., Koyama, K., Iwamatsu, A., Tsunasawa, S., Sakiyama, F., Matsui, H., Takahara, T., Taniguichi, T. and Kishimoto, T. (1986) *Nature* **324**, 73–75.

Howard, M., Farrar, J., Hilfiker, M., Johnson, B., Takatsu, K., Hamaoka, T. and Paul, W. (1982) *J. Exp. Med.* **155**, 214–219.

Hudak, S., Gollnick, S., Conrad, D. and Kehry, M. (1987) *Proc. Natl. Acad. Sci. USA* **84**, 4606–4610.

Isakson, P., Pure, E., Vitetta, E. and Krammer, P. (1982) *J. Exp. Med.* **155**, 734–748.

Jabara, H., Ackerman, S., Vercelli, D., Yokota, T., Arai, K., Abrams, J., Dvorak, A., Lavigne, M., Banchereau, J., DeVries, J., Leung, D. and Geha, R. (1988) *J. Clin. Immunol.* **8**, 437–446.

Jelinek, D. F., Splawski, J. B. and Lipsky, P. E. (1986) *Eur. J. Immunol.* **16**, 925–932.

Johnson, W., Stephlewski, Z., Koprowski, H. and Adams, D. (1985) In *Mechanisms of Cell-Mediated Cytotoxicity II.* Ed. by Henkart, P. and Martz, E. Plenum, New York, pp. 75–123.

Kehrl, J., Roberts, A., Wakefield, L., Jakolew, S., Sporn, M. and Fauci, A. (1986a) *J. Immunol.* **137**, 3855–3860.

Kehrl, J., Wakefield, L., Roberts, A., Jakolew, S., Alvarerz-Mon, M., Derynck, R., Sporn, M. and Fauci, A. (1986b) *J. Exp. Med.* **163**, 1037–1050.

Killar, L., MacDonald, G., West, J., Woods, A. and Bottomly, K. (1987) *J. Immunol.* **138**, 1674–1679.

Kim, J., Woods, A., Becker-Dorn, E. and Bottomly, K. (1985) *J. Exp. Med.* **162**, 188–193.

Kinashi, T., Harada, N., Severinson, E., Tanabe, T., Sideras, P., Konishi, M., Azuma, C., Tominaga, A., Bergstedt-Lindqvist, S., Takahashi, M., Matsuda, F., Yaoita, Y., Takatsu, K. and Honjo, T. (1986) *Nature* **324**, 70–73.

Kishimoto, T., Hirano, T., Kikutani, H. and Muraguchi, A. (1987) *Adv. Exp. Med. Biol.* **213**, 177–188.

Kishimoto, T. and Hirano, T. (1988) *Ann. Rev. Immunol.* **6**, 485–512.

Krusemeier, M. A. and Snow, E. C. (1988) *J. Immunol.* **140**, 367–375.

Kunimoto, D. Y., Nordan, R. and Strober, W. (1989) *J. Immunol.* **143**, 2230–2235.

Lanzavecchia, A. and Parodi, B. (1984) *Clin. Exp. Immunol.* **55**, 197–203.

Layton, J., Vitetta, E. S., Uhr, J. W. and Krammer, P. H. (1984) *J. Exp. Med.* **160**, 1850.

Lebman, D. and Coffman, R. (1988a) *J. Immunol.* **141**, 2050–2056.

Lebman, D. A. and Coffman, R. L. (1988b) *J. Exp. Med.* **168**, 853–862.

Lee, F., Yokota, T., Otsuku, T., Meyerson, T., Villaret, D., Coffman, R., Mosmann, T., Renrick, D., Roehm, N., Smith, C., Zlotnik, A. and Arai, K. (1986) *Proc. Natl. Acad. Sci. USA* **83**, 2061–2065.

Lowenthal, J., Cerottini, J. and MacDonald, H. (1988) *J. Immunol.* **137**, 1226–1231.

Lundgren, M., Persson, U., Larsson, P., Magnusson, C., Edvard Smith, C. I., Hammarstrom, L. and Severinson, E. (1989) *Eur. J. Immunol.* **19**, 1311–1315.

Lutzker, S. and Alt, F. W. (1988) *Mol. Cell Biol.* **8**, 1849–1852.

Lutzker, S., Rothman, P., Pollock, R., Coffman, R. and Alt, F. (1988) *Cell* **53**, 177–184.

Maggi, E., Del Prete, G., Macchia, D., Parronchi, P., Tiri, A., Chretien, I., Ricci, M. and Romagnani, S. (1988) *Eur. J. Immunol.* **18**, 1045–1050.

Malek, T. R., Robb, R. J. and Shevach, J. M. (1983) *Proc. Natl. Acad. Sci. USA* **80**, 5694–5698.

Matsui, K., Nakanishi, K., Cohen, D., Hada, T., Furuyama, J., Hamaoka, T. and Higashino, K. (1989) *J. Immunol.* **142**, 2918–2923.

Matsumoto, R., Matsumoto, M., Mita, S., Hitoshi, Y., Ando, M., Araki, S., Yamaguchi, N., Tominaga, A. and Takatsu, K. (1989) *Immunology* **66**, 32–37.

Matthews, T. J., Collins, J. J., Roloson, G. J., Thiel, H. J. and Bolognesi, D. P. (1981) *J. Immunol.* **126**, 2332–2336.

Mingari, M. C., Gerosa, F., Carra, G., Acolla, R. S., Moretta, A., Zubler, T. H., Waldman, T. A. and Moretta, L. (1984) *Nature* **312**, 641–643.

Moller, G. (1988) *Immunol. Rev.* **102**, 1–239.

Mosmann, T. and Coffman, R. (1989) *Ann. Rev. Immunol.* **7**, 145–173.

Mosmann, T. R., Cherwinski, H., Bond, M. W., Giedlin, M. A. and Coffman, R. L. (1986) *J. Immunol.* **136**, 2348–2357.

Mountz, J., Smith, J., Snapper, C., Mushiaski, J. and Finkelman, T. (1987) *J. Immunol.* **139**, 2172–2178.

Muraguchi, A., Hirano, T., Tang, B., Matsuda, T., Horii, Y., Nakajima, K. and Kishimoto, T. (1988) *J. Exp. Med.* **167**, 332–344.

Murray, P., McKenzie, D., Swain, S. and Kagnoff, M. (1987) *J. Immunol.* **139**, 2669–2674.

Nakanishi, K., Malek, T., Smith, K., Hamaoka, T., Shevach, E. and Paul, W. E. (1984) *J. Exp. Med.* **160**, 1605–1621.

Noelle, R., Krammer, P., Ohara, J., Uhr, J. and Vitetta, E. (1984) *Proc. Natl. Acad. Sci. USA* **81**, 6149–6153.

Noelle, R., McCann, J., Marshall, L. and Bartlett, W. (1989) *J. Immunol.* **143**, 1807–1814.

Noma, Y., Sideras, P., Naito, T. *et al.* (1986) *Nature* **319**, 640–646.

Ohara, J. and Paul, W. (1987) *Nature* **325**, 537–540.

Osawa, H. and Diamanstein, T. (1984) *J. Immunol.* **132**, 2445–2450.

Pace, J., Russell, S., Torres, B., Johnson, H. and Gray, P. (1983) *J. Immunol.* **130**, 2011–2013.

Paliard, X., de Waal Malefijt, R., Yssel, H., Blanchard, D., Chretien, I., Abrams, J., deVries, J. and Spits, H. (1988) *J. Immunol.* **141**, 849–855.

Pene, J., Rousset, F., Briere, F., Chretien, I., Bonnefoy, J., DeVries, J. (1988) *Proc. Natl. Acad. Sci. USA* **85**, 6880–6884.

Pistoia, V., Cozzolino, F., Rubartelli, A., Torcia, M., Roncella, S. and Ferrarini, M. (1986) *J. Immunol.* **136**, 1688–1692.

Philips, N. and Parker, D. (1984) *J. Immunol.* **132**, 627–632.

Powers, G. D., Abbas, A. K. and Miller, R. A. (1988) *J. Immunol.* **140**, 3352–3357.

Purkerson, J., Newberg, M., Wise, G., Lynch, K. and Isakson, P. (1988) *J. Exp. Med.* **168**, 1175–1180.

Raynal, M., Liu, Z., Hirano, T., Mayer, L., Kishimoto, T.. and Chen-Kiang, S. (1989) *Proc. Natl. Acad. Sci. USA* **86**, 8024–8028.

Rimsky, L., Wakasugi, H., Ferrara, P., Robin, P., Capdeveille, J., Tursz, T., Fradelizi, D. and Bertoglio, J. (1986) *J. Immunol.* **136**, 3304–3310.

Roehm, N., Liebson, J., Zlotnik, A., Kappler, J., Marack, P. and Cambier, J. (1984) *J. Exp. Med.* **160**, 679–694.

Rothman, P., Lutzger, S., Cook, W., Coffman, R. and Alt, F. (1988) *J. Exp. Med.* **168**, 2385–2389.

Rudd, C., Morimoto, C., Wong, L. and Schlossman, S. (1987) *J. Exp. Med.* **161**, 1758–1764.

Sanderson, C., Campbell, H. and Young, I. (1988) *Immunol. Rev.* **102**, 29–50.

Sarfati, M. and Delepese, G. (1988) *J. Immunol.* **141**, 2195–2199.

Savelkoul, H. F. J., Lebman, D., Benner, R. and Coffman, R. L. (1988) *J. Immunol.* **141**, 749–755.

Schimpl, A. and Wecker, B. (1975) *Transpl. Rev.* **23**, 176–188.

Schoenbeck, S., McKenzie, D. and Kagnoff, M. (1989) *Eur. J. Immunol.* **19**, 965–969.

Scott, P., Natovitz, P., Coffman, R. L., Pearce, E. and Sher, A. (1988) *J. Exp. Med.* **168**, 1675–1684.

Shields, J., Smith, S., Levinsky, R., DeFrance, T., DeVries, J., Banchereau, J. and Callard, R. (1987) *Eur. J. Immunol.* **17**, 535–540.

Shields, J. G., Armitage, R. J., Jamieson, B. N., Beverley, P. C. L. and Callard, R. E. (1989) *Immunology* **66**, 224–227.

Sidman, C. and Unanue, E. (1986) *J. Exp. Med.* **144**, 882–896.

Smeland, E. B., Blomhoff, H. K., Funderad, S., Shalaby, M. R. and Espevik, T. (1989) *J. Exp. Med.* **170**, 1463–1468.

Snapper, C. and Paul, W. (1987) *J. Immunol.* **139**, 10–17.

Snapper, C., Peschel, C. and Paul, W. (1988a) *J. Immunol.* **140**, 2121–2127.

Snapper, C. M., Finkelman, F. D. and Paul, W. E. (1988b) *J. Exp. Med.* **167**, 183.

Snapper, C., Hornbeck, P., Atasoy, U., Pereira, M. and Paul, W. (1988c) *Proc. Natl. Acad. Sci. USA* **85**, 6107–6111.

Snapper, C., Hooley, J., Atasoy, U., Finkelman, F. and Paul, W. E. (1989) *J. Immunol.* **143**, 2133–2141.

Solid, L., Kvale, D., Brandtzaeg, P., Markussen, G. and Thorsby, E. (1987) *J. Immunol.* **138**, 4303–4306.

Sonoda, E., Matsumoto, R., Hitoshi, Y., Ishii, T., Sugimoto, M., Araki, S., Tominaga, A., Yamaguchi, N. and Takatsu, K. (1989) *J. Exp. Med.* **170**, 1415–1420.

Splawski, J. B., Jelinek, D. F. and Lipsky, P. E. (1989) *J. Immunol.* **142**, 1569–1575.

Sporn, M., Roberts, A., Wakefield, L. and Associan, R. (1986) *Science* **233**, 532–534.

Stavnezer-Nordgren, J. and Sirlin, S. (1986) *EMBO J.* **5**, 95–102.

Stevens, T., Bossie, A., Sanders, V., Fernandez-Botran, R., Coffman, R., Mosmann, T. and Vitetta, E. (1988) *Nature* **334**, 255–258.

Suematsu, S., Matsuda, T., Aozasa, K., Akira, S., Nakano, N., Ohno, S., Miyazaki, J., Yamamura, K., Hirano, T. and Kishimoto, T. (1989) *Proc. Natl. Acad. Sci. USA* **86**, 7547–7551.

Swain, S. and Dutton, R. (1982) *J. Exp. Med.* **156**, 1821–1834.

Swain, S. L., McKenzie, D. T., Dutton, R. W., Tonkonogy, S. L. and English, M. (1988) *Immunol. Rev.* **102**, 77–105.

Swain, S. L., McKenzie, D. T., Weinberg, A. D. and Hancock, W. (1988b) *J. Immunol.* **141**, 3445–3455.

Takatsu, K., Tanaka, A., Tomingaga, A., Kumahara, Y. and Hamaoka, T. (1980) *J. Immunol.* **125**, 2646–2653.

Takatsu, K., Tominaga, A., Harada, N., Mita, S., Matsumoto, M., Takahashi, T., Kikuchi, Y. and Yamaguchi, N. (1988) *Immunol. Rev.* **102**, 107–135.

Taylor, R. B. and Wortis, H. H. (1968) *Nature* **220**, 927–929.

Teale, J. (1983) *J. Immunol.* **131**, 2170–2175.

Teale, J. and Abraham, K. (1987) *Immunol. Today* **8**, 122–126.

Teranishi, T., Hirano, T., Lin, B. and Onoue, K. (1983). *J. Immunol.* **133**, 3062–3074.

Thyphronitis, G., Tsokos, G. C., June, C. H., Levine, A. D. and Finkelman, F. D. (1989) *Proc. Natl. Acad. Sci. USA* **86**, 5580–5584.

Tonkonogy, S., McKenzie, D. and Swain, S. (1989) *J. Immunol.* **142**, 4351–4360.

Tony, H. and Parker, D. (1985) *J. Exp. Med.* **161**, 223–229.

Torrigiani, G. (1972) *J. Immunol.* **108**, 161–164.

Tsudo, M., Uchiyama, T. and Uchino, H. (1984) *J. Exp. Med.* **160**, 612–617.

Umetsu, D., Leung, D., Siraganian, R., Jabara, H. and Geha, R. (1985) *J. Exp. Med.* **162**, 202–214.

Unkeless, J., Scigliano, E. and Freedman, V. (1988) *Ann. Rev. Immunol.* **6**, 251–282.

Valentine, M., Lotz, M., Dinarello, A., Carson, D. and Vaughan, J. (1986) *Lymphokine Res.* **5**, 173–178.

Van Snick, J. A., Cayphas, S., Vink, A., Uyttenhove, C., Coulie, P. G., Ruira, M. R. and Simpson, R. J. (1986) *Proc. Natl. Acad. Sci. USA* **83**, 9679–9683.

Vercelli, D., Jabara, H., Arai, K. and Geha, R. (1989a) *J. Exp. Med.* **169**, 1295–1307.

Vercelli, D., Jabara, H. H., Arai, K., Yokota, T. and Geha, R. S. (1989b) *Eur. J. Immunol.* **19**, 1419–1424.

Vink, A., Coulie, P., Wauters, P., Nordan, R. and Van-Snick, J. (1988) *Eur. J. Immunol.* **18**, 607–612.

Vitetta, E., Ohara, J., Myers, S., Layton, C., Krammer, P. and Paul, W. (1985) *J. Exp. Biol.* **162**, 1726–1735.

Winter, J., Duncan, J., Santisteban, C., Douglas, J. and Adams, L. (1989) *Infect. Immun.* **57**, 3438–3444.

Yokota, T., Coffman, R., Hagiwara, R., Rennick, D., Takebe, T., Yokota, K., Gemmel, L., Shrader, B., Yang, G., Meyerson, P., Luh, J., Hoy, P., Pene, J., Briere, F., Spits, H., Bauchereau, J., deVries, J., Lee, F., Arai, N. and Arai, K. (1987) *Proc. Natl. Acad. Sci. USA* **84**, 7388–7392.

Yuan, D. and Vitetta, E. (1983) *Mol. Immunol.* **20**, 367–375.

Zubler, R. H., Lowenthal, J. W., Erard, F., Hashimoto, N., Devos, R. and MacDonald, H. R. (1984) *J. Exp. Med.* **160**, 1170–1183.

8
Autocrine aspects of the B lymphocyte response

JOHN GORDON

Introduction

The previous chapters have highlighted and focused upon those external influences which direct and modify the passage of the antigen-primed B lymphocyte to undergo regulated waves of clonal expansion and to fulfill its ultimate destiny by generating large numbers of antibody-secreting plasma cells. With such scenarios, the B lymphocyte is often viewed as a passive carrier with no direct input into how it (or indeed other cells) will be instructed to handle the complex series of events that eventually serve to eliminate antigen from the system.

Several observations, gathered over the last few years, have begun to challenge the notion of B cells being simple passengers in an active immune response. First, there is the notion that B cells can serve as highly efficient antigen-presenting cells (APC) once they have been activated by routes that involve more conventional APC and specific T helper cells. Both the level and the specificity of antigen-binding to specific immunoglobulin (Ig) on appropriately stimulated B cells have led some to argue that, *in vivo*, the B cell may be among the most important APC available to the immune response (reviewed in Weaver and Unanue, 1990). A second contribution to the postulate of the B lymphocyte as an immunoregulatory cell is the realization that secreted Ig, the end-products of a B cell response, are themselves important modulators at several stages in the development of antigen-specific immunity (for example, see Sinclair and Panoskaltsis, 1989); regulation via secretory Ig occurs through its interaction with a diverse range of Fc-receptors that are distributed on a wide variety of immune cells. Finally, following the initial observation in 1984 that B cells can produce an autocrine B cell growth factor (BCGF; Gordon *et al.*, 1984b), it is becoming clear that B cell products, acting either as membrane

CYTOKINES AND B LYMPHOCYTES
ISBN 0–12–155145–8

constituents in intimate cell-to-cell contacts or as released cytokines, have an important rôle to play, not only in autogenous reactions but also in directing the behaviour of non-B cells to generate a more efficacious immune response to an appropriate antigen.

The purpose of this chapter is to develop the thesis of the B lymphocyte as a regulatory cell in the immune response, with an emphasis on B cell-derived soluble factors; this focus does not preclude a discussion of those other features discussed above, which will be highlighted, as appropriate, within the framework described. A model that exemplifies these considerations is that of B cell transformation by the Epstein–Barr virus (EBV).

Epstein–Barr virus activation of B lymphocytes

The special relationship existing between EBV and the B lymphocyte was recently reviewed in some detail (Gordon, 1989b); the following constitutes a brief discussion of the more salient points. It is now clear that EBV gains entry into the B lymphocyte through its ability to bind to CD21 (Fingeroth *et al.*, 1984), which normally serves as the receptor for the C3d fragment of complement (CR2). Internalization of the virus is known to occur rapidly, and recent evidence indicates that this process may be mediated by an influx of extracellular Ca^{2+} following receptor activation (B. Dugas, personal communication). By using either inactivated EBV or certain monoclonal antibodies within the CD21 cluster that map the EBV binding domain, it has been shown that this initial event is sufficient to prime human B cells to reach an "excited" state but not to enter the growth cycle proper (Nemerow *et al.*, 1985; Gordon *et al.*, 1986a). Factors that are supplied by T cells are required for this to occur.

Receptors for EBV (CD21) are relatively widespread on B cells and all seem to be capable of internalization (Aman *et al.*, 1984). By contrast, the resulting transformation of a cell following viral entry is more restricted. Among both peripheral blood and tonsillar B lymphocytes, it is the small, dense, resting B cells that are most efficiently transformed (Aman *et al.*, 1984). Nevertheless, even within this population, not all the infected cells are able to establish growth. A recent study has indicated that once it has gained entry, the internalized EBV must undergo a process of circulariz-ation in order for effective transformation to proceed (Hurley and Thorley-Lawson, 1988). It is known that the circularization process generates, *de novo*, a fused gene which has an open reading frame that codes for the so-called "terminal protein" (Laux *et al.*, 1988). Interestingly, cells in which the

EBV does undergo successful circularization express the cellular gene product, CD23 (Hurley and Thorley-Lawson, 1988). The same workers had already shown earlier that the expression of CD23 following early EBV infection was a permissive marker for cellular transformation to proceed (Thorley-Lawson and Mann, 1985). What is not clear at present is whether the circularization *per se* is the central event, and only when this occurs is CD23 expressed, or whether it is the expression of CD23 that is the key, and the capacity for circularization is restricted to those B cells which have that particular capability.

It is important to note that not all strains of EBV are capable of immortalizing human B cells. Those that cannot, such as the P3HR-1 strain, contain a major deletion within the Epstein-Barr nuclear antigen 2 (EBNA2) coding region that precludes its expression (Dambaugh *et al.*, 1986; Knutson and Sugden, 1989). Nevertheless, such defective viruses are capable of activating resting B cells to the early G_1 phase of the cell cycle, a point beyond that which is reached by fully inactive EBV (Gordon *et al.*, 1986c; Ho *et al.*, 1986). This observation implies that the expression of non-EBNA2 genes can themselves serve a function in the activation process of the infected B cell. The *EBNA2* gene product is, however, clearly necessary in order to provide the full stimulus for B cells to proceed into and through the S phase of cell cycle; eventually, many infected cells establish immortalized lines that continually harbour and replicate the virus.

It is of interest to note that tumour-promoting esters that are direct activators of protein kinase C (PKC), such as phorbol myristic acetate (PMA), can partially replace EBNA2 in this process in that they will allow P3HR-1 infected B lymphocytes arrested in G_1 to proceed fully into DNA synthesis (Gordon *et al.*, 1986a). Furthermore, a recent study demonstrated that intact EBV delivers its mitogenic signal to B cells by directly activating Ca^{2+}-dependent PKC and generating a Ca^{2+} (and phospholipid) independent proteolytically cleaved fragment, protein kinase M (PKM) (Guy and Gordon, 1989). This is quite different from what is observed on the physiological signalling of B cells through antigen receptors, but it is strikingly similar to the way in which PMA is known to activate B cells (Guy and Gordon, 1989). An important difference that has been noted between PMA and EBV, however, is that whereas the PKM activity in B cells treated with the former eventually declines, that of cells infected with the latter appears to increase steadily. It has recently been suggested that EBV may transform B cells by by-passing the normally receptor-regulated inositol lipid hydrolytic pathway and constitutively activating PKC and elevating Ca^{2+} levels through the expression of EBNA2 and the membrane-spanning latent membrane protein, respectively (Lindholm *et al.*, unpublished).

EBV transformation of B cells and autostimulatory BCGF

It has long been apparent to all those working in the field that EBV-transformed B cells, while growing efficiently in bulk cultures, are notoriously difficult to clone. This empirical observation always strongly suggested that these cells required and produced a "companion" factor to maintain their growth at high cell number. To the best of our knowledge, the first demonstration that EBV-transformed B cells were capable of producing an activity that was stimulatory for lymphocytes was from a study by Vesole *et al.* (1979). In this study, it was shown that a panel of lymphoid lines, which could be either B or T cell derived, released soluble factors that would either enhance or inhibit mitogen-driven stimulations of normal peripheral blood lymphocytes. The stimulatory activity had a molecular weight in the region of 30 kD and could be separated from the inhibitory factor which was of larger size. More detailed investigations followed in 1980 on the stimulatory activities that were present in supernatant that had been conditioned by the EBV-carrying lymphoblastoid line RPMI 8866 (Sanderson *et al.*, 1980). The RPMI 8866 line had apparently been found to be a particularly high producer of the stimulating activity which could cross the species barrier into mice and was effective on both T and B lymphocytes.

A landmark report then appeared in 1983, with Blazar and colleagues demonstrating that the stimulatory activity present in medium conditioned by human B cell lines could be autocrine in nature (Blazar *et al.*, 1983). This was demonstrated by taking medium that had been conditioned by cells growing optimally at a relatively high cell density and supplying it to the same cells cultured at lower cell numbers; it was noted that there was a significant enhancement of their growth kinetics, most notably a reduction of the familiar lag phase that is usually observed. In other experiments performed in parallel, serum-free conditions of culture were used to investigate the requirements for autocrine growth (Gordon *et al.*, 1984a). It was found that in a selenium-rich medium (such as Iscove's modified MEM), optimal growth at high cell numbers could be obtained by supplementing cultures with bovine serum albumin (BSA) and human transferrin (30% Fe^{3+}-saturation). In short-term assays, the BSA could be omitted. On plating cells at low numbers, EBV-transformed cells were seen to stop growing whether or not BSA and transferrin were present. Their growth could be restored, however, on the addition of serum-free medium that had been conditioned from bulk cultures of autogenous cells. Cell-cycle analysis indicated that, in the absence of autostimulatory activity, cells were arrested in the G_1 phase of cycle, while in the absence of transferrin, the arrest occurred at the G_1/S transition stage. The results clearly demonstrated that although the B cells that had been transformed by EBV had escaped many of the usual environmental constraints on their growth, they were still strictly dependent upon the utilization of a soluble factor that could be supplied autogenously (Gordon *et al.*, 1984a). Separation of the activity responsible for autostimulatory growth using S-200 sizing chromatography revealed that the bulk of activity resided in the 25–35 kD range (Gordon *et al.*, 1984b). Importantly, the autostimulatory activity was coincident with activity that was positive in co-stimulation assays for normal tonsil B cells. Thus, by the criteria then operating, the autocrine factor was a "BCGF" and thus represented the first partially characterized B-cell-derived BCGF (B-BCGF).

Do normal B cells produce BCGF activity?

Following the observations on immortalized B lymphoblasts, it was tempting to speculate that the production of BCGF by transformed B cells was an ectopic event; this could account, at least in part, for the association of EBV with malignancy. It soon became apparent that such a simple notion would not hold. Thus, it was shown that normal B cells, when appropriately activated, also produced a BCGF-like activity (Jurgensen *et al.*, 1986; Muraguchi *et al.*, 1986). In addition, studies of large numbers of B lymphoma lines, many of which lacked the EBV genome, revealed that production of a "BCGF" was a common event among continually growing B cells and could not, therefore, be attributed to any specific attribute of the EB-virus (Gordon *et al.*, 1985a).

In the study by Jurgensen and colleagues describing the production of BCGF by normal B cells, the B cells were first stimulated with fixed particles of *Staphylococcus Aureus* Cowan Strain I (SAC) to provoke entry of the cells into active cycle. The BCGF subsequently released was purified to apparent homogeneity and shown to have a molecular weight of 30 kD and an isoelectric point (pI) of 8.0 (Jurgensen *et al.*, 1986). These properties make this B-BCGF distinct from any of the T cell-derived cytokines that have been described to act on B cells. In other studies, it was found that resting B cells responding to SAC utilize a soluble BCGF-activity to support their own growth. That study also showed that the soluble activity alone was not sufficient, but that an activity which could only be supplied by cell-to-cell contact was also required for optimal B cell growth to proceed (Gordon *et al.*, 1985d).

Interleukin-1 and B cell autostimulation

Activated B cells, particularly as exemplified by EBV-transformed cells, are extremely efficient at processing and presenting antigen to T lymphocytes (Wakasugi *et al.*, 1985). Associated with this function is the ability of the stimulating B cells to synthesize IL-1. Scala *et al.* reported in 1984 that an EBV-transformed cell line not only produced IL-1 but also utilized this product in an autostimulatory mode (Scala *et al.*, 1984). The IL-1 described had a molecular weight of 17 kD and a pI of 7, properties similar to those of monocyte-derived IL-1α. Other studies have now shown that EBV-transformed B-cell lines can produce either IL-1α or the more acidic IL-1β form (Acres *et al.*, 1987). However, it has not been determined whether these products are always autostimulatory. Responses of B cells to IL-1 are discussed in chapters 4 and 5. In a wider survey of cell lines, Matsushimi *et al.* (1985a) found that 8/8 EBV-transformed B-lymphoblastoid cell lines produced IL-1 activity while only 3/4 EBV-positive B lymphoma lines, 3/7 EBV-negative B lymphoma lines and 0/3 myeloma lines were positive for this phenotype. IL-1 from one of the EBV-transformed B cell lines was found to have a pI of 5.5 and an unusual molecular weight of 25 kD. Both those properties are, however, shared by the major soluble fragment of CD23 which has been shown to be functional as an IL-1-like activity (Swendeman and Thorley-Lawson, 1986). Normal B cells have also been reported to produce IL-1, in response to lipopolysaccharide (Matsushimi *et al.*, 1985b). Subsequent investigations have confirmed the notion that IL-1 can contribute to the autocrine profile of virally-transformed B cells (Gordon *et al.*, 1986d).

Wakasugi and colleagues (1987) described a subclone of an EBV-transformed line (3B6) that secreted an autocrine IL-1-like molecule, apparently with novel physical properties, having a molecular weight of 13.5 kD and a pI of 5 (Rimsky *et al.*, 1986). Analysis of the first 27 NH$_2$-terminal amino acids revealed no similarity with either IL-1α or IL-1β, suggesting that a unique B cell-associated IL-1 was involved. A cDNA from the 3B6 line, coding for the novel protein, was cloned and subsequently identified as a gene encoding a thioredoxin. When this gene was expressed, the product had no demonstrable IL-1 activity. It now seems that the initial activity in the cell supernatants was due to contaminating IL-1α that co-purified with the thioredoxin. Indeed, it has now been shown that the subclone did indeed express RNA for IL-1α (Bertoglio *et al.*, 1988). Interestingly, however, thioredoxin itself is now being claimed to serve as an efficient "BCGF" of 12 kD size, particularly when used together with other cytokines (K. Nilsson and A. Rosen, personal communication).

CD23 and B cell autostimulation

The 45 kD glycoprotein now defined by its reactivity with the CD23 panel of monoclonal antibodies was first described by Kintner and Sugden (1981) as the EBVCS ("CS" for cell surface) antigen. This designator reflected an apparently restricted expression of the antigen on B cells that had been transformed by EBV. We now know that appropriately activated normal B cells can also express the CD23 antigen (Walker *et al.*, 1986). However, high-level constitutive expression of CD23 remains a hallmark of the EBV-transformed B lymphoblast (Thorley-Lawson *et al.*, 1985). As discussed earlier, on infection of B cells by EBV, only those subsequently expressing CD23 proceed to transform. This phenotypic shift appears, in turn, to relate to the ability of the EBV DNA to circularize. Nevertheless, the direct introduction of the *EBNA2a* gene into some EBV-negative Burkitt's lymphoma lines leads to a super-induction of the CD23 antigen (Wang *et al.*, 1987). There is evidence indicating that this occurs through *trans*-activation of the CD23 gene.

Further observations suggest CD23 expression and the transforming activity of EBV are linked, with a major rôle for EBNA2 being implied. First, it has been found that sporadic, EBV-negative Burkitt's lymphomas produce none or very low levels only of the CD23 antigen (personal observation). While the rate of production does not alter on conversion of these lines with the EBNA2-defective P3HR-1 strain of virus, it increases dramatically on converting them with intact B95-8 virus. Second, studies by Rowe and Gregory (1989) show that while established lines from EBV-positive Burkitt's lymphoma display a surface marker profile similar to that of memory B cells, subsequent long-term culture leads to a progression, or "drift", toward a phenotype resembling that of activated B-lymphoblastoid cells. This is exemplified by the appearance of surface CD23. The change in cellular antigens correlates closely with the expression of both the *EBNA2* and *LMP* latent genes which appear to be down-regulated in the newly established Burkitt's lymphoma lines (Rowe and Gregory, 1989).

While the requirement for and association of CD23 expression with the transformation of B cells by EBV suggest that this antigen is involved in growth stimulation, the observations are indirect. A direct growth-related function for CD23 was first demonstrated by Gordon *et al.* (1986b), who found that restricted antibodies within the CD23 cluster were able to enhance DNA synthesis occurring in appropriately activated (phorbol ester) normal B cells; some CD23-expressing Burkitt's lymphoma cells can also be stimulated to increase DNA synthesis on the addition of these antibodies (Gordon *et al.*, 1988a). Recently it was found that normal B cells primed

Complexity of CD23 processing

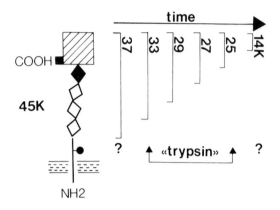

Biological heterogeneity of CD23 species

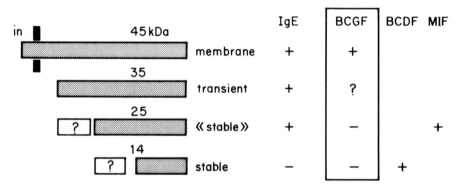

Figure 1 A synthesis on CD23 Processing and Function. Upper panel: CD23 is shown in membrane form and subsequent cleavage fragment indicated with the type of protease responsible where known. Lower panel: The different activities which have been attributed to CD23 forms are indicated schematically (see text for details).

with "physiological" signals that include IL-4, show enhanced stimulation when confronted with the CD23 antibody MHM6 (Gordon *et al.*, 1989a). A major contribution to the study of CD23 came in 1987 when Swendeman and Thorley-Lawson showed that shed "Blast-2" (that is, CD23), released from EBV-transformed cells with a half life of 1–2 hours (Thorley-Lawson *et al.*,

1986), was capable of promoting stimulation either in the autogenous transformed B cells or in activated normal B cells. Further studies indicated that stimulation by CD23 antibodies may reflect their ability either to generate more, or to stabilize, the active extracellular fragment of CD23 (Guy and Gordon, 1987). Addition of a partially purified "commercial" BCGF that had been derived from mitogen-stimulated T cells was found also to cleave surface CD23 and provide a growth signal (Guy and Gordon, 1987). Although a recombinant BCGF has been found not to possess this activity, a factor present in commercial BCGF that does cleave surface CD23 was recently identified (J. Shields and J-Y. Bonnefoy, personal communication).

The processing of membrane-bound CD23 is complex, and not all fragments are necessarily active in "BCGF" assays. It now seems that proteolytic cleavage of the membrane-bound molecule first yields fragments of 37 kD and 33 kD (Letellier *et al.*, 1989). These species are transient, however, and break down further to give rise to a more stable 25 kD fragment (Gordon *et al.*, 1988b). Eventually, this product degrades to a fully stable 14 kD molecule, possibly even via a short-lived 18 kD intermediate (reviewed by Gordon *et al.*, 1989b; Delespesse *et al.*, 1989). Current evidence suggests the BCGF-activity is contained within the short-lived 37 and 33 kD forms but may be lost on further breakdown to the 25 kD form (Uchibayashi *et al.*, 1989). Interestingly, recent studies have shown that the intact 45 kD molecule isolated from membranes is consistently active at supporting the stimulation of both normal and transformed B cells (Cairns and Gordon, 1990). Whether the intact molecule exerts its effect directly or needs to be processed further is unclear. Preliminary data from A. Ghaderi in Birmingham, indicate that the latter may be operative as a neutralizing antibody which is specific for cleaved CD23; this antibody appears to inhibit the growth-promoting activity of the 45 kD molecule. It will be important to identify the proteases that are responsible for the successive fragmentation of CD23; Figure 1 attempts a synthesis on the processing and biological function of CD23 as understood from present data.

Other autostimulatory factors for virally-transformed B cells

Apart from IL-1 and CD23, several other molecules have been implicated in the autostimulatory growth of EBV-transformed B cells. Buck *et al.* (1987) have described an autocrine growth factor (termed aBCGF) that is present in serum-free medium conditioned by an EBV-transformed line (5/2). They found that the major autostimulatory activity was associated with a 16 kD protein of pI 7–8. It appeared that the 16 kD molecule was in equilibrium with dimeric and tetrameric forms. All seven EBV-transformed B cell lines examined were found to be capable of responding by enhanced growth to the factor. The authors found that while the cell lines could respond to exogenous IL-1, the abCGF itself did not display IL-1 activity.

Another important soluble mediator that might be implicated in autocrine growth of EBV-transformed cells is IL-6. Originally, IL-6 was termed IFN-β_2 (although it is now known to possess no anti-viral activity) and it has also been referred to as 26-kD protein and B cell differentiation factor (BSF-2) (Billiau, 1987). Monocytes are known to provide good feeder layers for EBV-transformed B cells and, in 1988, Tosato *et al.* demonstrated that a soluble product of activated monocytes that contributed to their growth-supporting capacity was indeed IL-6. Production of IL-6 by haemopoetic cells is almost ubiquitous and has been shown for some B cells (Biondi *et al.*, 1989). Thus, in some situations, IL-6 may be able to serve as an autostimulatory factor for EBV-transformed cells.

Autocrine growth in B cell neoplasia

Chronic lymphocytic leukaemia

There are now several studies which indicate that B-CLL cells can produce IL-1. For example, in one study all but four of 17 leukaemic populations were found to produce IL-1 spontaneously (Morabito *et al.*, 1987)—all of the IL-1 producing populations were positive for certain surface markers that are typically associated with myelomonocytic cells. In another study, spontaneous IL-1 production from B-CLL cells was shown to be comprised of IL-1β by immunoassay and neutralization with the appropriate anti-IL-1 antiserum (Uggla *et al.*, 1987). It should be noted, however, that no study has demonstrated enhanced growth of autologous B-CLL cells resulting from their released IL-1. This may be because the B-CLL cell in circulation is generally refractory to growth-factor-promoted stimulation (Ghaderi *et al.*, 1988)—it remains possible, however, that the leukaemic progenitor cells might be using such activities to support autocrine growth. Similar arguments may hold for IL-6. Thus, it has been shown in one study that of 11 B-CLL populations, six were found to express mRNA for IL-6 and production of the factor was confirmed in biological assays (Biondi *et al.*, 1989). IL-6, therefore, has at least a potential rôle to play in the regulation and development of B-CLL.

Despite a general refractoriness, B-CLL cells can sometimes respond to certain exogenous growth factors (Ghaderi *et al.*, 1988). In a study by Diget *et al.* (1989), B-CLL populations displayed an enhanced DNA synthesis of two- to 104-fold in the presence of tumour necrosis factor (TNF) α. This observation is important in view of the known capacity of B cells to produce TNF-β, which displays similar function to TNF-α and which binds to identical receptors.

Other B cell malignancies

In primary malignancies other than B-CLL, little information is available concerning autocrine growth potential. In one report, a cytoplasmic 60 kD protein found within the cells of a patient with immunoblastic B cell lymphoma supported the growth of both the autologous tumour cells and of normal B cells (Sahasrabuddhe *et al.*, 1989). A similar 60 kD factor had been found in normal B cells, and antibodies raised against this were used to isolate immunoreactive 60 kD material and also 14 kD molecules from culture supernatants of the B lymphoma. The affinity-purified material was found to have BCGF activity. It was suggested that the 60 kD cytoplasmic molecule might be a precursor of the released 14 kD factor. These observations are reminiscent of those made previously on an autocrine factor synthesized by cells from a patient with hairy-cell leukaemia (Ford *et al.*, 1986). The Burkitt's lymphoma cell line Namalwa has also been found to produce a 60 kD BCGF (Ambrus and Fauci, 1985) of pI 6.7–7.8 that acts preferentially on large "pre-activated" B cells. Interestingly, an antibody raised against the Namalwa-BCGF cross-reacted with T cell-derived 60 kD BCGF, also known as "high molecular weight" BCGF (Ambrus *et al.*, 1985).

In 1988, Kawano *et al.* reported that multiple myeloma cells isolated from bone marrow could produce and bind IL-6, while an antibody to IL-6 inhibited the *in vitro* proliferation of these cells. It remains possible, however, that a few contaminating stromal cells in the bone marrow preparation could have been responsible for the production of the IL-6, which has an extremely high specific activity. Nevertheless, IL-6 should now be viewed as an important cytokine in the pathogenesis of this aggressive disease.

Autocrine growth-inhibitory factors

The establishment of an immortalized cell line or tumour will depend not only on the level of growth stimulation but also on the potential counteracting influence of growth inhibitory factors. The simultaneous presence of inhibitory and stimulatory factors found in crude conditioned medium often makes it an unsatisfactory source of growth-promoting activity. Vesole *et al.*

(1979), in their studies first describing stimulatory factors from B cell lines, noted an inhibitory activity present in high molecular weight material that was readily separable from the 30 kD stimulatory activity. Blazar *et al.* (1983) similarly noted inhibitory activity in B-cell line conditioned medium which led to a biphasic titration curve for the growth-enhancing effect. Gordon *et al.* (1984a,b) found that to minimize such negative factors, supernatants needed to be generated over a short period (24 h) from cells plated at non-saturating cell densities (2×10^5 to 4×10^5 per millilitre). In their study of autocrine IL-1 activity from virally-transformed B cells, Scala *et al.* (1984) described the concomitant production of a factor that could negate the IL-1-stimulatory effect. This factor was termed contra-IL-1 and had a molecular weight of 70–80 kD. Recently, an IL-1 inhibitor has been described which binds to the IL-1 receptor but has no IL-1-like activity (Hannum *et al.*, 1990). Cloning of this IL-1 receptor antagonist has shown it to be structurally related to IL-1β (Eisenberg *et al.*, 1990). Growth-inhibitory activity is most apparent in medium conditioned by cells in the plateau phase of growth and this, along with cell contact inhibition, may be responsible for the cessation of growth which occurs under these conditions.

Mechanisms of growth inhibition are poorly understood although several possibilities exist.

(i) Inactive molecules could compete with the receptor for an autostimulatory factor—the former could represent a degradation product of the latter or a distinct molecule, but one sharing a common receptor-binding site.

(ii) Growth factor "binding" or "carrier" proteins could effectively neutralize biological activity by either preventing receptor binding or inactivating a functional site—one obvious example for such a mechanism would be that of shed receptors for the growth factors.

(iii) Another possibility for promoting growth inhibition would be by having two factors that bind to different receptors but, owing to the nature of the second messenger invoked, the positive signal might be interrupted on its route to the nucleus—such a situation would be akin to the antagonism observed between interferons and IL-4 and between IL-4 and IL-2 as discussed in earlier chapters.

Recent evidence obtained in my own laboratory points to yet another potential mechanism to account for opposing influences between two cytokines. Simply, B cell-conditioned medium that had been depleted of soluble CD23 was seen to become toxic for activated normal B cells. Previously it had been noted that the inhibition of B cell stimulation seen to occur in crowded cultures could be overcome by the addition of purified B cell-derived BCGF (unpublished observation). It is possible, therefore, that a positive factor may be operating by its ability to counteract, or neutralize, inhibitory or toxic substances. Clearly, these considerations would be important in areas of high B cell density as encountered in the germinal centre reaction (see below).

A final mechanism whereby the growth-transformation of a B cell could disrupt the normal balance between positive and negative growth influences comes from observations on the broad-acting and widely expressed cytokine, transforming growth factor (TGF) β. Kehrl *et al.* (1987) first demonstrated that activated B cells could not only express TGF-β message but were also capable of releasing the soluble factor. In serum-free medium, TGF-β was found to be inhibitory for B cell stimulations. The degree of inhibition was seen to be dependent not only on the concentration of the TGF-β but also on the amount of stimulatory activity available. While normal activated B cells expressed high affinity receptors for TGF-β, an EBV-transformed B-cell line investigated lacked receptors—naturally, the latter failed to be affected by TGF-β. Smeland *et al.* (1987) later found that, for normal B cells, the inhibitory action of TGF-β was restricted to the G_1 to S transition stage—little or no effect was seen during the early activation phase from G_0 to G_1. Then it was shown that EBV-negative Burkitt's lymphoma cells, which are sensitive to the inhibitory actions of TGF-β, became refractory on their conversion with EBV (Blomhoff *et al.*, 1987). Thus, EBV may be responsible for down-regulating a normally inhibitory action of TGF-β through receptor shut-off.

Teleology of autocrine growth

Is autocrine growth stimulation of B lymphocytes simply an ectopic event restricted to abnormal populations encountered in malignancy, or is this phenotype a transient part of normal B cell physiology but one that is exaggerated in neoplasia? The observation that normal B cells can be provoked to release factors that are B-lymphotropic clearly indicates that autocrine growth at least has the potential to be operative in physiological processes. Perhaps the most compelling evidence for a normal rôle comes from the studies on IL-4 promoted growth stimulation of B cells. Several groups have noted the impressive link between the level of growth that can be stimulated by IL-4 and the release of the soluble CD23 molecule (reviewed in Gordon *et al.*, 1989b); however, it is the demonstration that IL-4 triggered B cell-stimulation is effectively neutralized by certain CD23 antibodies that provides the most convincing evidence for a rôle for CD23 in normal B cell growth. Three groups have now generated monoclonal antibodies with this property (Delespesse *et al.*, 1989; Tadmori *et al.*, 1989; Ghaderi and Stanworth, unpublished observations).

In the study by Tadmori *et al.*, they referred to an antibody that was capable of neutralizing an IL-4 promoted B-BCGF from a B cell line. This antibody also can deplete the B-BCGF from IL-4 conditioned medium (W. Tadmori, personal communication) and we have recently verified its CD23 reactivity on tissue sections (G. D. Johnson and J. Gordon, unpublished observations). Perhaps most important, however, is the demonstration of neutralization of IL-4 triggered stimulation by the Ghaderi antibody, which reacts exclusively with soluble CD23 and therefore could not be acting through its binding to cell membrane CD23 and transmitting a disruptive signal on the IL-4 promoted second messenger cascade. As discussed in an earlier chapter, IL-4 also turns on IL-6 production in human B cells; data obtained from my own laboratory, however, provide no evidence that IL-6 contributes to B cell growth in these circumstances nor that it synergizes with CD23 to this end (unpublished observations).

How do these *in vitro* observations relate to B cell function *in vivo*? As discussed in a recent review (Gordon *et al.*, 1989b), the likely site for CD23 induction in a primary response to TD-antigen will be on interdigitating cells within the paracortex of secondary lymphoid organs. Here, B cells bearing antigen will congregate with cognate T cells—release of IL-4 from the T cells would not only up-regulate major histocompatibility complex (MHC) class II, allowing for tighter association with the B cell, but would also efficiently induce CD23. Following activation at this site, a bifurcation occurs to generate an extrafollicular response and germinal centre formation, respectively. With the latter arm, the initial follicular B-blast reaction has been shown to generate in the order of 40,000 B cells from one to three starting cells in a matter of days (MacLennan *et al.*, 1988)—the follicle becomes completely occupied and crowded by antigen-specific B cells. It is clear that under such conditions the B cells themselves must be exerting very potent controls over their own proliferation.

We do not yet know the nature of the potential soluble and cell surface molecules involved in these processes, but it is possible that the CD23 that would have been induced following cognate interaction at the interdigitating cell is shed as the B cells move into the follicles, at least to initiate the blast reaction. The space occupied by the proliferating B cells is formed on a network of follicular dendritic cells (FDC), at least a subset of which can show very striking expression of CD23; it is conceivable that the proliferating B-blast cells continue to "feed-off" CD23 expressed on FDC as they undergo their extensive and rapid proliferation. The form of CD23 expressed by FDC is unknown, but one possibility is that the activated B cells express a high level of endogenous proteases at their surfaces which are able to cleave off FDC-associated CD23 to a stimulatory form. The signals that lead to differentiation of the B-blasts, initially to centroblasts and then to centrocytes, might be triggered by the shear crowding of the B cells and the subsequent cell contacts that would result. Centrocytes are the progeny of memory cells (MacLennan and Gray, 1986) and undergo programmed cell death by apoptosis unless selected for by antigen expressed in the form of immune complexes on FDC (Liu *et al.*, 1989). The FDC of mature germinal centres, which are located within the area where selection takes place, are extremely rich in CD23, and preliminary data suggest a rôle for soluble CD23 in the survival and/or differentiation of centrocytes. CD23-rich supernatants from RPMI 8866 B-lymphoblastoid cells can rescue germinal centre B cells from apoptosis and promote plasmacytoid differentiation— depletion of the CD23 results in a reduction of these activities (Liu *et al.*, in preparation). Alternatively, or additionally, CD23 on FDC may serve as an adhesion molecule for rescued centrocytes. The importance of these obser- vations is that B cell-derived factors might not only be stimulating growth but may also be promoting survival in tumour counterparts that normally would be destined to die. Figure 2 illustrates these concepts schematically.

Concluding remarks

This chapter has attempted to survey the data that indicate that B cells themselves have a contributory rôle to play in their own fate, and how disruption of this normal physiological process could be one facet of the multi-step scenarios that can result in B cell malignancies. A major question that arises is whether knowledge gained in these areas will find any practical application in the treatment of B cell related disease. The answer must be: perhaps! Maybe some clues will be provided from observations on the treatment of hairy-cell leukaemia by IFN-α, where there is evidence to suggest that phenotypic changes occur which render the tumour cells refractory to stimulation by (autocrine?) BCGF (Paganelli *et al.*, 1986).

I have not considered in any depth during this review the influence of B cells and their products on other cells of the immune system. Given the potential of B cells to produce IL-1, IL-6, TNFs and TGF-β, this possibility must be high. Evidence is also emerging to implicate B cell-derived CD23 as a multi-functional cytokine in immune regulation and modulation (reviewed in Gordon *et al.*, 1989b; see also Figure 1). Clearly, both the autocrine and paracrine aspects of B cell-derived cytokine should be of continuing interest in the years ahead.

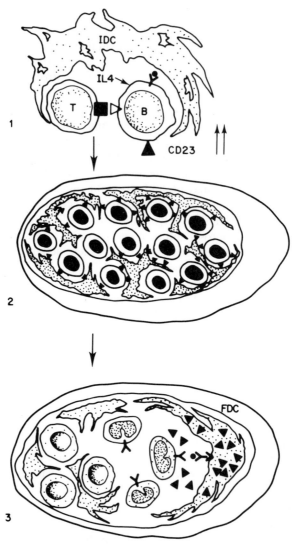

Figure 2   Model for rôle of CD23 in germinal centre reactions. 1. B cells are first activated on IDC with TH cells and the IL4 subsequently released upregulates CD23 (and MHC Class II). Induced CD23 may then be used in autocrine mode as B cells undergo: (i) extrafollicular proliferation in primary response; (ii) entry into follicles. 2. B cells undergo follicular blast reaction at rapid rate on FDC expressing surface CD23 (noted on a subset of FDC; Y-J. Liu, personal communication). 3. Centroblasts differentiating from B-blasts undergo somatic mutation on Ig and give way to centrocytes expressing mutated Ig (Y) which vies for antigen (●): cells are rescued from apoptosis on FDC that are expressing extremely high levels of CD23 cytoplasmically (Y-J. Liu, personal communication). This CD23 may also provide signal for further differentiation. CD23 indicated by filled triangles.

Acknowledgements

The work of John Gordon is supported by the Medical Research Council (U.K.) and the Leukaemia Research Fund. I wish to thank my colleagues whose work and ideas have contributed to some of the principles outlined in this chapter: Drs M. Melamed, P. Aman, A. Rosen, J. A. Cairns, L. Flores-Romo and Y-J. Liu. Special thanks are extended to Professor I. C. M. MacLennan for informing me that B lymphocytes have a life outside of tissue-culture flasks; warm thanks are also extended to Professor G. Klein for introducing me to the fascinations of EBV, and for his continual guidance, encouragement and stimulation over the last decade.

References

Acres, R. B., Larsen, A., Gillis, S and Conlon, P. J. (1987) *Mol. Immunol.* **24**, 479–485.
Aman, P., Ehlin-Henriksson, B. and Klein, G. (1984) *J. Exp. Med.* **159**, 208–220.
Ambrus, J. L. and Fauci, A. S. (1985) *J. Clin. Invest.* **75**, 732–739.
Ambrus, J. L., Jurgensen, C. H., Brown, E. J. and Fauci, A. S. (1985) *J. Exp. Med.* **162**, 1319–1335.
Billiau, A. (1987) *Immunol. Today* **8**, 84–87.
Biondi, A., Rossi, V., Bassan, R., Barbui, T., Bettoni, S., Mantovani, A. and Rambaldi, A. (1989) *Blood* **73**, 1279–1284.
Blazar, B. A., Sutton, L. M. and Strome, M. (1983) *Cancer Res.* **43**, 4562–4568.
Blomhoff, H. K., Smeland, E., Mustafa, A. S., Godal, T. and Ohlsson, R. (1987) *Eur. J. Immunol.* **17**, 299–301.
Buck, J., Hammerling, U., Hoffmann, M. K., Levi, E. and Welte, K. (1987) *J. Immunol.* **138**, 2923–2928.
Cairns, J., Flores-Romo, L. C., Millsum, M. J., Guy, G. R., Gillis, S., Ledbetter, J. A. and Gordon, J. (1988) *Eur. J. Immunol.* **18**, 349–353.
Cairns, J. and Gordon, J. (1990) *Eur. J. Immunol.* **20**, 539–543.
Dambaugh, T., Hennessy, K., Chamnankit, L. and Kieff, E. (1984) *Proc. Natl. Acad. Sci. USA* **81**, 7632–7636.
Delespesse, G., Sarfati, M. and Hofstetter, H. (1989) *Immunol. Today* **10**, 159–163.
Digel, W., Stefanic, M., Schoniger, W., Buck, C., Raghavachar, A., Frickhofen, N., Heimpel, H. and Porzsoltr, F. (1989) *Blood* **73**, 1242–1246.
Eisenberg, S. P., Evans, R. J., Arend, W. P., Verderber, E., Brewer, M. J., Hannum, C. H. and Thompson, R. C. (1990) *Nature* **343**, 341–346.
Fingeroth, J. D., Weis, J. J., Tedder, T. F., Strominger, J. L., Biro, P. A. and Fearon, D. T. (1984) *Proc. Natl. Acad. Sci. USA* **81**, 4510–4514.
Flores-Romo, L., Foster, D., Guy, G. R. and Gordon, J. (1989) *Immunology* **66**, 228–232.
Ford, R. J., Kwok, D., Quesada, J., Sahasrabuddhe, C. G. (1986) *Blood* **67**, 573–577.
Ghaderi, A. A., Richardson, P., Cardona, C., Millsum, M. J., Ling, N., Gillis, S., Ledbetter, J and Gordon, J. (1988) *Leukemia* **2**, 165–170.

Gordon, J., Ley, S. C., Melamed, M. D., Aman, P. and Hughes-Jones, N. C. (1984a) *J. Exp. Med.* **159**, 1554–1559.

Gordon, J., Ley, S. C., Melamed, M. C., English, L. S. and Hughes-Jones, N. C. (1984b) *Nature* **310**, 145–147.

Gordon, J., Aman, P., Rosen, A., Ernberg, I. Ehlin-Henriksson, B. and Kelin, G. (1985a). *Int. J. Cancer* **35**, 251–256.

Gordon, J., Guy, G. and Walker, L. (1985b) *Immunology* **56**, 329–335.

Gordon, J., Walker, L., Guy, G., Brown, G., Rowe, M. and Rickinson, A. (1986a) *Immunology* **58**, 591–595.

Gordon, J., Rowe, M., Walker, L. and Guy, G. (1986b) *Eur. J. Immunol.* **16**, 1075–1080.

Gordon, J., Guy, G. and Walker, L. (1986d) *Immunology* **57**, 419–423.

Gordon, J., Millsum, M. J. Finney, M. Cairns, J. A., Guy, G. R., Gregory, C. D., Abbot, S. D., Rickinson, A. B. Wang, F. and Kieff, E. (1988a) *Curr. Top. Microbiol. Immunol.* **4**, 149–156.

Gordon, J., Cairns, J. A., Flores-Romo, L., Millsum, M. J. and Guy, G. R. (1988c) *Blood* **72**, 367–368.

Gordon, J., Millsum, M. J., Flores-Romo, L. and Gillis, S. (1989a) *Immunology* **68**, 526–531.

Gordon, J., Flores–Romo, L., Cairns, J. A., Millsum, M. J., Lane, P. L., Johnson, G. D. and MacLennan, I. C. M. (1989b) *Immunol. Today* **10**, 153–157.

Guy, G. R. and Gordon, J. (1987) *Proc. Natl. Acad. Sci. USA* **84**, 6239–6243.

Guy, G. R. and Gordon, J. (1989) *Int. J. Cancer* **43**, 703–708.

Guy, G. R., Gordon, J. and Mitchell, R. H. (1989) *Inositol Lipids in Cell Signalling*, Ed. by R. H. Mitchell, pp. 433–458. Academic Press, New York.

Hannum, C. P., Wilcox, C. J., Arend, W. P., Joslin, F. G., Dripps, D. J., Heimdal, P. L., Armes, L. G., Sommer, A., Eisenberg, S. P. and Thompson, R. C. (1990) *Nature* **343**, 336–340.

Ho, C. P., Aman, P., Masucci, M-G., Klein, E. and Klein, G. (1986) *Eur. J. Immunol.* **16**, 841–845.

Hurley, E. A. and Thorley-Lawson, D. A. (1988) *J. Exp. Med.* **168**, 2059–2076.

Jurgensen, C. H., Ambrus, J. L. and Fauci, A. S. (1986) *J. Immunol.* **136**, 4542–4547.

Kawano, M., Hirano, T., Matsudo, T., Taga, T., Horii, Y., Iwato, Y., Asaoku, H., Tang, B., Tanabe, O., Tanake, H. and Kishimoto, T. (1988) *Nature* **331**, 83–85.

Kehrl, J. H., Alvarez-Mon, M., Delsing, G. A. and Fauci, A. S. (1987) *Science* **238**, 1144–1146.

Kitner, C. and Sugden, B. (1981) *Nature* **294**, 458–460.

Knutson, J. C. and Sugden, B. (1989) *Adv. Viral. Oncol.* **8**, 151–172.

Laux, G. Perricaudet, M. and Farrel, P. (1988) *EMBO J.* **7**, 769–778.

Letellier, M., Sarfati, M. and Delespesse, G. (1989) *Mol. Immunol.* **26**, 1105–1112.

Liu, Y-J., Joshua, D. E., Williams, G. T., Smith, C. A. and Maclennon, I. C. M. (1989) *Nature* **342**, 929–931.

MacLennan, I. C. M. and Gray, D. (1986) *Immunol. Rev.* **91**, 61–83.

MacLennan, I. C. M., Liu, Y-J. and Ling, N. R. (1988) *Curr. Topics Microbiol. Immunol.* **141**, 138–148.

Matsushima, K., Kuang, Y-D., Tosato, G., Hopkins, S. J. and Oppenheim, J. J. (1985a). *Cell. Immunol.* **94**, 406–417.

Matsushima, K., Procopio, A., Abe, H., Scala, G., Ortaldo, J. R. and Oppenheim, J. J. (1985b) *J. Immunol.* **135**, 1132–1136.

Morabito, F., Prasthofer, E. F., Dunlap, N. E., Grossi, C. E. and Tilden, A. B. (1987) *Blood* **70**, 1750–1757.

Muraguchi, A., Nishimoto, H., Kawamura, N., Hori, A. and Kishimoto, T. (1986) *J. Immunol.* **137**, 179–186.

Nemerow, G. R., McNaughton, M. E. and Cooper, N. R. (1985) *J. Immunol.* **135**, 3068–3073.

Paganelli, K. A., Evans, S. S., Han, T. and Ozer, H. (1986). *Blood* **67**, 937–942.⁄

Rimsky, L., Wakasugi, H., Ferrara, P., Robin, P., Capdevielle, J., Tusrsz, T., Fradelizi, D. and Bertoglio, J. (1986) *J. Immunol.* **136**, 3304–3310.

Rowe, M. and Gregory, C. (1989) *Adv. Viral Oncol.* **8**, 237–259.

Sahasrabuddhe, C. G., Sekhsaria, S., Yoshimura, L. and Ford, R. J. (1989) *Blood* **73**, 1149–1156.

Sanderson, R., Vesole, D., Jakway, J. and Talmage, D. (1980) *Immunol. Rev.* **51**, 177–190.

Sinclair, N. R. and Panoskaltsis, A. (1989) *Clinical Immunol. Immunopathol.* **52**, 133–146.

Scala, G., Kuang, Y. D., Hall, R. E., Muchmore, A. V. and Oppenheim, J. J. (1984) *J. Exp. Med.* **159**, 1637–1652.

Sharma, S., Mehta, S., Morgan, J. and Maizel, A. (1987) *Science* **235**, 1489–1492.

Smeland, E. N., Blomhoff, H. K., Holte, H., Ruud, E., Beiske, K., Funderud, S., Godal, T. and Ohlsson, R. (1987) *Exp. Cell Res.* **171**, 213–222.

Swendeman, S. and Thorley-Lawson, D. A. (1987) *EMBO J.* **6**, 1637–1642.

Tadmori, W., Lee, H-K., Clark, S. C. and Choi, Y. S. (1989) *J. Immunol.* **142**, 826–832.

Thorley-Lawson, D. A. and Mann, K. P. (1985) *J. Exp. Med.* **162**, 45–59.

Thorley-Lawson, D. A., Nadler, L. M., Bhan, A. K. and Schooley, R. T. (1985) *J. Immunol.* **134**, 3007–3012.

Tosato, G., Seamon, K. B., Goldman, N. D., Sehgal, P. V., May, L. T., Washington, G. C., Jones, K. D. and Pike, S. E. (1988) *Science* **239**, 502–504.

Uchibayashi, N., Kikutani, H., Barsumian, E. L., Hauptmann, R., Schneider, F-J., Schwendenwein, R., Sommergruber, W., Spevak, W., Maurer-Fogy, I., Suemara, M. and Kishimoto, T. (1989) *J. Immunol.* **142**, 3901–3908.

Uggla, C., Aguilar-Santelises, M., Rosen, A., Mellstedt, H. and Jondal, M. (1987) *Blood* **70**, 1851–1857.

Vesole, D. H., Goust, J. M., Fett, J. W. and Fudenberg, H. H. (1979) *J. Immunol.* **123**, 1322–1328.

Wakasugi, H., Dokhelar, M. C., Garson, D., Harel-Bellan, A., Fradelizi, D. and Tursz, T. (1985) *Eur. J. Immunol.* **15**, 256–261.

Wakasugi, H., Rimsky, L., Mahe, Y., Mahmoud, A., Fradelizi, D., Tursz, T. and Bertoglio, J. (1987) *Proc. Natl. Acad. Sci. USA* **84**, 804–808.

Walker, L., Guy, G., Brown, G., Rowe, M., Milner, A. E. and Gordon, J. (1986) *Immunology* **58**, 583–589.

Wang, R., Gregory, C. D., Rowe, M., Rickinson, A. B., Wang, D., Birkenbach, M., Kikutani, H., Kishimoto, T. and Kieff, E. (1987) *Proc. Natl. Acad. Sci. USA* **84**, 3452–3456.

Weaver, C. T. and Unanue, E. R. (1990) *Immunol. Today* **11**, 49–55.

9
Cytokine action on B cells in disease

SERGIO ROMAGNANI

Introduction

Over the past few years several factors that regulate the growth and differentiation of human B lymphocytes have been described. Initially, they were identified simply as activities present in culture supernatants, a situation which has generated considerable confusion. More recently, the genes for most of these factors have been cloned, and recombinant molecules are now available.

The most important cytokines acting on human B cells seem to be interleukin 4 (IL-4), IL-2 and IL-6 (reviewed by Romagnani, 1989). IL-4 probably acts on B cells several times during, and in most stages of, their differentiation process. First, it is an activation factor for resting B cells, being able to induce and/or enhance the expression of cell surface molecules, such as major histocompatibility complex (MHC) class II determinants and the FcεRII/CD23. In addition, IL-4 behaves as a true growth factor for activated B cells and represents an essential mediator for the induction of IgE synthesis. Finally human IL-4 seems to exert a regulatory rôle on the synthesis of other immunoglobulin (Ig) classes, such as IgM and IgG (particularly IgG4).

IL-2 plays a critical rôle in both growth and differentiation of human B cells. Besides promoting the proliferation of both *in vivo* and *in vitro* activated B lymphocytes, IL-2 is able to induce their differentiation into IgM-, IgG- and IgA-secreting cells. Furthermore, IL-2 can even replace T cells in the antigen-induced antibody response by memory B cells *in vitro*.

IL-6 also participates in the process of Ig production by human B cells. This highly pleiotropic cytokine selectively promotes the terminal differentiation of human B lymphocytes, but compared with IL-4 and IL-2 it appears to play a less important rôle, which merely consists of amplification of Ig secretion.

Other cytokines, such as IL-1, tumour necrosis factor α (TNF-α) and

CYTOKINES AND B LYMPHOCYTES
ISBN 0–12–155145–8

interferon γ (IFN-γ) are also involved in the induction of human B cell growth and differentiation, displaying a synergistic effect on the activity of IL-2. Conversely, IFN-γ exerts a negative regulatory rôle on IL-4 dependent IgE synthesis. The activity on human B cells of IL-5, the so-called low molecular weight B cell growth factor (LMW BCGF) (at least in its recombinant form) and the soluble FcεRII/CD23 antigen is still controversial.

The availability of cloned and purified B cell-tropic cytokines has led not only to better understanding of how they control B cell responses, but also to the exciting possibility of investigating their rôle in the pathogenesis of some human diseases and testing this new-found knowledge *in vivo*. Abnormal B cell function does indeed occur in a number of disorders including immunodeficiency, autoimmunity and allergy. Evidence is now accumulating for alterations of cytokine production or responses to cytokines in abnormalities of B cell function.

Our current knowledge of B cell-tropic cytokines in such diseases is reviewed in this chapter. Major emphasis is placed on discussing mechanisms that regulate the synthesis of human IgE and possible cytokine abnormalities in allergy, as well as on other pathological conditions characterized by hyperproduction of IgE. This choice of emphasis is for two obvious reasons: first, IgE production and allergy represent my basic area of interest in research; second, in the last two years, progress in this field has been enormous and complete revolution of previous interpretations has been achieved.

Immune deficiency syndromes

Immune deficiency syndromes (IDS) represent a heterogeneous group of disorders affecting specific and/or non-specific immunity, resulting in impairment of host defences against infections and a high incidence of autoimmune diseases and neoplasias (Rosen *et al.*, 1986). Some IDS are genetically determined (primary IDS), whereas others result from damage of the immune system due to malnutrition, infectious agents, metabolic diseases or treatment with radiation or immunosuppressive drugs (secondary IDS). In IDS where humoral immunity is exclusively or mainly affected, several studies have found more or less pronounced defects of B lymphocyte or both B and T lymphocyte numbers and functions.

The rôle of cytokines active on B cell function in IDS is probably important, but so far there has been no convincing evidence for an inherited defect in this area (Saiki *et al.*, 1984; Perri and Weisdorf, 1985; Mayer *et al.*, 1986; Matheson and Green, 1987). In only two IDS, common variable hypogammaglobulinaemia (CVH) and the acquired immune deficiency syndrome (AIDS), is less anecdotal information available on possible alterations that may occur in the network of cytokines active on B cells.

Common variable hypogammaglobulinaemia (CVH)

CVH is a heterogeneous group of diseases characterized by functional antibody deficiency. The degree of serum immunoglobulin (Ig) deficiency varies widely, but there is often some IgM, a little IgG and negligible IgA. The level of the defect responsible for reduced or lack of Ig production in patients with CVH is still obscure. When mononuclear cells (MNC) or B cells from peripheral blood (PB) of CVH patients were assayed for proliferation to anti-IgM antibodies, or to *Staphylococcus aureus* Cowan I strain (SAC) bacteria (T cell-independent B cell mitogens), and for differentiation to Ig-secreting cells of IgM, IgG and IgA classes in the presence of SAC and pokeweed mitogen (PWM) or T cell factors, three distinct groups of CVH patients were identified:

(1) CVH patients, whose B cells proliferated and secreted IgM but not IgG,
(2) patients showing B cell proliferation but not Ig production,
(3) patients without any response.

The latter group of patients are in the minority and may completely lack recirculating B cells (Saiki *et al.*, 1982). The ability of B cells from virtually all CVH patients who show normal numbers of recirculating B cells, to proliferate normally has recently been confirmed using a range of cytokines (IL-2, IL-4 and IL-6) and solid-phase anti-IgM. Under these experimental conditions, no IgG was produced by cells from any patient and in only one patient was IgM production observed (Farrant *et al.*, 1989). These data suggest that B cells from the majority of CVH patients (at least those showing normal numbers of circulating B cells) have the ability to proliferate, but that they usually fail to differentiate into Ig (particularly IgG and IgA) producing cells.

Interestingly, however, Epstein–Barr virus (EBV) can partially bypass the defect in CVH patients having B cells and can induce secretion of IgM and, sometimes, of IgG (Pereira *et al.*, 1982). Human immunodeficiency virus-1 (HIV-1) is also capable of overcoming the block in CVH B cell differentiation. Some cases of recovery of Ig production, including specific antibody, following HIV-1 infection have been reported (Morrell *et al.*, 1986; Wright *et al.*, 1987). In addition to viruses, retinoic acid can bypass the IgM secretion defects in some hybridomas prepared from CVH B cells (Sherr *et al.*, 1988). Thus, it is not yet clear whether the B cell defect in CVH is intrinsic or due to a lack of appropriate signals. So a simplistic explanation for the B cell failure in CVH could be the failure of production and/or response to the appropriate cytokines.

In 19 patients with CVH, Paganelli *et al.* (1988a, 1988b) found low or absent production of IL-2 and IFN-γ following stimulation with phytohaemagglutinin (PHA). Likewise, peripheral blood lymphocytes (PBLs) of 11 patients with CVH produced reduced levels of IL-2, IL-4 and IFN-γ upon activation with mitogens, compared with those secreted by PBL of healthy donors (Pastorelli *et al.*, 1989a).

More recently, the ability of MNC from 26 patients with CVH to produce cytokines active on B cell growth (such as IL-2, IFN-γ, IL-4 and TNF-α) following stimulation with PHA was examined. MNC from the majority of

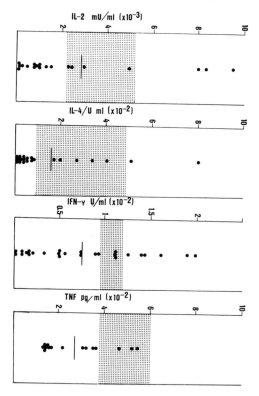

Figure 1 Production of cytokines by PBMNC from patients with CVH. PBMNC were stimulated with PHA for the appropriate time for each cytokine, and cytokine concentrations measured in the supernatants. Bars indicate mean values of cytokines found in CVH patients. Shaded areas represent 2 SD above and below mean values of contemporarily assessed PBMNC from controls.

patients showed defective production of one or more cytokines in comparison with age- and sex-matched controls (Figure 1). In two of these patients, the defect in the ability of T cells to produce cytokines active on B cells was confirmed at a clonal level by using a high efficiency cloning technique, based on stimulation with PHA of single PB T cells in the presence of irradiated feeder cells and IL-2 (Moretta *et al.*, 1983). Both patients showed significantly lower proportions of T cells able to produce IFN-γ, TNF-α, IL-2 and IL-4 compared with the control T cell clones (data not shown).

Obviously, these findings do not mean that defective Ig production in such patients is due to the inability of their T cells to produce cytokines active on B cells. However, they do strongly suggest that, at least in some patients, impaired function of, and response to, cytokines may contribute to the immune defects. This possibility has been further supported by other experiments in which the ability of a CD4$^+$ helper T cell clone (TCC) to induce Ig synthesis by B cells from patients with CVH was assessed.

Table 1   *In vitro* Ig production (μg ml^{-1}) by B cells from patients with CVH induced with SAC plus IL-2 or with activated T blasts of a selected helper T cell clone.[a]

	SAC + IL-2			Activated helper TCC		
	IgM	IgA	IgG	IgM	IgA	IgG
Patients						
A	<1	<1	<1	1.8	1.7	<1
B	<1	<1	<1	1.5	1.6	<1
C	1.3	<1	<1	3.0	9.4	2.9
D	1.2	<1	<1	5.4	2.3	1.3
E	3.8	<1	<1	2.5	1.6	1.4
F	2.4	<1	<1	3.5	3.4	1.5
G	2.9	<1	<1	3.9	5.7	1.8
H	2.8	1.3	1.2	2.4	2.3	4.7
I	6.7	8.9	5.4	3.9	3.7	2.8
J	3.4	2.7	3.2	3.3	8.6	4.5
K	2.8	4.2	2.9	3.9	10.0	7.3
Controls						
Mean	5.4	6.7	4.9	5.1	8.4	4.8
S.D.	±1.2	±1.1	±1.3	±1.5	±2.2	±1.2

[a]B cells (5×10^5) were cultured in 1 ml in the presence of SAC bacteria (final concentration 1/10,000) plus IL-2 (25 U ml^{-1}) or in the presence of T blasts (1×10^5) of a selected helper T cell clone previously activated with anti-CD3 and IL-2. After 10 days culture supernatants were assayed for the IgM, IgG and IgA content by appropriate radioimmunoassays.

Following stimulation with anti-CD3 monoclonal antibody, this clone (TR46) had been found to be capable of inducing the synthesis of IgG, IgM, IgA and IgE by B cells from virtually all normal donors tested (Parronchi *et al.*, 1990). Under analogous experimental conditions, the same TCC enabled B cells from all 11 CVH patients tested to produce IgM and IgA; B cells from nine of the patients also producing IgG. In contrast, eight of the 11 patients produced IgM, and only four produced IgG and IgA in response to stimulation with SAC plus IL-2 (Table 1). Similar results have also been reported by Pastorelli *et al.* (1989b), who showed that supernatants of activated TCCs can induce IgM production in B cells of all five and IgG and IgA production in B cells of two out of the five patients with CVH.

A comparison of the data obtained by the study of *in vitro* Ig production by B cells stimulated with the anti-CD3-activated TCC with those emerging from assessment of cytokine production by T cells from the same patients, supports the view that different and complex pathogenic mechanisms are operating in patients with CVH. It also suggests that the utilization of new technologies, such as cloning procedures and assays for quantitation of different cytokines, may help to discriminate between cytokine abnormalities in individual patients.

AIDS

The human immunodeficiency virus, the aetiological agent of AIDS, has the capability of selectively infecting $CD4^+$ T lymphocytes, resulting in a derangement of the immune system which renders the body highly susceptible to opportunistic infections and neoplasms. The critical basis for the immunopathogenesis of HIV infection is the depletion of the helper/inducer T cell subset (which express the CD4 phenotypic marker), resulting in profound immunosuppression (Fauci, 1988). Additionally, people infected by HIV have significant abnormalities of B cell function, as manifested by polyclonal activation, hypergammaglobulinaemia, circulating immune complexes and autoantibodies (Lane *et al.*, 1983). The polyclonal hyperactivity of the B cell limb of the immune response is probably due to multiple factors. The high incidence of infection with EBV and cytomegalovirus (CMV), both of which are polyclonal B cell activators, certainly contributes to this phenomenon. Also of importance is the fact that HIV itself, or subunits of the virus, can polyclonally activate B cells *in vitro* (Schnittman *et al.*, 1986). Whether alterations in the network of cytokines regulating the growth and differentiation of B cells is responsible for polyclonal B cell activation in HIV-infected individuals is still unclear. TNF-α and IL-6, which up-regulate HIV replication in HIV-infected lines (Rosenberg and Fauci, 1989), also act as B cell growth factor (Kehrl *et al.*, 1987) and B cell differentiation factor

1987) and B cell differentiation factor (BCDF; Hirano *et al.*, 1985; Muragu-chi *et al.*, 1988), respectively, for human B cells. On the other hand, increased IL-6 mRNA levels and increased IL-6 secretion have been observed soon after exposure of MNC isolated from healthy donors to both "live" and inactivated HIV. HIV-induced IL-6 was seen in monocyte/mac-rophages, which also produce TNF-α in response to HIV and represent an important reservoir for the virus, but not in T cells (Nakajima *et al.*, 1989). This may explain, at least in part, the enhanced Ig production which occurs ' in HIV-infected individuals. The enhanced synthesis of IgE detectable in about one-third of patients with AIDS is discussed later.

Autoimmune diseases

There is increasing clinical and experimental evidence that many auto-immune diseases develop as a result of abnormalities in T lymphocyte-mediated immunity. These diseases include systemic rheumatic diseases, such as systemic lupus erythematosus (SLE) and rheumatoid arthritis (RA). Included also are the organ specific diseases, such as insulin-dependent diabetes mellitus (IDDM), Hashimoto's thyroiditis, Graves' disease, idio-pathic Addison's disease, idiopathic hypopituitarism, pernicious anaemia, multiple sclerosis, coeliac disease, active chronic hepatitis, and some fibrotic skin, liver and lung diseases. T cell-mediated immune reactions are initiated and controlled by cytokines produced by either T or B lymphocytes as well as other cells involved in these reactions.

Systemic lupus erythematosus (SLE)

SLE is a representative autoimmune disease characterized by B cell hyper-reactivity resulting in the production of large amounts of Ig and various kinds of autoantibodies. B cells from SLE patients also show enhanced Ig production in *in vitro* culture without any stimulation (Blaese *et al.*, 1980). The possibility that such B cell hyperactivation, leading to enhanced antibody (and autoantibody) formation, is associated with states of hyper-function of cytokine–cytokine receptor systems has recently been suggested.

In the lupus-prone MRL-1pr/1pr murine strain, lymph node cells spon-taneously proliferate and produce IL-2 when cultured *in vitro*, even prior to the manifestations of autoimmunity, whereas such cells from control mice do not (Weston *et al.*, 1987). In addition, while unfractionated B cells from immunologically normal control mice respond to IL-2 only after stimulation with lipopolysaccharide (LPS) plus anti-Ig antibody, MLR-1pr/1pr cells respond to IL-2 following exposure to LPS alone and (NZB × NZF)F1 B cells proliferate with IL-2 in the absence of additional mitogens (Lehmann *et al.*, 1986). B cell hyperresponsiveness to IL-2 was also found in young NZB × NZW (B/W)F1 mice. With ageing, activation of the B cells progressed and they appeared to downregulate both the IL-2 hyper-response of B cells and IL-2 synthesis by T cells (Sekigawa *et al.*, 1989).

Initial reports suggested defective peripheral T-cell function due to an incapacity of T helper cells to produce IL-2 in patients with SLE (Altman *et al.*, 1981; Linker-Israeli *et al.*, 1983). However, subsequent studies have clearly demonstrated that genetically conferred autoimmunity may be associated with states of hyperactivation of the IL-2/IL-2 receptor (IL-2R) system. Increased IL-2 and IL-2R serum levels have been found in patients with SLE and appear to correlate significantly with IgG hypersecretion by PBL from the same patients (Huang *et al.*, 1988). This suggests that T cells of the helper type (TH) are activated *in vivo* and that their persistent production of IL-2 could play a rôle in the B cell hyperactivity of this disease (Kroemer and Wick, 1989).

Besides IL-2, other cytokines active on B cell growth and differentiation are also probably involved in the B cell hyperactivation of SLE. Spontaneous anti-histone and anti-DNA IgM autoantibody production by spleen cells from young NZB/NZW mice was strongly potentiated by supernatants from TH_2 helper clones, which contain IL-4 and IL-5, whereas supernatants from TH_1 clones, which contain IL-2 and IFN-γ, had no effect (Herron *et al.*, 1988). IL-5 has recently been shown to be responsible for B cell hyperresponsiveness in NZB/W, but not in BXSB or MRL/1 lupus prone murine strains (Umland *et al.* 1989). Human IL-5, however, although showing eosinophil differentiation activity as in mice, does not possess growth and differentiating activity on B cells (Clutterbuck *et al.*, 1987). Thus, at present, results showing increased responsiveness of B cells to IL-5 in lupus prone mice cannot be extrapolated to the human disease. Cytokines different from IL-5 are probably involved in B cell hyperresponsiveness in human SLE. SLE B cells have indeed been found to be able to produce spontaneously IL-1, IL-4 and IL-6, and to express receptors for these cytokines, suggesting that an autocrine mechanism is involved in the enhanced proliferation and differentiation into Ig-producing cells of SLE B cells (Tanaka *et al.*, 1988). Interestingly, the heterogeneity of B cell responsiveness to B cell-tropic cytokines, such as IL-4, IL-6 and LMW BCGF, appeared to result from discrete stages of B cell activation found in SLE (Kitani *et al.*, 1989).

Rheumatoid arthritis (RA)

Several cytokines have been reported to be elevated in synovial effusions of patients with RA, including IL-1 (Buchan *et al.*, 1988; Gitter *et al.*, 1989),

TNF-α (Gitter *et al.*, 1989), granulocyte and macrophage colony stimulatory factors (GM-CSF; Alvaro-Garcia *et al.*, 1989), TGF-β (Fava *et al.*, 1989) and IL-6 (Hirano *et al.*, 1988; Houssiau *et al.*, 1988). In particular, high levels of IL-6 were detected in synovial fluids from the joints of patients with active RA and the synovial fluid cells were found to express IL mRNA. Although synovial fluid monocytes are surely involved in the production of IL-6, synoviocytes and mononuclear cells of the pannus or synovial lining seem to represent the main source of IL-6. *In vitro*, synoviocytes spontaneously release IL-6 which is increased by IL-1 and TNF-γ (Bhardwaj *et al.*, 1989; Guerne *et al.*, 1989; Harigai *et al.*, 1989; Miyasaka *et al.*, 1989). However, IL-6 may also be synthesized systematically and become concentrated within the joint space as an effusion develops, Houssiau *et al.* (1988) have shown that there is elevation of IL-6 in sera of many RA patients and this appears to correlate with serum levels of acute phase proteins (APP). Since it has been shown that IL-6 can function as a hepatocyte-stimulating factor to produce APP (Gauldie *et al.*, 1987), as an endogenous pyrogen (Nijstein *et al.*, 1987) and as a BCDF (Hirano *et al.*, 1985; Muraguchi *et al.*, 1988), both the local and several of the generalized symptoms in RA patients— such as hypergammaglobulinaemia, increase in APP and fever—might be explained by excessive IL-6 production (Hirano and Kishimoto, 1989). Furthermore, since IL-6 may be a BCGF for EBV-transformed B lympho- blastoid cell lines, the abnormal secretion of IL-6 might also explain the presence of abnormally elevated numbers of circulating EBV-infected B cells in RA patients (Hirano and Kishimoto, 1989). However, increased production of IL-6 is not unique to RA, and may also be found in other inflammatory joint conditions, such as psoriatic arthritis, Behçet's syn- drome, hydroartrosis, pseudogout, joint disease of unknown aetiology or traumatic joint disease (Houssiau *et al.*, 1988; Bhardwaj *et al.*, 1989; Miyasaka *et al.*, 1989) (Figure 2). These findings raise questions as to the crucial role of IL-6 in RA.

Other autoimmune disorders

Involvement of IL-6 has also been suggested in other autoimmune dis- orders. Cardiac mixoma is a benign intra-atrial heart tumour and one-third of patients show clinical abnormalities such as hypergammaglobulinaemia, presence of various types of autoantibodies, and an increase in APP (Hirano and Kishimoto, 1989). Furthermore, these symptoms disappear upon surgi- cal removal of the tumour, suggesting that the myxoma itself or its products are responsible for the clinical picture. In fact, the culture supernatants of tumour cells were found to contain high IL-6 activity (Hirano *et al.*, 1987) and IL-6 mRNA could be detected in myxoma cells (Hirano *et al.*, 1986).

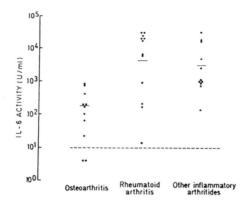

Figure 2 IL-6 activity in synovial fluid of patients with osteoarthritis, rheumatoid arthritis, and other inflammatory arthitides. Bars represent the log of the mean; broken line represents the limit of detection. (From Houssiau *et al.*, 1988).

IL-6 may also play a role in the pathogenesis of insulin-dependent diabetes mellitus. Murine pancreatic islet or rat insulinoma cells were found to produce IL-6 after their exposure to IFN-γ or TNF-α (Campbell *et al.*, 1989). On the basis of these data, it has been suggested that in addition to an effect on the pancreatic β-cell function, IL-6 produced by the pancreatic β-cell may also act as a co-stimulator for autoreactive B and T lymphocytes in autoimmune diabetes (Campbell *et al.*, 1989).

Despite the injuring activity of cytokines such as IL-1, IFN-γ and TNF-α on endocrine tissues in either autoimmune type I diabetes (Mandroup-Pulsen *et al.*, 1989) or in autoimmune thyroid diseases (Del Prete *et al.*, 1987, 1989a), the pathogenetic importance of IL-6 in these diseases, as well as that of other cytokines active on B cells, still remains to be proved.

Allergy and other pathological conditions characterized by hyperproduction of IgE

The IgE antibody system is among the most sophisticated of immune defence mechanisms. Although its specific function is still partially unknown, this system probably protects against offending agents coming from the respiratory and gastrointestinal tracts. IgE molecules bind specifically and avidly to receptors localized on the surface of tissue mast cells and circulating basophils, which are capable of producing and releasing several potent mediators via the interaction of the antigen with a small number of

IgE molecules. However, because of its complexity and unusual amplification power, the IgE antibody system is highly susceptible to perturbations resulting in exaggerated IgE production. The highest IgE levels (excluding IgE myelomas) have been found in patients with hyper-IgE (or Buckley's) syndrome, parasitic infestations, some primary or secondary immune deficiencies (such as Di George, Nezelof and Wiskott–Aldrich syndromes, Hodgkin's disease and AIDS) and in bone marrow transplanted patients during the acute phase of graft-versus-host-disease (GVHD). Finally, the human condition most commonly associated with increased IgE antibody production is atopy, the familial allergic disorder of immediate-type hypersensitivity to environmental allergens.

Regulatory mechanisms of IgE synthesis

IgE regulation by T cells and T cell-derived cytokines in experimental animals. Earlier studies in rodents suggested that IgE production could be regulated not only by antigen-specific helper and suppressor T cells, but also through isotype-specific factors showing affinity for IgE, the so-called IgE-binding factors (reviewed in Ishizaka and Ishizaka, 1989). More recently, a different pathway of IgE regulation essentially based on the reciprocal activity of IL-4 and IFN-γ, has been disclosed. LPS-stimulated spleen B cells (which usually produce IgM and IgG3) were induced to produce IgG1 and IgE in the presence of BSF-1/IL-4 (Coffman *et al.*, 1986), and such a phenomenon was inhibited by addition to the cultures of IFN-γ (Coffman and Carty, 1986). IL-4 stimulated IgE production has been shown to be due to isotype switching (Lebman and Coffman, 1989). The essential rôle of IL-4 and IFN-γ in regulating IgE synthesis in mice has been confirmed by *in vivo* studies. Injection of mice with an anti-IL-4 antibody completely suppressed polyclonal IgE production induced by treatment with anti-IgD antibody or infestation with *Nyppostrongilus brasiliensis* (NB), as well as primary antigen-specific IgE antibody responses (Finkelman *et al.*, 1986). In addition, it strongly reduced secondary antibody responses. *In vivo* injection of IFN-γ also resulted in the inhibition of IgE production (Finkelman *et al.*, 1988; Jardieu *et al.*, 1989).

T cell- and cytokine-mediated regulation of human IgE synthesis. Until recently, little was known of the mechanisms responsible for the control of human IgE synthesis since *in vivo* studies analogous to those performed in rodents are not feasible. In the last few years, however, information has emerged from *in vitro* studies performed in several laboratories, including my own.

Spontaneous and T cell clone-induced in vitro *IgE synthesis.* Initial attempts to induce the synthesis of IgE by signals delivered *in vitro* were unsuccessful. IgE synthesis was never detectable in cultures of MNC or purified B cells stimulated with different polyclonal B cell activators such as PWM, EBV or SAC (Romagnani *et al.*, 1980b; Sarjan *et al.*, 1983). Only PBL from a proportion of atopic patients, studied during or immediately after the allergen challenge, showed the ability to synthesize spontaneously detectable amounts of IgE *in vitro* (Fiser and Buckley, 1979; Tjio *et al.*, 1979; Romagnani *et al.*, 1980b). Cells spontaneously producing IgE were found to bear surface IgE but not surface IgM (Romagnani *et al.*, 1980c). By contrast, spontaneous or induced IgE synthesis was never detectable in cultures of normal B cells (Fiser and Buckley, 1979; Romagnani *et al.*, 1980b).

The first unambiguous demonstration of *in vitro* induced IgE synthesis in normal B cells was provided by the use of alloreactive human TTC (Romagnani *et al.*, 1983; Lanzavecchia and Parodi, 1984; Umetsu *et al.*, 1985; Ricci *et al.*, 1985). The alloreactive TCC used was able to induce synthesis of IgM, IgG, IgA and IgE in B cell cultures from either normal or atopic individuals provided that they shared the appropriate alloantigen (Romagnani *et al.*, 1983; Ricci *et al.*, 1985). Autoreactive TCCs also appeared to be capable of inducing IgE synthesis in B cells (Leung *et al.*, 1986).

In subsequent years, it was shown that a proportion of PHA-induced TCCs obtained from either tonsil or PBMNC from normal and atopic individuals, were able to support IgE synthesis by autologous or allogeneic normal B cells, regardless of their auto- or allo-antigen specificity (Del Prete *et al.*, 1986; Romagnani *et al.*, 1987). Addition of heterogeneous T cell populations to such cultures suppressed TCC-induced IgE synthesis, suggesting that some T cells were able to induce the synthesis of IgE in B cells, whereas other T cells delivered strong inhibitory signals for IgE synthesis (Romagnani *et al.*, 1987).

IL-4 and IFN-γ produced by TCCs reciprocally regulate in vitro *human IgE synthesis.* Attempts were then made to generate soluble factor(s) from TCCs which were able to induce or enhance IgE production. Upon stimulation with PHA or anti-CD3 antibody, supernatants of TCC selected for helper function for IgE synthesis were found to induce the production of IgE in both normal and atopic B cell enriched populations, whereas supernatants from TCC unable to provide helper function for IgE synthesis consistently failed to elicit or enhance production of IgE (Maggi *et al.*, 1987a, 1988b). Interestingly, the IgE helper activity of supernatants was strongly inhibited by addition of recombinant IFN-γ (Maggi *et al.*, 1987a, 1988a). Subsequently, many (109) PHA-induced CD4$^+$ TCCs were assessed for their ability to induce IgE synthesis by human B cells *in vitro*, and for

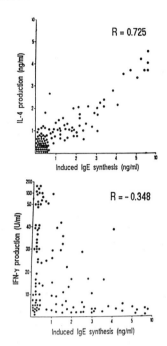

Figure 3 Ability of human TCCs to induce IgE synthesis vs. their secretion of IL-4 or IFN-γ. Each clone was stimulated with PHA and its supernatant assessed for the content of IL-4 and IFN-γ. T cell blasts were cultured for 10 days with B cells from two different donors and supernatants from these cultures assayed for their IgE content. Mean values from duplicate IL-4 or IFN-γ determinations were plotted against mean IgE values of duplicate determinations performed on B cell cultures from two different donors. (From Del Prete *et al.*, 1988).

ability to produce IL-2, IL-4 and IFN-γ following stimulation with PHA. A significant positive correlation between the ability to induce IgE synthesis and to secrete IL-4 was found (Del Prete *et al.*, 1988; Maggi *et al.*, 1988b) (Figure 3). In contrast, there was a significant inverse correlation between the IgE helper activity of TCCs and their ability to produce IFN-γ (Del Prete *et al.*, 1988; Maggi *et al.*, 1988b).

The ability to induce IgE synthesis in PB B cell-enriched suspensions by supernatants from 71 of these CD4$^+$ TCC was also investigated. Twenty-nine supernatants induced production of substantial amounts of IgE by target B cells. Again, there was a correlation between the amount of IgE synthesized by B cells in response to these supernatants and their IL-4 content (Del Prete *et al.*, 1988). An even higher correlation was found between the ability of these supernatants to induce IgE synthesis and the ratio between their IL-4 and IFN-γ content, providing additional evidence that IL-4 and IFN-γ had opposite regulatory effects on *in vitro* human IgE synthesis (Del Prete *et al.*, 1988). This was confirmed by testing the activity of human recombinant IL-4 and IFN-γ on cultures of PBMNC. Like IL-4 containing supernatants from TCC, recombinant IL-4 was found to induce the synthesis of IgE (Del Prete *et al.*, 1988; Pene *et al.*, 1988a), and this effect was inhibited by addition to the cultures of recombinant IFN-γ (Del Prete *et al.*, 1988; Pene *et al.*, 1988b) IFN-α or prostaglandin E2 (Pene *et al.*, 1988b). More importantly, an anti-IL-4 antibody virtually abolished not only the IgE synthesis induced by recombinant IL-4 but also that stimulated by active TCCs and their supernatants (Del Prete *et al.*, 1988). In contrast, the IgG synthesis induced by supernatants was not inhibited or was only slightly inhibited by addition to the cultures of anti-IL-4 antibody or IFN-γ (Del Prete *et al.*, 1988). Taken together, these data indicate that IL-4 and IFN-γ play a decisive (reciprocal) rôle in the regulation of IgE synthesis in humans as well as in mice.

A two signal model for in vitro *human IgE synthesis.* It was then necessary to ask whether IL-4 was a sufficient mediator for the induction of human IgE synthesis. Both recombinant IL-4 and IL-4 containing supernatants, which had been found to induce the synthesis of IgE in unfractionated MNC or B cell-enriched PB suspensions, were consistently ineffective when tested on highly purified tonsillar B cells containing less than 1% T lymphocytes and monocytes (Del Prete *et al.*, 1988). Production of IgE in response to IL-4 could be restored by re-addition of autologous or allogeneic T cells (Romagnani *et al.*, 1989b). Adherent cells alone (mainly monocytes) were unable to reconstitute IgE synthesis in purified B cells stimulated with IL-4, but they potentiated the IgE synthesis induced by IL-4 in the presence of appropriate concentrations of T lymphocytes (Romagnani *et al.*, 1989b). These data suggest that (i) the presence in culture of T cells is essential for IL-4 dependent IgE synthesis, and (ii) monocytes are able to potentiate the activity of IL-4.

How might T cells and monocytes collaborate with IL-4 in the induction of IgE synthesis? To answer this question, the effect of antibodies against different cytokines on IL-4 stimulated IgE synthesis was tested. Both anti-IL-2 and anti-IL-6 antibodies inhibited the synthesis of IgE, whereas anti-IL-1 antibody was usually without effect (Romagnani *et al.*, 1989b; Maggi *et al.*, 1989a). These results suggest that IL-2 and IL-6 collaborate with IL-4 in the induction of IgE synthesis. Other investigators have shown that endogenously produced IL-6 is essential for the synthesis of IgE (Vercelli *et al.*, 1989a), a finding that might explain the potentiating effect of monocytes in this response. Nevertheless, the fact that both IL-2 and IL-6 act on T and B cells makes it difficult to establish whether these cytokines act directly on

B cells, or merely increase the survival, or enhance the secretion of other cytokines by T cells. Several studies have been unable to reconstitute the synthesis of IgE in highly purified B cells with combinations of IL-4, IL-2 and IL-6 (Romagnani *et al.*, 1989b; Vercelli *et al.*, 1989b; Parronchi, 1990). This suggests that T cells and monocytes do not support the IL-4 dependent IgE synthesis merely by producing IL-2 and IL-6.

More direct demonstration that a physical interaction between T and B cells was needed for IL-4 dependent IgE synthesis to occur was provided by experiments using a double chamber assay. When T and B cells were cultured in different chambers separated by a millipore membrane permeable to molecules but not to cells, IL-4 was unable to induce the synthesis of IgE. In contrast, IgE synthesis occurred when T and B cells were cultured in the same chamber (Maggi *et al.*, 1989a; Parronchi *et al.*, 1990) (Figure 4). Kinetic studies then provided evidence that physical interaction with T cells was required by B cells prior to the signal delivered by IL-4. When B cells were cultured with IL-4 and the addition of T cells delayed until day 4 of culture, IgE synthesis did not occur. In contrast, when B cells were cultured with T cells from the beginning and IL-4 added to the culture after 4 days,

Culture condition in double chamber	IgE production (ng/ml)		
	Exp.1	Exp.2	Exp.3
IL-4 / B cells	< 0.3	0.4	0.3
IL-4 / B cells + T cells	6.5	10.7	2.4
T cells / B cells + IL-4	0.4	0.8	0.7
B cells / T cells + IL-4	0.3	0.7	0.4

Figure 4 Physical interaction between T and B cells is required for IL-4 dependent IgE synthesis. Highly purified tonsillar B cells were stimulated with IL-4 in the presence of autologous T cells cultured in the same or in a distinct compartment separated by a 0.4 μm membrane. After 10 days supernatants were collected and assayed for their IgE content.

IgE synthesis was unchanged or even enhanced (Parronchi *et al.*, 1990). These data suggest a two-signal model for the induction of *in vitro* human IgE synthesis: the first signal is provided to the B cells by a physical interaction with T cells, and the second signal is provided by T cell-derived IL-4. The essential rôle of LMW BCGF as additional (third) signal for IgE synthesis has also been claimed (DeKruyff *et al.*, 1989). However, using a recombinant molecule, this factor does not appear to be essential (unpublished results). Such a difference may be due to the fact that the above investigators made use of the commercial LMW BCGF preparation, rather than a recombinant molecule. IL-5 has also been shown to enhance IgE synthesis induced by suboptimal concentrations of IL-4 (Pene *et al.*, 1988b). However, IL-5 does not seem to play a critical rôle in induction of IgE synthesis *in vivo*: injection of anti-IL-5 antibody in mice infected with NB inhibited hypereosinophilia, but did not influence the synthesis of IgE (F. D. Finkelman, personal communication). Recently, it has been shown that infection of B cells with EBV in the presence of IL-4 can also enable B cells to produce IgE (Thyphronitis *et al.*, 1989). Such a mechanism of IgE synthesis induction might be operating *in vivo* in some pathological conditions, such as AIDS and Hodgkin's disease (see later).

Both cognate and non cognate T–B cell interaction can support IL-4 dependent in vitro *IgE synthesis.* It has been claimed that cognate interaction between T and B cells (recognition by the TCR of MHC class II antigens in association with self or foreign peptides) is absolutely required for IL-4 dependent IgE synthesis to occur (Vercelli *et al.*, 1989b). Several data obtained in the author's laboratory, however, do not substantiate this conclusion. First, the great majority, if not all, PHA-induced CD4$^+$ T cell clones were able to support the synthesis of IgE in B cells from randomly selected donors provided that exogenous IL-4 was added to the culture. Second, some CD8$^+$ TCCs, which do not bind MHC class II antigens, were also able to induce IgE secretion under the same experimental conditions. Additional evidence was provided by the use of an alloreactive TCC. This IL-4 secreting clone (TR46) induced the synthesis of IgE in B cells possessing the appropriate alloantigen (HLA-DR4). When DR4-positive B cells were irradiated, IgE synthesis no longer occurred, but it could be restored by addition of unirradiated DR4-negative B cells. Under each of these experimental conditions, IgE synthesis was consistently inhibited by addition to the cultures of either anti-IL-4 antibody, or IFN-γ (Table 2). Moreover, the TR46 TCC, in the presence of exogeneously added IL-4, enabled B cells from all donors tested to produce IgE, irrespective of whether they possessed the DR4 antigen (Romagnani *et al.*, 1989b; Parronchi *et al.*, 1990).

Table 2 Alloreactive TR46 TCC triggers bystander B cells to IgE synthesis in the presence of endogenous or exogenously added IL-4.

Stimulator B cells (DR 4,5)	Bystander B cells (DR 3,7)	DR4-specific TR46 TCC	Exogenous IL-4	IgE synthesis (ng ml^{-1})		
				Medium	IFN-γ	Anti-IL-4 antibody
+	−	+	−	11.0	1.3	2.5
−	+	+	−	<0.3	<0.3	<0.3
+**	+	+	−	5.0	0.6	0.8
+**	−	+	−	<0.3	<0.3	<0.3
−	+	+	+	7.5	1.2	0.9

** Irradiated.

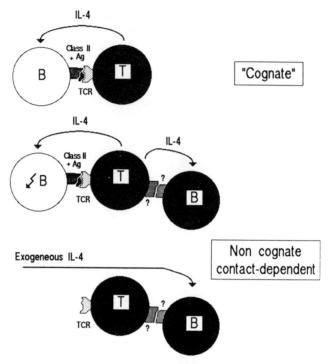

Figure 5 Schematic representation of three different ways by which physical interaction (both cognate and noncognate) between T and B cells in the presence of IL-4 can result in induction of *in vitro* IgE synthesis (see text for explanations).

Thus, at least three different ways can be identified by which *in vitro* human IgE synthesis can be induced (Figure 5):

(a) cognate interaction which involves both the T–B cell contact and production of IL-4,

(b) cognate interaction with irradiated B cells resulting in the production of IL-4 and non-cognate interactions between the IL-4 producing TCC and DR-unrelated B cells, and

(c) non-cognate interaction between the TCC and DR-unrelated B cells in the presence of exogenously added IL-4.

In the last two pathways, non-cognate interactions between T and B cells provides the first signal for IL-4 dependent IgE synthesis to occur. The latter possibility has recently been substantiated by experiments showing that thymocytes from murine EL4 thymoma are also able to support IgE synthesis in human B cells in the presence of phorbol myristate acetate

Table 3 EL-4 murine thyoma cells can support IL-4 dependent *in vitro* IgE synthesis by human B cells.[a]

EL-4	IL-4	PMA	IgE synthesis (ng ml^{-1} per 200 B cells)
−	−	−	<0.1
+	−	−	<0.1
−	+	−	<0.1
+	+	−	3.5
+	+	+	12.3
+(CysA)[a]	+	+	22.7

[a] EL4 cells were incubated overnight with cyclosporin A (CysA) and then extensively washed before adding to the cultures.

(PMA) and exogenously added IL-4 (Lundgren *et al.*, 1989). Similar results have been obtained in the author's laboratory, as well. As shown in Table 3, as few as 200 human B cells were able to produce detectable amounts of IgE in the presence of both 5×10^4 murine EL4 T cells and IL-4, and such production was further potentiated by addition of PMA to the culture, or by preincubation of T cells with PMA. Pre-treatment of EL4 cells with cyclosporin A (in order to inhibit release of cytokines) had no inhibitory effect, and in some cases enhanced IgE synthesis (Table 3).

Taken together, these data clearly show that cognate interactions are needed for production of endogenous IL-4 by T cells, but they may not be required for the first signal to B cells. Non cognate, contact-dependent, activation of the B cells can also function as an efficient signal for IL-4 dependent IgE synthesis (Romagnani *et al.*, 1989b; Parronchi *et al.*, 1990). This conclusion is consistent with recently reported findings showing that both MHC class II-restricted and MHC class II-unrestricted physical interaction with helper T cells can lead B cells into cell cycle, thus rendering them susceptible and responsive to the subsequent action of cytokines (Sekita *et al.*, 1988; Brian, 1988; Noelle *et al.*, 1989).

The nature of the molecule(s) responsible for non-specific physical interaction occurring between T and B cells is still obscure. Our experiments have shown that such a molecule is resistant to the treatment of cells with 0.05% paraformaldehyde, is distinct from the TCR/CD3 complex, but it is fully (and transiently) expressed on the membrane of TCR/CD3 activated T cells (Parronchi *et al.*, 1990).

The physiopathological implications of these findings are noteworthy. When a B cell presents antigen to T helper cells, cognate interactions provide the first signal to the B cell, and if the T cell is able to produce IL-4, but not inhibitory amounts of IFN-γ, production of antigen-specific IgE

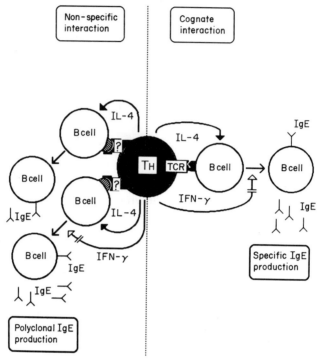

Figure 6 Schematic representation of the network of cellular and molecular interations leading to specific and polyclonal IgE production and its possible regulation. TH = helper T cell; TCR = T cell receptor. (From Romagnani, 1989a).

occurs. Other B cells, showing different antigen-specificity, present in the microenvironment can also respond to the physical non-specific signal by the activated T cell, and to the influence of T cell derived IL-4, thus being induced to produce IgE. This might explain why polyclonal IgE production occurs in some pathological conditions, such as parasitic infestations or the acute phase of GVHD (Romagnani *et al.*, 1989b) (Figure 6).

Possible rôle of the soluble FcεRII/CD23 antigen in IgE regulation. A still unsolved question is whether isotype-specific (IgE) factors similar to those described in rodents (Ishizaka and Ishizaka, 1989) play some additional rôle in regulation of human IgE synthesis. It has been hypothesized that the so-called soluble CD23/FcεRII or Blast 2 antigen (see chapter 8) is involved in the regulation of human IgE synthesis. However, the demonstration that HTLV-1-infected, but not normal, T cells express mRNA for FcεRII (Kikutani *et al.*, 1986) argues against the possibility of a T cell mediated isotype-specific (IgE) regulation. Since supernatants from FcεRII-positive cells or semi-purified soluble CD23, enhance IgE synthesis (Sarfati *et al.*, 1984), while anti-CD23 antibodies inhibit both IL-4 induced and spontaneous *in vitro* IgE synthesis (Sarfati and Delespesse, 1988), it has been suggested that IL-4 (a strong inducer of the FcεRII/CD23 antigen on B cells) exerts its IgE-inducing activity through the release of the sCD23/FcεRII by B cells (Delespesse *et al.*, 1989). However, the addition of affinity-purified FcεRII fragments or anti-FcεRII antibody does not affect the IL-4 induced IgE synthesis in mice (Keegan *et al.*, 1989). In addition, human recombinant sCD23, although displaying low affinity for IgE, does not display B cell growth promoting activity (Uchibayashi *et al.*, 1989) and does not significantly influence the IL-4 dependent human IgE synthesis (T. Kishimoto, personal communication).

Cytokine release by mast cells: a possible new pathway of IgE regulation. It has been known for many years that mast cells play a central rôle in IgE-mediated diseases. The binding of IgE to the high affinity or type I receptor for IgE (FcεRI) on mast cells and basophils enables these cells to react specifically with allergens. Such contact leads to the activation of mast cells and to the release of histamine and other pharmacological mediators, causing immediate hypersensitivity and acute inflammatory reactions, accompanied by the development of allergic symptoms.

Recently, it has been shown that murine mast cell lines can release cytokines such as IL-1, IL-3, GM-CSF, IL-4, IL-5 and IL-6, following FcεRI-activation (Plaut *et al.*, 1989; Wodnar-Filipowicz *et al.*, 1989). In addition, non-T, non-B cells isolated from bone marrow, spleen and peritoneal exudate of mice infested with NB were able to produce IL-4 in response to stimulation with complexed IgE (Le Gros *et al.*, 1989). These data suggest that mast cells and perhaps some myeloid precursors may play a far more important part in allergic and immune responses than has been assumed so far.

Disregulation of cytokine production in disorders characterized by hyperproduction of IgE

The mechanisms that regulate *in vitro* human IgE synthesis may be involved in the pathogenesis of human diseases characterized by hyperproduction of IgE. Some promising results have recently been obtained in patients with hyper-IgE syndrome, parasitic infestations, vernal conjunctivitis or common atopic diseases.

Hyper-IgE syndrome. Patients with the hyper-IgE (or Buckley's) syndrome have recurrent severe infections secondary to *Staphylococcus aureus*, or to other bacteria or fungi, and a history of pruritic dermatitis earlier in life

Table 4   Reduced proportions of TCCs able to produce IFN-γ and TNF-α in PB of patients with the hyper-IgE syndrome.

Subjects	No. of CD4$^+$ TCCs tested	No. of TCCs producing:		
		IFN-γ	TNF-α	IL-4
Hyper-IgE syndrome (4)	142	15 (11%)[a]	19 (15%)[b]	68 (48%)
Healthy controls (8)	294	159 (54%)[a]	141 (48%)[b]	118 (40%)

[a] $= P < 0.0005$.
[b] $= P < 0.0005$.

(Buckley *et al.*, 1972). Laboratory findings include exceedingly high serum IgE, depressed delayed-type cutaneous hypersensitivity (DCH), lymphocyte proliferation to recall antigens, altered chemotaxis of neutrophils and monocytes, and deficient T cell suppressor activity (Buckley *et al.*, 1972; Buckley and Becker, 1978). However, the nature of defect(s) responsible for these abnormalities is still unclear. We have recently examined the ability of circulating T cells from four children with the hyper-IgE syndrome to produce different cytokines in response to stimulation with PHA. MNC from all four children produced significantly lower concentrations of IFN-γ than did MNC from eight age-matched healthy controls. Clonal analysis revealed that patients with the hyper-IgE syndrome had markedly lower proportions of circulating T cells able to produce IFN-γ and TNF-α in comparison with controls (Romagnani *et al.*, 1989c; Del Prete *et al.*, 1990) (Table 4). All the four patients with hyper-IgE syndrome showed high proportions of circulating CD4$^+$ T helper cells able to induce IgE synthesis in allogenic B cells. Such helper activity for IgE synthesis appeared to be positively correlated with IL-4 production by T cells and inversely related to the ability of the same T cells to produce IFN-γ (Romagnani *et al.*, 1989b; Del Prete *et al.*, 1990). Since IFN-γ inhibits IgE synthesis and both IFN-γ and TNF-α play an important rôle in cell-mediated immune reactions, it can reasonably be suggested that the defective production of IFN-γ is responsible for hyperproduction of IgE, and that the combined defect of IFN-γ and TNF-α may contribute to the undue susceptibility of patients with hyper-IgE syndrome to infections. Indeed it has recently been reported that *in vivo* injection of IFN-γ (Leung *et al.*, 1989) or IFN-α (Souillet *et al.*, 1989) dramatically reduces serum IgE levels and results in improvement of clinical manifestations in such patients.

AIDS and Hodgkin's disease (HD). Elevated IgE levels have been detected in the serum of a proportion of patients with HD (Romagnani *et al.*, 1980a) or AIDS (Maggi *et al.*, 1989b). Most AIDS patients with elevated IgE levels showed the presence in their serum of IgE specific for uncommon allergens, such as *Candida albicans*, *Penicillium fumigatus* and other fungal antigens (Maggi *et al.*, 1989b). Frequent occurrence of drug hypersensitivity and exacerbation of clinical manifestations in AIDS patients with a previous history of atopy have also been reported (Parkin *et al.*, 1987; Pedersen *et al.*, 1987). The significance of these findings, as well as the mechanisms possibly responsible for IgE hyperproduction in such diseases, are at present unknown. Lymphocytes of some HIV-infected individuals have been found to produce IgE-binding factors (Carini *et al.*, 1988), but the role of these factors in regulating human IgE synthesis is controversial.

Among residual circulating CD4$^+$ T cells from most patients with AIDS, a strong reduction in the proportion of TCCs able to produce IFN-γ has been found (Maggi *et al.*, 1987b). More recently my colleagues and I have evaluated the frequency of CD4$^+$ TCCs able to produce IL-2, IL-4 and IFN-γ in the PB of some AIDS patients showing high levels of serum IgE. The proportion of IL-2 and IL-4 producing TCCs appeared normal in contrast to the reduced proportion of IFN-γ producing TCCs (data not shown). Such an imbalance between IL-4 and IFN-γ production may explain why production of IgE in response to different environmental antigens, such as those derived from fungi, can easily occur in patients with AIDS.

On the other hand, it is well known that EBV infection is very common in patients with AIDS. Since EBV infection in the presence of IL-4 leads human B cells to synthesize IgE (Thyphronitis *et al.*, 1989), both EBV infection and the reduced proportion of IFN-γ producing T cells (due to the cytolytic activity of HIV) may contribute to the IgE hyperproduction seen in a proportion of patients with AIDS.

The latter mechanism (EBV infection) may be operating in patients with HD, as well. EBV in episomal form has recently been documented in Reed–Sternberg (R–S) cells from some patients with HD (Boiocchi *et al.*, 1989; Weyss *et al.*, 1989). These findings suggest that, at least in some HD patients, R–S represents a monoclonal B cell and EBV probably plays an aetiopathogenic role in such disease. It will be of interest to establish whether patients with HD showing EBV in their R–S cells display the same high levels of serum IgE. Spontaneous IgE-producing cells have been detected in mesenteric lymph nodes histologically involved in HD, whose activity was strongly reduced or abolished by radiation therapy (unpublished data). On the other hand, it is well known that R–S cells are often in strict physical association and sometimes form rosettes with CD4$^+$ T cells in involved tissues (Poppema *et al.*, 1979). Thus, the EBV-infected R–S cells themselves, following association with IL-4 producing but not IFN-γ producing CD4$^+$ T cells in involved tissues, may be the source of IgE in such patients.

GVHD. Strong elevations in serum IgE levels were unexpectedly found during the acute phase of GVHD in bone-marrow transplanted patients (Ringden *et al.*, 1983) and attributed to impairment in the function of suppressor T cells (Ringden *et al.*, 1983). Interestingly, increased serum levels of soluble FcεRII/CD23 antigen (which is induced/enhanced by IL-4) have recently been reported to precede the increase in IgE levels in serum of autologous bone marrow-transplanted patients (J. Gordon, personal communication). In addition, IL-4 has recently been found to be the main mediator of chronic GVHD in mice, which in some aspects resembles both AIDS and HD. In these animals, GVHD is associated with a two- to four-fold increase in the expression of Ia antigens on B cells and a 30- to 400-fold increase in IgE serum levels. These changes are associated with the appearance of an IL-4 like activity in culture supernatants of GVHD spleen cells, which can be prevented by *in vivo* administration of an anti-IL-4 antibody during the first 12 days after GVHD induction (Doutrelepont *et al.*, 1989). These results suggest that increased production of IL-4 may be responsible for IgE hyperproduction associated with GVHD.

Vernal conjunctivitis (*VC*). This is a seasonally recurrent, bilateral inflammation of the conjunctiva, It is distinguished by cobblestone papillae, usually on the tarsal conjunctiva (Figure 7) and by a papillary hypertrophy,

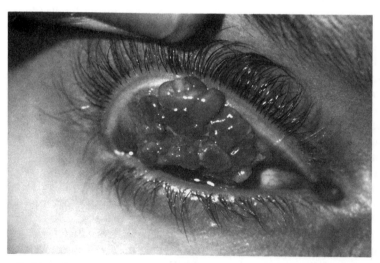

Figure 7 Vernal conjunctivitis showing typical "cobblestone" papillary hypertrophy on everted superior tarsal plate, from which CD4[+] T cells were isolated and TCCs established.

discrete or confluent, on the limbal conjunctiva. Histologic examination reveals infiltration in the substantia propria of lymphocytes, plasma cells, basophils, mast cells and, especially, eosinophils. Elevated levels of IgE are usually present both in serum and tears from these patients. An allergic aetiology has been suggested, but little is known about its specific pathogenesis (Friedlaender, 1985).

My colleagues and I have recently established TCCs from cell suspensions of conjunctival biopsies of three children with VC and then studied their helper activity for IgE synthesis, as well as their ability to produce cytokines. The results of these experiments are summarized in Table 5. Unusually high proportions of CD4$^+$ TCCs showing helper function for IgE synthesis and the ability to produce IL-4 were obtained from the conjunctival infiltrates of all the three patients. In contrast, only very few CD4$^+$ TCCs had the ability to produce IFN-γ, and the majority of them failed to produce this cytokine even when subject to maximal stimulation with PMA plus anti-CD3 anti-

Table 5 Reduced ability of TCCs established from suspensions of biopsies of patients with vernal conjunctivitis to produce IFN-γ.

	IFN-γ (U ml^{-1})		IL-4 (pg ml^{-1})	
TCC	PHA	PMA + anti-CD3	PHA	PMA + anti-CD3
Conjunctival infiltrate				
1	<10	<10	1,230	3,700
2	<10	<10	<200	n.d.
3	<10	15	260	20,000
6	<10	<10	<200	1,060
9	<10	<10	2,550	20,000
10	<10	<10	240	920
11	<10	<10	<200	20,000
12	<10	18	680	20,000
13	<10	<10	550	20,000
Control[a]				
1	36	136	520	1,560
2	10	144	<200	<200
3	57	156	250	820
4	30	154	<200	<200
5	18	80	1,050	12,000
6	25	195	2,200	20,000

[a]Control TCCs were contemporarily established from PB suspensions of the same patient.

body (Table 5). These data indicate that selective accumulation of TH_2-type TCCs occurs in the conjunctiva of patients with VC, suggesting their possible rôle in the pathogenesis of lesions. Interestingly, VC is often associated with hyper-IgE syndrome (Butrus et al., 1984), where similar alterations of the helper T cell profile in PB were found (see above). More importantly, eye alterations resembling those of VC have recently been observed in mice transfected with murine IL-4 (R. Tepper, personal communication). Thus, abnormal T cell subsets showing the ability to produce IL-4 but not IFN-γ seem to play an important role in the pathogenesis of VC.

Parasitic infestations. It has been known for many years that parasites induce marked production of IgE in infested animals. Interestingly, most IgE produced in response to parasite infestation are not directed against parasite antigens. Parasite-specific IgE proteins play an important role in the defence against parasites by arming eosinophils, macrophages and platelets, for antibody-dependent cell cytotoxicity (ADCC) against parasites (Capron et al., 1980). The mechanisms by which parasites stimulate IgE production in infested hosts are still largely unknown. Filarial parasite-specific T cell lines secrete soluble factors able to induce IgE synthesis in normal B cells (Nutman et al., 1985), but the nature of such factors has not been investigated. More recently, it has been reported that mesenteric lymph nodes from mice infested with NB contain significantly higher proportions of IL-4 producing and significantly lower proportions of IFN-γ producing, T cells (T. Mosmann, personal communication). In addition, my colleagues and I have found that MNC from patients with filariasis spontaneously release detectable amounts of IL-4, whereas MNC from control subjects do not (unpublished results).

On the basis of these latter results, TCCs were established from PB of two patients with filariasis and one patient with toxocariasis, by PHA stimulation of single PB T cells. One hundred and fifteen CD4$^+$ TCCs from patients were then compared with 373 CD4$^+$ TCCs established from 10 controls for their ability to produce IL-4 and IFN-γ in response to PHA-stimulation. Patients infested by parasites showed significantly higher proportions of IL-4 producing and significantly reduced proportions of IFN-γ producing CD4$^+$ TCCs in comparison with controls (Table 6). Supernatants from two out of six IL-4 producing TCCs also induced selective differentiation of eosinophil colonies from bone marrow precursors (R. Ackerman, personal communication), suggesting that they were probably able to produce IL-5 as well. Taken together, these data suggest that parasites can stimulate specific subsets of helper T cells and/or alter the potential of helper T lymphocytes to produce/secrete cytokines. Following parasite infestation, the secretion of

Table 6 Increased proportions of IL-4- and decreased proportions of IFN-γ-producing TCCs in PB of patients with parasitic infestations.[a]

Diagnosis	No. of CD4$^+$ TCCs tested[b]	No. of TCCS producing:	
		IL-4	IFN-γ
Parasitic infestation (3)	115	67 (58%)[c]	42 (36%)[d]
Normal subjects (10)	373	138 (37%)[c]	214 (57%)[d]

[a] Two patients with filariasis and one patient with toxocariasis.
[b] TCCs were established with a high efficiency cloning technique (Moretta *et al.*, 1983).
[c] & [d] Differences were statistically significant.

cytokines such as IFN-γ is markedly inhibited, whereas the capacity to secrete IL-4 is greatly augmented. The mechanisms by which parasites induce such alterations in helper T cells is still unclear.

Atopic diseases. Patients with common atopic diseases also show increased production of IgE, but this is usually limited to antibodies specific for environmental allergens, such as those derived from pollens, house dust mites, pets or fungal spores. The reason why allergens preferentially induce production of IgE is unknown. Antibody responses against minute amounts of purified antigens appear to be under the control of MHC class II (*Ir*) genes (Marsh *et al.*, 1981). Several significant associations have been observed between particular HLA haplotypes and responsiveness toward different purified allergens (HLA-DR2/Dw2 in the case of Amb V and DR3/Dw3 for the Lo1 p molecules) (Marsh *et al.*, 1982; Freidhoff *et al.*, 1988). To date, there is no molecular evidence for regarding allergens as a unique subset of antigens; the key issues in allergy seem to relate to the genetic make-up of the individual. The reason why B cells in individuals genetically determined to recognize allergenic epitopes switch to IgE synthesis remains unclear. One possibility is that allergens differ from other antigens in their ability to "select" T helper cells with a particular profile of cytokine production. To explore such a possibility, my colleagues and I have recently established *Dermatophagoides pteronyssinus* (DP) and tetanus toxoid (TT) specific TCCs from PB T cells of one atopic donor showing both mite-allergy and DCH to TT (Figure 8). A total number of 25 TT- and 17 DP-specific TCCs were obtained and assessed for their ability to produce IL-4 and IFN-γ in response to stimulation by PMA plus anti-CD3 antibody or by the specific antigen, as well as their ability to provide helper function for IgE synthesis by autologous B cells in the presence of the same antigen.

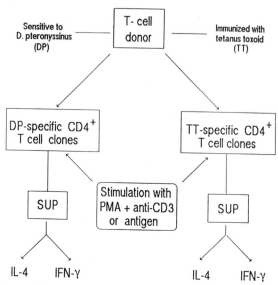

Figure 8 Schematic representation of the experimental approach used to assess the functional capability of DP- and TT-specific TCCs established from one individual showing both immediate-type hypersensitivity to DP and DCH to TT. SUP = supernatant.

Virtually all TT-specific TCCs produced both IL-4 and IFN-γ in response to PMA plus anti-CD3 antibody. The great majority of DP-specific TCCs also produced IL-4, but five out of 17 DP-specific TCCs (30%) failed to produce IFN-γ in response to the same stimuli (Table 7). When assayed with the specific antigen, the great majority of TT-specific TCCs (86%) still produced IFN-γ with or without production of IL-4, whereas only 37% of DP-specific TCCs displayed this ability. The majority of these TCCs (63%) produced IL-4 but not IFN-γ in response to DP (Table 7). All but one of these DP-specific T cell clones were able to induce the synthesis of IgE in autologous B cells following stimulation with DP (Table 8), whereas only two out of six TT-specific T cell clones were able to induce the synthesis of IgE in autologous B cells following TT-stimulation (data not shown). These data indicate that in a given (atopic) individual DP-specific T cells have a higher probability of belonging to the T$_{H2}$-like helper T cell subset than TT-specific TCCs. If confirmed with other allergens, this feature might explain why allergens induce production of IgE more easily than other antigenic molecules.

The mechanisms responsible for the apparent selection of T$_{H2}$-like cells by allergenic determinants is at present unclear.

Table 7 Profile of cytokine production following stimulation with PMA plus anti-CD3 antibody or with the specific antigen by DP- or TT-specific TCCs established from the same donor.

Antigen-specificity of TCCs	No. of TCCs	Stimulation with PMA plus anti-CD3 antibody			Stimulation with the specific antigen		
		IFN-γ[a]	IL-4[b]	IFN-γ + IL-4	IFN-γ	IL-4	IFN-γ + IL-4
TT	26	1	1	24	6	3	14
DP	17	0	5	12	1	5	2

[a]Values higher than 10 U ml^{-1}.
[b]Values higher than 200 pg ml^{-1}.

Table 8 Induction of IgE synthesis by DP-specific TCCs following stimulation with DP.

TCC	Cytokine production		IgE synthesis (ng ml^{-1})
	IL-4 (pg ml^{-1})	IFN-γ (U ml^{-1})	
None			0.5
DP47	790	<10	2.3
DP35	325	<10	4.1
DP18	435	<10	3.3
DP10	5,170	15	0.4
DP14	3,220	<10	15.0
DPA/21	4,125	<10	9.8

Whether atopic subjects are equipped with higher numbers of these allergen-specific T helper cells, showing such a peculiar profile of cytokine production, than non-atopics remains to be established. However, recent findings support such a possibility. DP-specific activation of DP-specific TCCs obtained from one non-atopic donor resulted in considerable production of IFN-γ and low production of IL-4, in sharp contrast to DP-specific TCCs from one atopic donor which showed relatively high production of IL-4 and low or undetectable production of IFN-γ (Wierenga *et al.*, 1989).

Concluding remarks

Evidence is accumulating to suggest that B cell tropic cytokines play a rôle in the pathogenesis of some human diseases, including immune deficiencies, autoimmune diseases and allergic disorders. At least in some patients with CVH, impaired function of, and/or response to, cytokines may be responsible for the immune defects. Increased production of IL-6 by HIV-infected macrophages may contribute to the enhanced antibody formation in patients with AIDS. Excessive IL-6 production may also account for the local, and several of the generalized, symptoms in patients with RA, including fever, production of APP and hypergammaglobulinaemia. B cell hyperactivity leading to enhanced antibody and autoantibody formation in patients with SLE or other systemic and organ-specific autoimmune disorders is probably associated with states of hyperfunction of some cytokine/cytokine receptor systems, such as IL-2, IL-4, IL-5 and IL-6. However, our understanding of the rôle and degree of cytokine alterations in such diseases is still very poor.

More clear and detailed evidence suggests a role for cytokine alterations in allergy and in other pathological conditions characterized by hyperproduction of IgE. It is well established that IL-4 and IFN-γ are the main regulatory cytokines of IgE production, with opposite effects on the synthesis of this Ig class. An imbalance (in favour of IL-4) in the production of these two cytokines seems to be responsible for polyclonal IgE synthesis in parasitic infestations and in the hyper-IgE syndrome, where reduced production of IFN-γ (and of TNF-α) may explain depression of DTH and undue susceptibility to infections. Preliminary *in vivo* findings suggest that administration of IFN-γ (or IFN-α) in patients with the hyper-IgE syndrome or severe atopic dermatitis results in dramatic reduction of serum IgE levels, as well as improvement of clinical manifestations. An altered balance between IL-4 and IFN-γ production in favour of IL-4 probably plays a role in the pathogenesis of VC, as well. CD4$^+$ T cells present in conjunctival infiltrates of these patients are indeed unable to produce IFN-γ, whereas all produce IL-4 and provide helper function for IgE synthesis. Finally, preliminary observations suggest that allergens may differ at least in part from other antigenic molecules for their ability in atopic donors to "select" TH cells inducible to relatively high production of IL-4 and low or undetectable production of IFN-γ. It is reasonable to suggest that accumulation of TH cells with peculiar profiles of cytokine production in target organs, and "selection" by allergens of TH cells with peculiar patterns of cytokine production, may be at least partly responsible for IgE-mediated disorders.

A detailed analysis of the therapeutical potential of B cell-tropic cytokines is now a major research priority. Indeed, not only may the cytokines be useful *in vivo*, but antibodies against them or their receptors may also have a therapeutic potential in some immunodeficiency syndromes, autoimmune diseases and hypersensitivity states. These cytokines are ushering in new and exciting possibilities for the investigation, diagnosis and treatment of many hitherto untreatable conditions. Over the next few years major progress both in the laboratory and in the clinic is anticipated.

Acknowledgements

The experiments reported in this chapter have been performed by funds from CNR (Finalized Project 'Oncology'), AIRC and Ministry of Health (AIDS project). I thank my coworkers Drs A. Alessi, F. Almerigogna, P. Biswas, R. Biagiotti, M. De Carli, G. F. Del Prete, L. Emmi, M. G. Giudizi, D. Macchia, E. Maggi, M. Mazzetti, P. Parronchi, A. Ravina, C. Simonelli, L. Stendardi and A. Tiri, whose contributions have been essential in the experiments here reported. I also wish to thank Professor M. Ricci for suggestions and helpful discussion; Drs J. Banchereau (Unicet, Dardilly), J. de Vries (DNAX, Palo Alto) and S. Gillis (Immunex, Seattle) for the generous gift of human recombinant IL-4 and anti-IL-4 antibody; Dr P. Falagiani (Lofarma, Milano) for the generous gift of *Dermatophagoides pteronyssinus* extract; Istituto Sieroterapico Sclavo (Siena) for the generous gift of tetanus toxoid.

References

Altman, A., Theofilopoulos, A., Weiner, R., Katz, D. A. and Dixon, F. J. (1981) *J. Exp. Med.* **154**, 791–808.

Alvaro-Gracia, J. M., Zvaifler, N. J. and Firestein, G. S. (1989) *J. Exp. Med.* **170**, 865–875.

Bhardwaj, N., Santhanam, U., Lau, L. L., Tatter, S. B., Ghrayeb, J., Rivelis, M., Steinman, R. M., Seghal, P. B. and May, L. T. (1989) *J. Immunol.* **143**, 2153–2159.

Blaese, R. M., Grayson, I. and Steinberg, A. D. (1980) *Am. J. Med.* **69**, 345–350.

Boiocchi, M., Carbone, A., De Re, V. and Dolcetti, R. (1989) *Tumori* **75**, 345–350.

Brian, A. (1988) *Proc. Natl. Acad. Sci. USA* **85**, 564–568.

Buchan, G., Barrett, K., Turner, M., Chantry, D., Maini, R. M. and Feldmann, M. (1988) *Clin. Exp. Immunol.* **73**, 449–455.

Buckley, R. H., Wray, B. B. and Belmaker, E. Z. (1972) *Pediatrics* **49**, 59–70.

Buckley, R. H. and Becker, W. G. (1978) *Immunol. Rev.* **41**, 288–314.

Butrus, S. I., Lleung, D. Y. M., Gelleis, S., Baum, J., Kenyon, K. R. and Abelson, M. B. (1984) *Ophthalmology* **91**, 1213–1216.

Campbell, I. L., Cutri, A., Wilson, A. and Harrison, L. C. (1989) *J. Immunol.* **143**, 1188–1191.

Capron, A., Capron, M. and Dessaint, J-P. (1980) *Immunology 80* (Eds M. Fougereau and J. Dausset), pp. 782–793. Academic Press, London.

Carini, C., Margolick, J., Yodoi, J. and Ishizaka, K. (1988) *Proc. Natl. Acad. Sci. USA* **85**, 9214–9218.

Clutterbuck, E. J., Shields, J., Gordon, J., Smith, S. H., Boyd, A., Callard, R. E., Campbell, H. D., Young, H. D. and Sanderson, C. J. (1987) *Eur. J. Immunol.* **17**, 1743–1750.

Coffman, R. L. and Carty, J. (1986) *J. Immunol.* **136**, 949–954.

Coffman, R. L., Ohara, J., Bond, M. W., Carty, J., Zlotnik, A. and Paul, W. E. (1986) *J. Immunol.* **136**, 4538–4541.

DeKruyff, R. H., Turner, T., Abrams, J. S., Palladino, M. A. and Umetsu, D. T. (1989) *J. Exp. Med.* **170**, 1477–1493.

Delespesse, G., Sarfati, M. and Peleman, R. (1989) *J. Immunol.* **142**, 134–138.

Del Prete, G. F., Maggi, E., Macchia, D., Tiri, A., Parronchi, P., Ricci, M. and Romagnani, S. (1986) *Eur. J. Immunol.* **16**, 1509–1514.

Del Prete, G. F., Tiri, A., Mariotti, S., Pinchera, A., Ricci, M. and Romagnani, S. (1987) *Clin. Exp. Immunol.* **69**, 323–331.

Del Prete, G. F., Maggi, E., Parronchi, P., Chretien, I., Tiri, A., Macchia, D.,

Ricci, M., Banchereau J., de Vries, J. and Romagnani, S. (1988) *J. Immunol.* **140**, 4193–4198.

Del Prete, G. F., Tiri, A., De Carli, M., Mariotti, S., Pinchera, A., Chretien, I., Romagnani, S. and Ricci, M. (1980a) *Autoimmunity* **4**, 267–276.

Del Prete, G. F., Tiri, A., Maggi, E., De Carli, M., Macchia, D., Parronchi, P., Rossi, M. E., Pietrogrande, M. C., Ricci, M. and Romagnani, S. (1989b) *J. Clin. Invest.* **84**, 1830–1835.

Doutrelepont, J-M., Moser, M., Abramowicz, D., Lambert, P., Vanderhaeghen, M-L., Urbain, J., Leo, O. and Goldman, M. (1989) *Seventh International Congress of Immunology Berlin*, p.643. G. Fischer, Stuttgart, New York.

Farrant, J., Bryant, A., Almandoz, F., Spickett, G., Evans, S. W. and Webster, A. D. B. (1989) *Clin. Immunol. Immunopathol.* **51**, 196–204.

Fauci, A. S. (1988) *Science* **239**, 617–622.

Fava, R., Olsen, N., Keski-Oja, J., Moses, H. and Pincus, T. (1989) *J. Exp. Med.* **169**, 291–296.

Finkelman, F. D., Katona, I. M., Urban, J. F., Snapper, C. M., Ohara, J. and Paul, W. E. (1986) *Proc. Natl. Acad. Sci. USA* **83**, 9675–9678.

Finkelman, F. D., Katona, I. M., Mosmann, T. M. and Coffman, R. L. (1988) *J. Immunol.* **140**, 1022–1027.

Fiser, P. M. and Buckley, R. H. (1979) *J. Immunol.* **123**, 1788–1794.

Freidhoff, L. R., Kautzky, E. E., Mayer, D. A., Hsu, S. H., Bias, W. B. and Marsh, D. G. (1988) *Tissue Antigens* **31**, 211–219.

Friedlaender, M. H. (1985) *J. Allergy Clin. Immunol.* **76**, 645–657.

Gauldie, J., Richards, C., Harnish, D., Lansdorp, P. and Baumann, H. (1987) *Proc. Natl. Acad. Sci. USA* **84**, 7251–7255.

Gitter, B. D., Lebus, J. M., Lees, S. L. and Scheetz, M. E. (1989) *Immunology* **66**, 196–200.

Guerne, P-A., Zuraw, B. L., Vaughan, J. H., Crason, D. A. and Lotz, M. (1989) *J. Clin. Invest.* **83**, 585–592.

Harigai, M., Hara, M., Norioka, K., Kitani, A., Hirose, T., Suzuki, K., Kawakami, M., Masuda, K., Shinmei, M., Kawagoe, M. and Nakamura, H. (1989) *Scand. J. Immunol.* **29**, 289–297.

Herron, L. R., Coffman, R. L. and Kotzin, B. L. (1988) *Clin. Immunol. Immunopathol.* **46**, 314–327.

Hirano, T. and Kishimoto, T. (1989) *Res. Clin. Lab.* **19**, 1–10.

Hirano, T., Taga, T., Nakano, N., Yasukawa, K., Kasjiwamura, S., Shimizu, K., Nakajima, K., Pyun, K. H. and Kishimoto, T. (1985) *Proc. Natl. Acad. Sci. USA* **82**, 5490–5494.

Hirano, T., Yasukawa, K., Harada, H., Taga, T., Watanabe, Y., Matsuda, T., Kashiwamura, S., Nakajima, K., Koyama, K., Iwamutu, A., Tsunasawa, S., Sakiyama, F., Matsui, H., Takahara, Y., Taniguchi, T. and Kishimoto, T. (1986) *Nature* **324**, 73–76.

Hirano, T., Taga, T., Yasukawa, K., Nakajima, K., Nakano, N., Takatsuki, F., Shimizu, M., Murashima, A., Tsunasawa, S., Sakiyama, F. and Kishimoto, T. (1987) *Proc. Natl. Acad. Sci. USA* **84**, 228–231.

Hirano, T., Matsuda, T., Turner, M., Miyasaka, N., Buchan, G., Tang, B., Sato, K., Shimizu, M., Maini, R., Feldmann, M. and Kishimoto, T. (1988) *Eur. J. Immunol.* **18**, 1797–1801.

Houssiau, F. A., Devogealer, J-P., Van Damme, J., Nagant de Deuxchaisnes, C. and Van Snick, J. (1988) *Arthr. Rheum.* **31**, 784–788.

Huang, Y-P., Perrin, L. H., Miescher, P. A. and Zubler, R. H. (1988) *J. Immunol.* **141**, 827–833.

Ishizaka, K. and Ishizaka, T. (1989) In *Fundamental Immunology*, 2nd edition (Ed. W. E. Paul), pp. 867–888. Raven Press, New York.

Jardieu, P., Thomsen, K. and Holmes, R. (1989) *Faseb J.* **3**, 967 (abstr.).

Keegan, A. D., Snapper, C. M., Van Dusen, R., Paul, W. E. and Conrad, D. H. (1989) *J. Immunol.* **142**, 3868–3874.

Kehrl, J. H., Miller, A. and Fauci, A. S. (1987) *J. Exp. Med.* **166**, 786–791.

Kikutani, H., Inui, S., Sato, R., Barsumian, E. L., Owaki, H., Yamasaki, K., Kaisho, T., Uchibayashi, N., Hardy, R. R., Hirano, T., Tsunasawa, S., Sakiyama, F., Suemura, M. and Kishimoto, T. (1986) *Cell* **47**, 657–665.

Kitani, A., Hara, M., Hirose, T., Norioka, K., Harigai, M., Hirose, W., Suzuki, K., Kawakami, M., Kawagoe, M. and Nakamura, H. (1989) *Clin. Exp. Immunol.* **77**, 31–36.

Kroemer, G. and Wick, G. (1989) *Immunol. Today* **10**, 246–251.

Lane, H. C., Masur, H., Edgar, L. C., Whalen, G., Rook, A. H. and Fauci, A. S. (1983) *N. Engl. J. Med.* **309**, 453–458.

Lanzavecchia, A. and Parodi, B. (1984) *Clin. Exp. Immunol.* **55**, 197–203.

Lebman, D. A. and Coffman, R. L. (1988) *J. Exp. Med.* **168**, 853–862.

Le Gros, G., Ben-Sasson, S. Z., Conrad, D., Finkelman, F. D. and Paul, W. E. (1989) *Seventh International Congress of Immunology, Abstracts*, p. 466. G. Fischer, Stuttgart, New York.

Lehmann, K. R., Kotzin, B. L., Portanova, J. P. and Santoro, T. J. (1986) *Eur. J. Immunol.* **16**, 1105–1110.

Leung, D. Y. M., Young, M. C. and Geha, R. S. (1986) *J. Immunol.* **136**, 2851–2857.

Leung, D. Y. M., Boguniewicz, M., Vercelli, D., Jabara, H. and Geha, R. S. (1989) *Clin. Research* **37**, 239a (abstr.).

Linker-Israeli, M., Bakke, A. C., Kitridou, R. C., Gendler, S., Gillis, S. and Horwitz, D. A. (1983) *J. Immunol.* **130**, 2651–2655.

Lundgren, M., Persson, U., Larsson, P., Magnusson, C., Edvard Smith, C. I., Hammarstrom, L. and Severinsson, E. (1989) *Eur. J. Immunol.* **19**, 1311–1315.

Maggi, E., Del Prete, G. F., Tiri, A., Macchia, D., Parronchi, P., Ricci, M. and Romagnani, S. (1987a) *Res. Clin. Lab.* **17**, 363–367.

Maggi, E., Macchia, D., Parronchi, P., Mazzetti, M., Ravina, A., Milo, D. and Romagnani, S. (1987b) *Eur. J. Immunol.* **17**, 1685–1690.

Maggi, E., Del Prete, G. F., Tiri, A., Macchia, D., Parronchi, P., Ricci, M. and Romagnani, S. (1988a) *Clin. Exp. Immunol.* **73**, 57–62.

Maggi, E., Del Prete, G. F., Macchia, D., Parronchi, P., Tiri, A., Chretien, I., Ricci, M. and Romagnani, S. (1988b) *Eur. J. Immunol.* **18**, 1045–1050.

Maggi, E., Del Prete, G. F., Parronchi, P., Tiri, A., Macchia, D., Biswas, P., Simonelli, C., Ricci, M. and Romagnani, S. (1989a) *Immunology* **68**, 300–306.

Maggi, E., Mazzetti, M., Ravina, A., Simonelli, C., Parronchi, P., Macchia, D., Biswas, P., Di Pietro, M. and Romagnani, S. (1989b) *Res. Clin. Lab.* **19**, 45–49.

Mandroup-Pulsen, T., Helqvist, S., Molvig, J., Dall Vogensen, L. and Nerup, J. (1989) *Autoimmunity* **4**, 191–218.

Marsh, D. G., Meyers, D. A. and Freidhoff, R. L. (1981) *Int. Archs. Allergy Appl. Immunol.* **66**, 48–55.

Marsh, D. G., Meyers, D. A., Freidhoff, R. L. (1982) *J. Exp. Med.* **155**, 1452–1463.

Matheson, D. S. and Green, B. J. (1987) *J. Immunol.* **138**, 2469–2472.

Mayer, L., Kwan, S. P., Thompson, C., Ko, H. S., Chiorazzi, N., Waldmann, T. and Rosen, F. (1986) *New Engl. J. Med.* **314**, 409–413.

Moretta, A., Pantaleo, G., Moretta, L., Cerottini, J. C. and Mingari, M. C. (1983) *J. Exp. Med.* **157**, 743–754.

Morrell, A., Barandun, S. and Locher, G. (1986) *New Engl. J. Med.* **316**, 456–457.

Miyasaka, N., Sato, K., Hashimoto, J., Kohsaka, H., Yamamoto, K., Goto, M., Inoue, K., Matsuda, T., Hirano, T., Kishimoto, T. and Nishioka, K. (1989) *Clin. Immunol. Immunopathol.* **52**, 238–247.

Muraguchi, A., Hirano, T., Tang, B., Matsuda, T., Horii, Y., Nakajima, K. and Kishimoto, T. (1988) *J. Exp. Med.* **167**, 332–344.

Nakajima, K., Martinez-Maza, O., Hirano, T., Breen, E. C., Nishanian, P. G., Salazar-Gonzalez, J. F., Fahey, J. L. and Kishimoto, T. (1989) *J. Immunol.* **142**, 531–536.

Nijstein, M. W. N., De Groot, E. R., Ten Duis, H. J., Klasen, H. J., Hack, C. E. and Aarden, L. A. (1987) *Lancet* **2**, 921.

Noelle, R. J., McCann, J., Marshall, L. and Bartlett, W. C. (1989) *J. Immunol.* **143**, 1807–1814.

Nutman, T. B., Withers, A. S., Ottesen, E. A. (1985) *J. Immunol.* **135**, 2794–2799.

Paganelli, R., Capobianchi, M. R., Ensoli, B., D'Offizi, G. P., Facchini, J., Dianzani, F. and Aiuti, F. (1988a) *Clin. Exp. Immunol.* **72**, 124–129.

Paganelli, R., Quinti, I., Capobianchi, M. R., D'Offizi, G. P., Scala, E., Giannini, G., Di Marco, P., Cherchi, M., Di Sabatino, A. and Aiuti, F. (1988b) In *Topics in Immunology* (Eds. F. Aiuti, L. Bonomo and G. Danieli), pp. 291–296. Il Pensiero Scientifico Editore, Roma.

Parkin, J. M., Eales, L. J., Galazka, A. R. and Pinching, A. J. (1987) *Br. Med. J.* **294**, 1185–1186.

Parronchi, P., Tiri, A., Macchia, D., Biswas, P., Simonelli, C., Maggi, E., Del Prete, G. F., Ricci, M. and Romagnani, S. (1990) *J. Immunol.*, in press.

Pastorelli, G., Roncarolo, M. G., Touraine, J. L., Peronne, G., Tovo, P. A. and de Vries, J. (1989a) *Clin. Exp. Immunol.* **78**, 334–340.

Pastorelli, G., Roncarolo, M. G., Touraine, J. L., Rousset, F., Pene, J. and de Vries, J. (1989b) *Clin. Exp. Immunol.* **78**, 341–347.

Pedersen, M., Permin, H., Jensen, C., Skov, P. S., Norn, S. and Feber, V. (1987) *Allergy* **42**, 291–297.

Pene, J., Rousset, F., Briere, F., Chretien, I., Bonnefoy, J-Y., Spits, H., Yokota, T., Arai, K., Banchereau, J. and de Vries, J. (1988a) *Proc. Natl. Acad. Sci. USA* **85**, 6880–6884.

Pene, J., Rousset, F., Briere, F., Chretien, I., Paliard, X., Banchereau, J. and de Vries, J. (1988b) *J. Immunol.* **141**, 1218–1224.

Pereira, S., Webster, D. and Platts-Mills, T. (1982) *Eur. J. Immunol.* **12**, 540–546.

Perri, R. T. and Weisdorf, D. J. (1985) *Blood* **66**, 345–349.

Plaut, M., Pierce, J. H., Watson, C. J., Hanley-hyde, J., Nordan, R. P. and Paul, W. E. (1989) *Nature* **339**, 64–67.

Poppema, S., Elema, J. D. and Halie, M. R. (1979) *Int. J. Cancer* **24**, 532–537.

Ricci, M., Del Prete, G. F., Maggi, E., Lanzavecchia, A., Sala, P. G. and Romagnani, S. (1985) *Int. Archs. Allergy Appl. Immunol.* **77**, 32–37.

Ringden, O., Persson, U. and Johansson, S. G. O. (1983) *Blood* **61**, 1190–1195.

Romagnani, S. (1989a) *J. Immunol. Res.* **1**, 41–51.

Romagnani, S., Biagiotti, R., Amadori, A., Maggi, E., Biti, G., Bellesi, G. and Ricci, M. (1980a) *Int. Archs. Allergy Appl. Immunol.* **63**, 64–72.

Romagnani, S., Maggi, E., Del Prete, G. F., Troncone, R. and Ricci, M. (1980b) *Clin. Exp. Immunol.* **42**, 167–174.

Romagnani, S., Del Prete, G. F., Maggi, E., Troncone, R., Giudizi, M. G., Almerigogna, F. and Ricci, M. (1980c) *Clin. Exp. Immunol.* **42**, 579–588.

Romagnani, S., Lanzavecchia, A., Del Prete, G. F., Maggi, E. and Ricci, M. (1983) In *Proc. XII Congress Eur. Acad. Allergol. Clin. Immunol.* (Eds. U. Serafini and E. Errigo), pp. 7–16. O.I.C. Medical Press, Firenze.

Romagnani, S., Del Prete, G. F., Maggi, E. and Ricci, M. (1987) *J. Immunol.* **138**, 1744–1749.

Romagnani, S., Del Prete, G. F., Maggi, E., Parronchi, P. and Ricci, M. (1989b) *Haematologica* **74**, 317–323.

Romagnani, S., Del Prete, G. F., Maggi, E., Parronchi, P., Tiri, A., Macchia, D., Guidizi, M. G., Almerigogna, F. and Ricci, M. (1989c) *Clin. Immunol. Immunopathol. (suppl.)* **50**, 13–23.

Rosen, F. S., Wedgwoof, R. J. and Eibl, M. (1986) *Clin. Immunol. Immunopathol.* **40**, 166–196.

Rosenberg, Z. F. and Fauci, A. S. (1989) *Clin. Immunol. Immunopathol. (suppl.)* **50**, 149–156.

Saiki, O., Ralph, P., Cunningham-Rundles, C. and Good, R. A. (1982) *Proc. Natl. Acad. Sci. USA* **79**, 6008–6012.

Saiki, O., Shimizu, M., Saeki, Y., Kishimoto, S. and Kishimoto, T. (1984) *J. Immunol.* **133**, 1920–1924.

Sarfati, M. and Delespesse, G. (1988) *J. Immunol.* **141**, 2195–2199.

Sarfati, M., Rector, E., Wong, K., Rubio-Trujillo, M., Sehon, A. H. and Delespesse, G. (1984) *Immunology* **53**, 197–205.

Sarjan, J. A., Leung, D. Y. M. and Geha, R. S. (1983) *J. Immunol.* **130**, 242–248.

Schnittman, S. M., Lane, C., Higgins, S. E., Folks, T. and Fauci, A. S. (1986) *Science* **233**, 1084–1086.

Sekigawa, I., Noguchi, K., Asegawa, K., Hirose, S., Sato, H. and Shirai, T. (1989) *Clin. Immunol. Immunopathol.* **51**, 172–184.

Sekita, K., Straub, C., Hoessli, D. and Zubler, R. H. (1988) *Eur. J. Immunol.* **18**, 1405–1410.

Sherr, E., Adelman, D. C., Saxon, A., Gilly, M., Wall, R. and Sidell, N. (1988) *J. Exp. Med.* **168**, 55–71.

Souillet, G., Rousset F. and de Vries J. (1989) *Lancet* **ii**, 1384–1385.

Tanaka, Y., Saito, K., Shirakawa, F., Ota, T., Suzuki, H., Eto, S. and Yamashita, U. (1988) *J. Immunol.* **141**, 3043–3049.

Thyphronitis, G., Tsokos, G. C., Levine, A. D. and Finkelman, F. D. (1989) *Proc. Natl. Acad. Sci. USA* **86**, 5580–5584.

Tjio, A. H., Hull, W. M. and Gleich, G. J. (1979) *J. Immunol.* **122**, 2131–2133.

Uchibayashi, N., Kikutani, H., Barsumian, E. L., Hauptamann, R., Schneider, F-J., Schwendenwein, R., Sommergruber, W., Spevak, W., Maurer-Fogy, I., Suemura, M. and Kishimoto, T. (1989) *J. Immunol.* **142**, 3901–3908.

Umetsu, D. T., Leung, D. Y. M., Siraganian, R., Jabara, H. H. and Geha, R. S. (1985) *J. Exp. Med.* **162**, 202–214.

Umland, S. P., Go, N. F., Cupp, J. E. and Howard, M. (1989) *J. Immunol.* **142**, 1528–1535.

Vercelli, D., Jabara, H. H., Arai, I., Yokata, T. and Geha, R. S. (1989a) *Eur. J. Immunol.* **19**, 1419–1424.
Vercelli, D., Jabara, H. H., Arai, K-I. and Geha, R. S. (1989b) *J. Exp. Med.* **169**, 1295–1307.
Weston, K. M., Yeh, E. T. H. and Sy, M. S. (1987) *J. Immunol.* **139**, 734–742.
Weyss, L. M., Movahed, L. A., Warnke, R. A. and Sklar, J. (1989) *New Engl. J. Med.* **320**, 502–531.
Wierenga, E. A., Snoek, M., de Groot, C., Chretien, I., de Vries, J. and Kapsenberg, L. (1989) *Seventh International Congress of Immunology, Berlin*, p.463. G. Fischer, Stuttgart, New York.
Wodnar-Filipowicz, A., Heusser, C. H. and Moroni, C. (1989) *Nature* **339**, 150–152.
Wright, J. J., Birx, D. L., Wagner, D. K. (1987) *New Engl. J. Med.* **317**, 1516–1520.

10
B Cell assays for growth and differentiation factors

JOHN G. SHIELDS AND JEAN-YVES BONNEFOY

Introduction

It is now well established that the production of antibodies by B lymphocytes is a complex process involving stimulation of the B cells by antigen, by direct cell–cell contact with other cell types, in particular T lymphocytes, and by cell-derived soluble mediators. In this chapter we will discuss the different ways of measuring B cell activation, growth and differentiation in response to cytokines, highlighting the merits and limitations of the various methods. In addition, we will attempt to reconcile some of the differing results obtained using different bioassays. This chapter is not meant as a "recipe book" for assays of B cell growth and differentiation factors. For details of the various methods the reader is referred to reviews by Hamblin and O'Garra (1987), Callard *et al.* (1987) or O'Garra and Defrance (1990).

Assays for B cell activation

Activation of the B cell is the first cellular event leading to proliferation and differentiation into antibody-secreting cells. In a normal immune response *in vivo*, the first activation signal transmitted to the B cell is by antigen via surface immunoglobulin. Due to the low frequency of B cells responding to any one antigen, this signal is usually mimicked *in vitro* by using $F(ab')_2$ fragments of anti-IgM or anti-IgD to activate the B cells polyclonally. Stimulation via surface immunoglobulin results in the hydrolysis of phosphatidylinositol bisphosphate to inositol trisphosphate and diacylglycerol (see chapter 3). These in turn lead to the mobilization of intracellular Ca^{2+} stores and activation of protein kinase C (PKC). A second signal is then delivered by T cells via direct cell–cell contact and/or the release of

CYTOKINES AND B LYMPHOCYTES
ISBN 0–12–155145–8

Table 1   Measurement of B cell activation by cytokines.

Parameter measured	Method used	Examples
Cell volume	Particle counting	Murine IL-4[a]
Second messenger generation		
IP$_3$	HPLC analysis	Human IL-4[b]
	Binding assay	Human IL-4[b]
[Ca^{2+}]$_i$	Fluorimetry	Human IL-4[b]
cAMP	Binding assay	Human IL-4[b]
Protein kinase activity	Protein phosphorylation	Murine IL-4[c]
Cell surface marker expression	Flow cytometry using specific monoclonal abs or ligand binding assay	Human IL-4 increases expression of MHC II,[d] CD23,[e] CD40,[d] sIgM,[f] CD25[g] Murine IL-4 increases expression of MHC II,[h] CD23,[i] Thy-1,[j] IL-2R p70 (β) chain[k] Murine IL-5 induces expression of IL-2R p55 chain[k]

[a] Rabin et al. (1985).   [b] Finney et al. (1990).   [c] Justement et al. (1986).
[d] Clark et al. (1989).   [e] Defrance et al. (1987a).   [f] Shields et al. (1989).
[g] Butcher et al. (1990).   [h] Noelle et al. (1984).   [i] Hudak et al. (1987).
[j] Snapper et al. (1988).   [k] Loughnan and Nossal (1989).

lymphokines. However, it is now clear that some cytokines can activate B lymphocytes before they are triggered via their antigen receptors.

The most commonly used methods for assessing B cell activation are listed in Table 1. In many cases, one factor can result in the activation of several different parameters which may be causally related; for instance, murine interleukin 4 (IL-4) causes an increase in B cell volume, in membrane-protein phosphorylation and in surface-marker expression. For the majority of cytokines, there is little or no information on the mechanisms of transmembrane signalling. Studies of the action of murine IL-4 on B cells have failed to detect the involvement of the phosphatidylinositol bisphosphate hydrolysis pathway (Justement et al., 1986; Mizugichi et al., 1986). Furthermore, levels of [Ca^{2+}]$_i$ and cAMP remain stationary after stimulation of murine B cells by IL-4 (G. Klaus, personal communication). In contrast, Finney et al. (1990) have shown a transient rise in IP$_3$ generation and a subsequent increase in $[Ca^{2+}]_i$, followed later by a sustained elevation of intracellular cAMP levels in human B cells stimulated with IL-4. It is not yet certain whether this difference between murine and human IL-4 signal transduction is due to the source of cells used in the assay or whether it is to a difference in the mode of action of IL-4 in these two species (see "Species differences", below).

The expression of activation antigens follows hours or days after the early signal transduction events, but the chain of biochemical events leading from one to the other is largely unknown. In some recent studies the activation of DNA binding proteins in B cells by IL-4 (Boothby *et al.*, 1988) and the characterization of early response genes in activated B cells (Murphy *et al.*, 1990) have been reported.

Assays for B cell proliferation

Proliferation of B lymphocytes takes place after the B cells have been activated via surface immunoglobulin, and it is dependent on the presence of soluble mediators. The B cell must be stimulated in order for the soluble cytokine to then be able to deliver its growth-promoting signal. Physiologically, this co-stimulation signal is delivered by antigen binding to surface immunoglobulin. *In vitro*, the requirement for antigen can be replaced by agents which either act via surface immunoglobulin (e.g. anti-IgM antibodies, protein-A containing *Staphylococcus aureus* Cowan I bacteria), by other less well-defined surface receptors (e.g. dextran sulphate, lipopolysaccharide or monoclonal antibodies such as CD20, G28.8, etc.), or by pharmacologically mimicking signal transduction pathways (e.g. phorbol ester plus calcium ionophore). The requirement for a co-stimulant may be obviated *in vitro* by using certain B cell growth factor responsive B cell lines (which are already activated) or by selecting for *in vivo* activated B cells on the basis of their lower buoyant density. There are some factors which may not need co-stimulation of the B cell for growth activity, such as nerve growth factor (NGF) and B cell activating factor (BCAF) described by Theze and co-workers (Roth *et al.*, 1988; Diu *et al.*, 1990). Until now, only partially purified BCAF has been available, and a source of recombinant protein is awaited to confirm that the activation and growth promoting activities of this preparation are due to a single factor.

Proliferation is most commonly measured by the uptake of tritiated thymidine into newly synthesized DNA (see Table 2). As this technique measures cells that are in S phase of the cell cycle during the time that the radiolabelled nucleotide is present, any factor which merely pushes the cells from G_0/G_1 into S phase but not into mitosis may also score as a B cell

Table 2   Measurement of B cell proliferation by cytokines.

Cytokine	Target cell[a]	Co-stimulant	Method[b]
IL-1	B cells (h)	Anti-IgM	A[c]
IL-2	B cells (h)	SAC	A[d]
	B cells (m)	LPS/anti-IgM	A[e]
	Hapten-specific B cells (m)	specific Ag	C[f]
IL-4	BCL1 line (m)	None	B[g]
	B cells (h)	Anti-IgM	A[h]
IL-5	BCL1 line (m)	None	A[i]
	B cells (m)	DxS	A[i]
IL-6	B cell hybridoma (m)	None	A[j]
	EBV-LCL	None	A[k]
IL-7	pre B cells (m)	None	—[l]
LMW-BCGF	B cells (h)	SAC	A[m]
	B cells (h)	Anti-IgM	A[n]
	P[3]HR1 (h)	None	A[o]
BCAF	Small resting B cells (m)	None	A[p]
IFN-gamma	B cells (h)	Anti-IgM	A[q]
TNF-alpha	B cells (h)	SAC	A[r]
TNF-beta	B cells (h)	SAC	A[s]
GM-CSF	BCL1 line (m)	None	B[g]
Factor B	B cells (h)	SAC	A[t]
Fragment Ba	B cells (m)	LPS	A[u]

[a] h = human; m = murine.
[b] A = ^{3}HTdR incorporation; B = MTT colorimetric assay; C = microscopic examination.
[c] Falkoff *et al.* (1983).   [d] Muraguchi *et al.* (1985).   [e] Zubler *et al.* (1984).
[f] Pike *et al.* (1984).   [g] O'Garra *et al.* (1989).   [h] Defrance *et al.* (1987b).
[i] Swain *et al.* (1983).   [j] Van Snick *et al.* (1986).   [k] Tosato *et al.* (1988).
[l] Namen *et al.* (1988).   [m] Jelinek and Lipsky (1987).   [n] Sharma *et al.* (1987).
[o] Vazquez *et al.* (1988).   [p] Roth *et al.* (1988).   [q] Romagnani *et al.* (1986).
[r] Kehrl *et al.* (1987a).   [s] Kehrl *et al.* (1987b).   [t] Peters *et al.* (1988).
[u] Praz and Ruuth (1986).

growth factor (BCGF), even if no cell division occurs. Cell-cycle analysis by flow cytometry can confirm that cells have traversed the full cell cycle. Proliferation may also be estimated by measuring enzymatic activity such as the MTT (Mosmann, 1983) or hexosaminidase (Landegren, 1984) assays, although a good correlation between enzymatic activity and cell number must first be established.

Assays for B cell differentiation

Differentiation of B lymphocytes is usually taken to mean the transition to high-rate immunoglobulin secretion. Table 3 lists the cytokines which have been shown to be B cell differentiation factors. They can be divided into two broad groups: those which selectively enhance the production of one or a small number of immunoglobulin classes/subclasses (e.g. IL-4) and those which show no class specificity (e.g. IL-6).

Table 3 Measurement of B cell differentiation by cytokines.

Cytokine	Target cell[a]	Method[b]	(Sub-)class specificity
IL-2	SAC-blasts (h)	ISC	None[c]
	SKW6.4 line (h)	ISC	—[d]
	PBL E⁻ (h)	Ag-specific ab (EIA)	None[e]
IL-3	JDA line (h)	EIA	—[f]
IL-4	B cells + LPS (m)	ISC	IgG1[g]
	B cells + LPS (m)	RIA	IgE[h]
	B cells + EBV (h)	EIA	IgE[i]
IL-5	BCL1 line (m)	ISC	None[j]
IL-6	CESS line (h)	ISC	—[k]
	SAC/IL-2 + B cells (h)	EIA	None[l]
IFN-α	B cells + LPS (m)	EIA	IgG2a[m]

[a] h = human; m = murine.
[b] ISC = Ig-secreting cell; EIA = enzyme immunoassay; RIA = radioimmunoassay.
[c] Jelinek *et al.* (1986).   [d] Ralph *et al.* (1984).   [e] Callard *et al.* (1986).
[f] Tadmori *et al.* (1989).   [g] Sideras *et al.* (1985).   [h] Coffman *et al.* (1986).
[i] Thyphronitis *et al.* (1989).   [j] Takatsu *et al.* (1988).   [k] Muraguchi *et al.* (1981).
[l] Splawski *et al.* (1990).   [m] Snapper and Paul (1987).

Cytokine-induced B cell differentiation may increase the amount of immunoglobulin produced per cell and/or increase the number of cells secreting Ig. This can be an important distinction as in some systems the rate of immunoglobulin production is increased without a concomitant increase in the number of cells secreting immunoglobulin (Splawski *et al.*, 1990). The methods used for determining Ig secretion are either: (a) measurement of total Ig in supernatant by radio- or enzyme immunoassay, or (b) estimation of the number of immunoglobulin-producing cells by reverse plaque or ELISPOTS assays.

Assay considerations

The source of B lymphocytes, their purity, and the type of co-stimulant used are important considerations in assays for measuring B cell responses to cytokines.

Source of cells

A major variable in the different assays employed for measuring B cell responses is the source of mononuclear cells used for B lymphocyte purification. In man, tonsils obtained from patients after tonsillectomy, usually as a result of recurrent infections, and venous blood are most commonly used. Occasional studies have also used splenic B cells, although this material is usually less readily available from humans. In mice, B lymphocytes are most commonly prepared from spleen or lymph node cells.

Each starting population may contain different subpopulations of B cells, and/or B cells in different states of activation. For example, staining with CD20 monoclonal antibodies has been shown to distinguish two subpopulations of human B cells derived from tonsils but not of B cells from blood or spleens (Gadol *et al.*, 1988). Antibodies against other cell-surface markers such as CD39 and IgD have similarly revealed different subpopulations within tonsillar B cell preparations (Liu *et al.*, 1989), whereas the same heterogeneity is not seen in B cells purified from venous blood. Immunohistological studies have also shown that differential expression of cell surface markers *in vivo* can identify B cell subpopulations, probably representing different stages of activation. For example, tonsillar mantle zone B cells expressing CD39 and surface IgD are very similar to blood B cells and are believed to be small, resting cells. On the other hand, germinal centre B cells that do not express CD39 or sIgD are actively proliferating. These two different subpopulations also show different behaviour in response to various stimuli *in vitro*: for example, mantle zone but not germinal centre B cells produced IgM *in vitro* in response to PWM (Gadol *et al.*, 1988), a process known to be IL-6 dependent.

Direct comparison of the *in vitro* response of human B cells from various tissue sources has revealed important functional differences. McCaughan *et al.* (1984), examining the production of IgA anti-influenza antibody *in vitro* using blood, tonsil and spleen cells, showed that only cells from secondary lymphoid tissue and not from blood were able to produce specific IgA. By a series of mixing experiments they determined that the difference lay in the B cell fraction, which in blood lacked antigen-specific IgA memory B cell precursors. In another study, Jelinek and Lipsky (1987) have shown that purified B cells from spleen (and blood) can be induced to secrete immunoglobulin *in vitro* by a combination of *Staphylococcus aureus* Cowan I mitogen plus IL-2, while B cells from lymph nodes require an additional stimulus provided by a partially purified preparation of low molecular weight B cell growth factor (LMW BCGF).

Different responses of B cells *in vitro* may reflect the proportion of *in vivo* activated cells. For example, the subpopulation of tonsillar B cells which responds to LMW BCGF has a low buoyant density and expresses the activation marker 4F2 (Richard *et al.*, 1987) and is found in greater numbers in tonsils than in venous blood. In the same series of experiments, it was also found that tonsillar but not blood B cells could respond to a partially purified 50 kD BCGF. This was not due to the presence of more activated B cells in the tonsils, but rather to the presence of a subpopulation of B cells expressing the cell surface marker CD5, which was virtually absent from the blood B cell preparations.

Preparation and purification of cells

In order to study the response of B lymphocytes to a given stimulus, it is important to start with as pure a population as possible. Many of the cytokines having an effect on B cells also stimulate other cell types; for example, IL-2, IL-4, IL-6 and IL-7 are all growth factors for both T and B lymphocytes (Zubler *et al.*, 1984; Yokota *et al.*, 1986). Consequently, the factor under study may be acting indirectly through non-B cells present in the culture. Contaminating T cells, macrophages or LGLs can also provide inhibitory signals to B cells (Lobo and Wright, 1988). On the other hand, non-B cells may be required for some responses; for example, some monocytes are necessary in the antigen-specific antibody response to influenza virus *in vitro*, presumably for the purpose of antigen presentation (Callard *et al.*, 1987).

B lymphocytes from tissue sources are obtained normally by mechanical disruption and occasionally by enzymatic digestion. The former method can result in cells being left trapped in the tissue debris while the use of enzymes can affect the subsequent response by removing cell-surface antigens. The cell suspensions obtained from various lymphoid tissues can be used to isolate B cells directly, as is usually the case with murine splenocytes, or they can first be enriched for mononuclear cells by density-gradient centrifugation over Ficoll-Metrizoate or Percoll. This latter step removes granulocytes, red cells and most of the dead cells.

Isolation of purified B cells from mixed mononuclear cell populations can be achieved by:

(i) Positive selection, usually with antibodies recognizing surface immunoglobulin, although it is possible to use monoclonal antibodies to other B cell-restricted cell-surface molecules such as CD19 or CD20 (Abts *et al.*, 1989). Hapten-specific B cells have also been purified by positive selection. Separation is achieved by panning, by rosetting or by FACS sorting. The main problems with these methods are that they can be slow to perform, the yield is often low and the antibodies (or other ligands) used may result in activation of the B cells.

(ii) Negative selection. Some depletion of monocyte/macrophages can be achieved by the ability of these cells to adhere to plastic surfaces. Better depletion can be achieved by adherence to microexudate-coated plastic surfaces, passage through Sephadex G10 columns or treatment of cells with the lysosomotropic agent L-leucine methyl ester. Removal of both monocytes and, more often, T cells can also be performed by using a cocktail of monoclonal antibodies against the relevant cell types and complement-mediated lysis. This method releases a large variety of intracellular enzymes and perhaps also cytokines. Although the cells are in contact with these products for only a brief period, it is possible that this exposure could activate some of the cells and alter their subsequent *in vitro* response. An alternative and commonly used method for depletion of both T cells and some natural killer (NK) cells from human cell populations is by rosetting of these cells with AET-treated sheep erythrocytes (E). In cases where the starting density of T cells is high (e.g. human peripheral blood mononuclear cells, PBMCs) a second round of rosetting is usually necessary.

The B cell fraction prepared by these techniques can be further subdivided by density gradient centrifugation into small, dense ("resting", G_0) and large, light ("activated", G_1) B cells. This distinction is particularly important when the effect of factors on B cell activation is being investigated, although it may also influence the results of assays examining B cell proliferation and/or differentiation (Callard and Smith, 1988; Almerigogna *et al.*, 1989).

No matter which method is used for purification of B cells, it is essential to assess the purity of the final population. This is most easily performed using a panel of monoclonal antibodies and either a fluorescence or enzyme-based detection system, although it is also possible to assess contamination using functional assays (e.g. response to the T cell mitogen concanavalin A, ConA; Ruuth *et al.*, 1989). In humans, the proportion of B cells is best estimated with pan B cell markers such as CD20 or CD19, whereas in mice it is more common to use sIg as a marker. Contaminating T cells can be estimated with CD3 antibodies in man and Thy1 in mouse. It is worth noting that E$^-$ cells prepared from human PBMC by AET E-rosetting typically contain only 20–30% CD20 (B cells), whereas E$^-$ from tonsillar mononuclear cells are usually 95–98% CD20$^+$.

Species differences

The response of B lymphocytes to cytokines has been studied most intensively in two species, mouse and man. It is important to realize that there may be significant inter-species variation in the responses of B cells, which could be due either to the use of different methods for assessing the action of these agents on B cell function or to a fundamental species difference in the regulation of B cell responses. For example, whereas IL-5 is a potent growth factor on dextran sulphate (DxS) -stimulated mouse B lymphocytes, and on the murine B cell leukaemia line BCL-1 (Swain *et al.*, 1983) and the PRO-B cell clone LyH7-B13 (Rolink *et al.*, 1989), human IL-5 was not a B cell growth factor when tested in all the standard assays on human B cells, even though it had activity on BCL-1 and on human eosinophils (Clutterbuck *et al.*, 1987). Moreover, IL-5 is a T cell-replacing factor in mice (Takatsu *et al.*, 1985) but not in humans (Clutterbuck *et al.*, 1987; Smith *et al.*, 1989).

Another example of species difference in response to cytokines can be seen with IL-4. In one of the original bioassays for IL-4, co-stimulation of B lymphocytes in the presence of anti-IgM and IL-4 led to proliferation (Howard *et al.*, 1982). In a similar bioassay using human cells, insolubilized anti-IgM and IL-4 cause B cell proliferation (Defrance *et al.*, 1987b), but the mode of action of IL-4 in this case may be fundamentally different. Preincubation of murine B cells with IL-4 primes the B cells to respond more readily to subsequent addition of anti-IgM (Oliver *et al.*, 1985). In contrast, human IL-4 functions as a growth factor for the human B cells after they have been activated by anti-IgM (Defrance *et al.*, 1987b; Almerigogna *et al.*, 1989). Indeed, prior stimulation with IL-4 may inhibit subsequent responses to anti-IgM (Gordon *et al.*, 1988; Shields *et al.*, 1989). This fundamental species difference in the mode of action of IL-4 is underlined by the observations that different second messengers are generated in B cells in response to human and murine IL-4 (see "Assays for B cell activation", above, and Table 1).

B cell lines and normal B cells

Many investigators have selected B cell lines as alternatives to normal B cells to investigate cytokine responses and receptors. The availability of quick, easy, reproducible bioassays using B cell lines has aided the purification and cloning of several cytokines including IL-5 (Kinashi *et al.*, 1986), IL-6 (Hirano *et al.*, 1986) and IL-7 (Namen *et al.*, 1988). Cell lines have also proved useful for cloning receptors of cytokines that stimulate B cells (Yamasaki *et al.*, 1988). The control of proliferation and differentiation in transformed B cell lines is a subject worthy of study in its own right as it may shed some light on those causative factors important in the appearance and development of B cell tumours. On the other hand, the study of cytokine action on B cell lines is limited in what it can tell us about the normal physiological response of B lymphocytes. Activities of B cell factors which have been investigated using cell lines have to be confirmed on normal B cells if the true physiological importance of such factors is to be determined.

Other assays

B cell responses to cytokines are informative in terms of B cell physiology but are usually too insensitive and/or not specific enough to be of much use as primary assays for cytokines. Bioassays based on other cell types are often preferable, although in some cases such as the response of the B9 line to IL-6 (Lansdorp *et al.*, 1986) B cells are used. More recently, ELISAs for all the main B cell cytokines except IL-5 and IL-7 (at the time of writing) have become commercially available. In general, these are more sensitive than bioassays and can detect cytokines down to concentrations of 25–100 pg ml^{-1}. Their main disadvantage is that they do not distinguish between biologically active and inactive material. Finally, cDNA probes for most cytokines are now available which can be used to detect cells synthesizing specific mRNA. When used together with the polymerase chain reaction (PCR) this is an extremely sensitive method for detecting cytokine production by small numbers of cells *in vitro* and *in vivo*.

References

Abts, H., Emmerich, M., Miltenyi, S., Radbruch, A. and Tesch, H. (1989) *J. Immunol. Methods* **125**, 19–28.

Almerigogna, F., Giudizi, M. G., Biagotti, R., Alessi, A., Defrance, T., Banchereau, J., Ricci, M. and Romagnani, S. (1989) *Immunology* **67**, 244–250.

Boothby, M., Gravallese, E., Liou, H-C., Glimcher, I. H. (1988) *Science* **242**, 1559–1562.

Butcher, R. D. J., McGarvie, G. M. and Cushley, W. (1990) *Immunology* **69**, 57–64.

Callard, R. E., Smith, S. H., Shields, J. G. and Levinsky, R. J. (1986) *Eur. J. Immunol.* **16**, 1037–1042.

Callard, R. E., Shields, J. G. and Smith, S. E. (1987) In *Lymphokines and Interferons: A Practical Approach*, Eds M. J. Clemens, A. G. Morris and A. J. H. Gearing, pp. 345–364. IRL Press, Oxford.

Callard, R. E. and Smith S. H. (1988) *Eur. J. Immunol.* **18**, 1635–1638.

Clark, E. A., Shu, G. L., Lüscher, B., Draves, K. E., Banchereau, J., Ledbetter, J. A. and Valentine, M. A. (1989) *J. Immunol.* **143**, 3873–3880.

Clutterbuck, E., Shields, J. G., Gordon, J., Smith, S. H., Boyd, A., Callard, R. E., Campbell, H. D., Young, I. G. and Sanderson, C. J. (1987) *Eur. J. Immunol.* **17**, 1743–1750.

Coffman, R. L., Ohara, J., Bond, M. W., Carty, J., Zlotnick, A. and Paul, W. E. (1986) *J. Immunol.* **136**, 4538–4542.

Defrance, T., Aubry, J. P., Rousset, F., Vanbervliet, B., Bonnefoy, J. Y., Arai, N., Takebe, Y., Yokota, T., Lee, F., Arai, K., de Vries, J. and Banchereau, J. (1987a) *J. Exp. Med.* **165**, 1459–1467.

Defrance, T., Vanbervliet, B., Aubry, J. P., Takebe, Y., Arai, N., Miyajima, A., Yokota, T., Lee, F., Arai, K. I., de Vries, J. and Banchereau, J. (1987b) *J. Immunol.* **139**, 1135–1141.

Diu, A., Fevrier, M., Mollier, P., Charron, D., Banchereau, J., Reinherz, E. L. and Theze, J. (1990) *Cell. Immunol.* **125**, 14–28.

Falkoff, R. J. M., Muraguchi, A., Hong, J-X., Butler, J. L., Dinarello, C. A. and Fauci, A. S. (1983) *J. Immunol.* **131**, 801–805.

Finney, M., Guy, G. R., Michell, R. H., Gordon, J. G., Dugas, B., Rigley, K. P. and Callard, R. E. (1990) *Eur. J. Immunol.* **20**, 151–156.

Gadol, N., Peacock, M. A. and Ault, K. A. (1988) *Blood* **71**, 1048–1055.

Gordon, J., Millsum, M. J., Guy, G. R. and Ledbetter, J. A. (1988) *J. Immunol.* **140**, 1425–1430.

Hamblin, A. S. and O'Garra, A. (1987) In *Lymphocytes: A Practical Approach*, Ed. G. G. B. Klaus, pp. 209–228. IRL Press, Oxford.

Hirano, T., Yasukawa, K., Harada, H., Taga, T., Watanabe, Y., Matsuda, T., Kashiwamura, S., Nakajima, K., Koyama, K., Iwamatsu, A., Tsunasawa, S., Sakiyama, F., Matsui, H., Takahara, Y., Taniguchi, T. and Kishimoto, T. (1986) *Nature* **324**, 73–76.

Howard, M., Farrar, J., Hilfiker, M., Johnson, B., Takatsu, K., Hamaoka, T. and Paul, W. E. (1982) *J. Exp. Med.* **155**, 914–923.

Hudak, S. A., Gollnick, S. O., Conrad, D. H. and Kehry, M. R. (1987) *Proc. Natl. Acad. Sci. USA* **84**, 4606–4610.

Jelinek, D. F. and Lipsky, P. E. (1987) *J. Immunol.* **139**, 1005–1013.

Jelinek, D. F., Splawski, J. B. and Lipsky, P. E. (1986) *Eur. J. Immunol.* **16**, 925–932.

Justement, L., Chen, Z., Harris, L., Ransom, J., Sandoval, V., Smith, C., Rennick, D., Roehm, N. and Cambier, J. (1986) *J. Immunol.* **137**, 3664–3670.

Kehrl, J. H., Miller, A. and Fauci, A. S. (1987a) *J. Exp. Med.* **166**, 786–791.

Kehrl, J. H., Alvarez-Mon, M., Delsing, G. A. and Fauci, A. S. (1987b) *Science* **238**, 1144–1146.

Kinashi, T., Harada, N., Severinson, E., Tanabe, T., Sideras, P., Konishi, M., Azuma, C., Tominaga, A., Bergstedt-Lindqvist, S., Takahashi, M., Matsuda, F., Yaoita, Y., Takatsu, K. and Honjo, T. (1986) *Nature* **324**, 70–73.

Landegren, U. (1984) *J. Immunol. Methods* **67**, 379–388.

Landsdorp, P. M., Arden, L. A., Calafat, J. and Zeijlemaker, W. P. (1986) *Current Topics Microbiol. Immunol.* **132**, 105–113.

Liu, Y. J., Joshua, D. E., Smith, C. A., Gordon, J. and Maclennan, I. C. M. (1989) *Nature* **342**, 929–931.

Lobo, P. I. and Wright, A. E. (1988) *J. Immunol. Methods* **115**, 239–246.

Loughnan, M. S. and Nossal, G. J. V. (1989) *Nature* **340**, 76–79.

McCaughan, G. W., Adams, E. and Basten, A. (1984) *J. Immunol.* **132**, 1190–1196.

Mizugichi, J., Beaven, M. A., Ohara, J. and Paul, W. E. (1986) *J. Immunol.* **137**, 2215–2219.

Mosmann, T. (1983) *J. Immunol. Methods* **65**, 55–63.

Muraguchi, A., Kishimoto, T., Miki, Y., Kuritani, T., Kaieda, T., Yoshizaki, K. and Yamamura, Y. (1981) *J. Immunol.* **127**, 412–416.

Muraguchi, A., Kehrl, J. H., Longo, D. L., Volkman, D. J., Smith, K. A. and Fauci, A. S. (1985) *J. Exp. Med.* **161**, 181–197.

Murphy, J. J., Trascz, M. and Norton, J. D. (1990) *Immunol.* **69**, 490–493.

Namen, A. E., Schmierer, A. E., March, C. J., Overell, R. W., Park, L. S., Urdal, D. R. and Mochizuki, D. Y. (1988) *J. Exp. Med.* **167**, 988–1002.

Noelle, R., Krammer, P. H., Ohara, J., Uhr, J. W. and Vitetta, E. S. (1984) *Proc. Natl. Acad. Sci. USA* **81**, 6149–6153.

O'Garra, A., Barbis, D., Wu, J., Hodgkin, P. D., Abrams, J. and Howard, M. (1989) *Cell. Immunol.* **123**, 189–200.

O'Garra, A. and Defrance, T. (1990) In *Bioassays for Interleukins*, Ed. H. Zola. CRC Press (in press).

Oliver, K., Noelle, R. J., Uhr, J. W., Krammer, P. H. and Vitetta, E. S. (1985) *Proc. Natl. Acad. Sci. USA* **82**, 2465–2467.

Peters, M. G., Ambrus, J. L., Fauci, A. S. and Brown, E. J. (1988) *J. Exp. Med.* **168**, 1225–1235.

Pike, B. L., Raubitschek, A. and Nossal, G. J. V. (1984) *Proc. Natl. Acad. Sci. USA* **81**, 7917–7921.

Praz, F. and Ruuth, E. (1986) *J. Exp. Med.* **163**, 1349–1354.

Rabin, E. M., Ohara, J. and Paul, W. E. (1985) *Proc. Natl. Acad. Sci. USA* **82**, 2935–2939.

Ralph, P., Jeong, G., Welte, K., Mertelsmann, R., Rabin, H., Henderson, L. E., Souza, L. M., Boone, T. C. and Robb, R. J. (1984) *J. Immunol.* **133**, 2442–2447.

Richard, Y., Leprince, C., Dugas, B., Treton, D. and Galanaud, P. (1987) *J. Immunol.* **139**, 1563–1567.

Rolink, A. G., Melchers, F. and Palacios, R. (1989) *J. Exp. Med.* **169**, 1693–1701.

Romagnani, S., Giudizi, M. G., Biagiotti, R., Almerigogna, F., Mingari, C., Maggi, E., Liang, C-M. and Moretta, L. (1986) *J. Immunol.* **136**, 3513–3517.

Roth, C., Moreau, J-L., Korner, M., Jankovic, D. and Theze, J. (1988) *Eur. J. Immunol.* **18**, 577–584.

Ruuth, E.; Couillin, I., Herbelin, A. and Praz, F. (1989) *Lymphokine Res.* **8**, 147–158.

Shields, J. G., Armitage, R. J., Jamieson, B. N., Beverley, P. C. L. and Callard, R. E. (1989) *Immunology* **66**, 224–227.

Sharma, S., Mehta, S., Morgan, J. and Maizel, A. (1987) *Science* **235**, 1489–1492.

Sideras, P., Bergstedt-Lindqvist, S. and Severinson, E. (1985) *Eur. J. Immunol.* **15**, 593–599.

Smith, S. H., Shields, J. G. and Callard, R. E. (1989) *Eur. J. Immunol.* **19**, 2045–2049.

Snapper, C. M. and Paul, W. E. (1987) *Science* **236**, 944–947.

Snapper, C. M., Hornbecj, P. V., Atasoy, U., Pereira, G. M. B. and Paul, W. E. (1988) *Proc. Natl. Acad. Sci. USA* **85**, 6107–6111.

Splawski, J. B., McAnally, L. M. and Lipsky, P. E. (1990) *J. Immunol.* **144**, 562–569.

Swain, S. L., Howard, M., Kappler, J., Marrack, P., Watson, J., Booth, R., Wetzel, G. D. and Dutton, R. W. (1983) *J. Exp. Med.* **158**, 822–835.

Tadmori, W., Feingeresh, D., Clark, S. C. and Choi, Y. S. (1989) *J. Immunol.* **142**, 1950–1956.

Takatsu, K., Harada, N., Hara, Y., Yamada, G., Takahama, Y., Dobashi, K. and Hamaoka, T. (1985) *J. Immunol.* **134**, 382–389.

Takatsu, K., Tominaga, A., Harada, N., Mita, S., Matsumoto, M., Takahashi, T., Kikuchi, Y. and Yamaguchi, N. (1988) *Immunol. Rev.* **102**, 107–135.

Thyphronitis, G., Tsokos, G. C., June, C. H., Levine, A. D. and Finkelman, F. D. (1989) *Proc. Natl. Acad. Sci. USA* **86**, 5580–5584.

Tosato, G., Seamon, K. B., Goldman, N. D., Sehgal, P. B., May, L. T., Washington, G. C., Jones, K. D. and Pike, S. E. (1988) *Science* **239**, 502–504.

Van Snick, J., Cayphas, S., Vink, A., Uyttenhove, C., Coulie, P. G., Rubira, M. R. and Simpson, R. J. (1986) *Proc. Natl. Acad. Sci. USA* **83**, 9679–9683.

Vazquez, A., Mills, S., Sharma, S. and Maizel, A. L. (1988) *Eur. J. Immunol.* **18**, 1647–1650.

Yamasaki, K., Taga, T., Hirata, Y., Yawata, H., Kawanishi, Y., Seed, B., Taniguchi, T., Hirano, T. and Kishimoto, T. (1988) *Science* **241**, 825–828.

Yokota, T., Otsuka, T., Mosmann, T., Banchereau, J., Defrance, T., Blanchard, D., de Vries, J., Lee, F. and Arai, K. I. (1986) *Proc. Natl. Acad. Sci. USA* **83**, 5894–5898.

Zubler, R., Lowenthal, J. W., Erard, F., Hashimoto, N., Devos, R. and MacDonald, H. R. (1984) *J. Exp. Med.* **160**, 1170–1183.

Index

The following abbreviations are used in the subheadings of this index:

B-CLL   B chronic lymphocytic leukaemia
BCGF   B cell growth factor
EBV   Epstein-Barr virus
IFN   interferon
IG   immunoglobulin
IL   interleukin
MHC   major histocompatibility complex
TGF   transforming growth factor
TNF   tumour necrosis factor

Activation of B cells
  accessory cells in, 73
  assays, 253–255
  C3d complement fraction in, 79
  EBV in, 72, 196–197
  IFN-γ in, 78
  IL-1 in, 78
  IL-4 in, 50–54, 73–78
    as competence factor, 73–74
    IFN antagonism, 75
    with IL-5, 78–79
    in phenotypic alterations, 74–75, 76
    signal transduction, 51–54
  IL-5 in, 78–79
  lipopolysaccharides in, 72
  MHC class II and, 5, 77
  proto-oncogene expression and, 57
  species differences, 7–8
  T-B interactions and, 71–72
Adenylate cyclase system, 40–41, 42
  G-proteins in, 41, 43
  IL-4 activation, 51, 52
AIDS, 220–221
  cytokine disregulation in, 236–237
Allergy, and cytokine disregulation,
    241–244, 245
cAMP production
  IL-2 in, 55

IL-4 in, 51, 53
Antibody response, see Cellular
    collaboration in antibody
    response; Differentiation of B
    cells
Arthritis, rheumatoid, 222–223
Assays, B cell, 253–265
  for activation, 253–255
  cell lines for, 262
  for differentiation, 257–258
  preparation/purification of cells, 259–
    261
  for proliferation, 255–257
  source of cells, 258–259
  and species differences, 261–262
Atopic disease, cytokine disregulation
    in, 241–244
Autocrine activity of B cells, 195–213
  autostimulation of EBV-transformed
    cells, 201–204
  autostimulatory growth factor
    (aBCGF), 203–204
  CD23 and autostimulation, 201–203
  IL-1 and autostimulation, 200
  BCGF activity
    in EBV-transformed cells, 198–199
    in normal cells, 199
  EBV activation, 196–197

Autocrine activity of B cells, *cont.*
growth inhibitory factors, 205–207
IL-6 in EBV-transformed cell
growth, 204
in neoplasia, 204–205
in normal B cell growth, 207–209
Autoimmune diseases
cardiac myxoma, 223
insulin dependent diabetes mellitus,
224
rheumatoid arthritis, 222–223
systemic lupus erythematosus, 221–
222
thyroid, 224

B cell activating factor (BCAF), 99
B cell growth factor (BCGF) *see also*
Interleukin 5
autostimulatory growth factor
(aBCGF), 203–204
B cell derived, 198–199
low molecular weight B cell growth
factor (LMW BCGF), 84, 87,
92–94
high molecular weight, 99
B chronic lymphocytic leukaemia (B-
CLL), *see* Leukaemic B cells
Buckley's syndrome, 235–236
Burkitt's lymphomas, CD23
expression, 201

C3 complement factors
in B cell proliferation, 98–99
in B cell activation, 79
Calcium ion, mobilization
anti-IG in, 46, 47
inositol phosphates in, 45
IL-4 in, 51, 53
Cardiac myxoma, 223
CD5 B-cell subpopulations, IL-5
stimulation of, 89–90
CD23
in activation of B cells, 77
in autostimulation of B cells, 201–
203
expression
in EBV infection, 197
IL-4 in, 53–54, 74–75, 76–77, 101

in growth of B cells, 81–82, 207–209,
210
in IgE regulation, 234–235
CD40
in activation of B cells, 77
expression on B cells, IL-4 in, 75
Cellular collaboration in antibody
response, 71–72, 143–172
'antigen-bridging' in, 144–145
antigen-specific interations, 146–
148
cell contact in, 149–158
antigen-specific responses, 149–
150
B cell surface molecules, 153
leucocyte function adhesion
antigen-1 (LFA-1), 156–158
MHC class II molecules, 153–156
physical interaction, 151–153
polyclonal responses, 150–151
MHC in, 145–146
mechanisms of T cell help, 148–149
T cells in, 158–166
IFN-γ secretion, 165–166
IL-2 secretion, 164–165
IL-4 secretion, 160–163
IL-5 secretion, 163–164
IL-6 secretion, 166
MTOC reorientation and
lymphokine release, 160
Th cell subsets, 158–160
Chronic lymphocytic leukaemia, B cell
autocrine growth in, 204–205 *see
also* Leukaemia; Leukaemic B
cells
Common variable
hypogammaglobulinaemia
(CVH), 217–220
Complement factors
in B cell proliferation, 98–99
in B cell activation, 79
Conjunctivitis, vernal, cytokine
disregulation in, 238–240
Corticosteroids, and leukaemia B cell
IgE secretion, 102
Corticotropin, 99
Cyclosporin A, and T cell lymphokine
secretion, 178
Cytokine synthesis inhibitory factor
(CSIF), 99

Dextran sulphate
  B cell activator, 72
  and IL-4 in B cell proliferation, 80
Diabetes mellitus, insulin dependent, 224
Differentiation of B cells, 65
  assays, 257–258
  IFN in, 124, 127–129
  IL-1 in, 129–130, 182
    IL-6 interaction, 126
  IL-2 in, 115, 116–119, 124, 129, 183
  IL-3 in, 130–131
  IL-4 in, 119–122
    IFN inhibition, 124
    IFN-γ interaction, 119–120, 121, 122
    IL-5 synergism, 123, 125
    IL-6 interaction, 121
  IL-5 in, 122–125
    IFN-γ interaction, 124
    IL-2 interaction, 124
    IL-4 synergism, 123, 125, 127
  IL-6 in, 116, 126–127, 184
  in vitro to *in vivo* extrapolation, 134–135, 136
  models, 2–5
  soluble interleukin receptors, 135–136
  TGF in, 131
  T-cell replacing factors in, 115–116
  Tн subsets, cytokines and immune response, 131, 134
  TNFs in, 130
Disease, cytokines and B cells in, 216–224, 235–251
  autoimmune diseases, 221–224
    cardiac myxoma, 223
    diabetes mellitus, insulin dependent, 224
    rheumatoid arthritis, 222–223
    systemic lupus erythematosus (SLE), 221–222
    thyroid disease, 224
  IgE hyperproduction disorders, 235–244
    in AIDS, 236–237
    in atopic diseases, 241–244
    in GVHD, 238
    in Hodgkin's disease, 236–237
    in hyper-IgE syndrome, 235–236

    in parasitic infection, 240–241
    in vernal conjunctivitis, 238–240
  immune deficiency syndromes, 216–221
    AIDS, 220–221
    common variable hypogammaglobulinaemia (CVH), 217–220

Early response genes (ERGs), 57
Endorphins, 99
Epstein-Barr virus (EBV)
  in AIDS, 237
  in B cell activation, 72, 196–197, 217
  and B cell transformation, 198
  BCGF, 198–199
  CD23 expression, 201
  cell lines, TGF growth inhibition, 97–98
  in Hodgkin's disease, 237
  IL-1, 200

Fc receptors
  in B cell activation inhibition, 47–49
  expression on B cells, IL-4 in, 75
  FcεRII/CD23 soluble antigen in IgE regulation, 234–235
Fibroblast growth factors, 99
Filariasis, cytokine disregulation in, 240

G proteins
  and phospoinositide-phosphodiesterase receptor, 45
  in second messenger systems, 41, 43
Genomic organization of human cytokines, 12, 13
Glucagon binding, 101

Hairy cell leukaemia
  IFNs for, 92
  TGF growth inhibition, 98
Helper T cells, *see* T helper cells
Hodgkin's disease, cytokine disregulation in, 236–237
Human immunodeficiency virus (HIV), 220–221
Hyper-IgE syndrome, 235–236

IgE hyperproduction, 235–244
  in AIDS, 236–237
  in atopic diseases, 241–244
  in GVHD, 238
  in Hodgkin's disease, 236–237
  in hyper-IgE syndrome, 235–236
  in parasitic infection, 240–241
  in vernal conjunctivitis, 238–240
IgE synthesis regulation, 225–235
  mast cell cytokine release in, 235
  soluble FcεRII/CD23 antigen in,
    234–235
  T-cell/cytokine regulation in animals,
    225
  T-cell/cytokine regulation in humans,
    225–234
    cognate/noncognate interactions,
      230–234
    IL-4/IFN-γ reciprocal regulation,
      226–228
    spontaneous/T cell clone induced,
      226
    two-signal model, 228–230
Immune deficiency syndromes, 216–221
  AIDS, 220–221
  common variable
    hypogammaglobulinaemia
    (CVH), 217–220
Immunoregulation, species differences,
  7–8
Inositol phosphates
  anti-Ig in release, 45, 48
  release by IL-4, 51
Interactions, cell–cell, in B cell
  development, 101
  see also Cellular collaboration in
    antibody response
Interferon
  see also Disease, cytokines and B
    cells in
  in B cell activation, 78
  in B cell differentiation, 124, 127–129
  in B cell proliferation, 4, 5, 90–92
    early stage action, 92
    leukaemic B cells, 91
    normal B cells, 91
    in vivo effect, 92
    IL-2 synergism, 87
    and IL-4, 82–83
  and IL-4 in B cell activation, 75

  and IL-4-induced B cell
    differentiation, 124
  and Ig secretion by B cells, IL-4
    interaction, 119–120, 121, 122
  in IgE regulation, and IL-4, 226–228
  in isotype regulation, 179–181
  receptor, 23–26
  in specific antibody responses, 165–
    166
  therapeutic effects, 92
Interleukin-1
  in B cell activation, 78
  in B cell autostimulation, 200
  in B cell differentiation, 129–130, 182
    IL-6 interaction, 126
  in B cell proliferation, 94–95, 96, 97,
    182
    and IL-4, 82
  from B-CLL cells, 204
  inhibitory factors, 206
  in isotype regulation, 182–183
  in lymphopoiesis, 69, 71
  physico-chemical properties, 12–16
  receptor in B cell signalling, 56
Interleukin-2, 215
  in cAMP production, 55
  in B cell differentiation, 115, 116–
    119, 183
    IL-1 synergism, 129
    IL-5 interaction, 124
  in B cell hyperactivation in lupus,
    221–222
  in B cell proliferation, 84–88, 183
    activation requirements, inter-
      specific, 84–85
    IL-4, 83–84, 86–87
    and IL-5, 87
    interactions with other cytokines,
      86–87
    leukaemic B cells, 86
    in vivo lack of effect, 87–88
    in vivo/in vitro responses, 85–86
  effects on B cells, 115
  and IgM secretion, 163
  in isotype regulation, 183–184
  physico-chemical properties, 16–17
  receptor in B cell signalling, 54–55
  in specific antibody responses, 164–
    165
  as T cell replacing factor, 5–6

Interleukin-3
  in B cell differentiation, 130–131
  in lymphopoiesis, 66–67
  physico-chemical properties, 17–19
Interleukin-4, 215
  see also Disease, cytokines and B
    cells
  in antibody responses, 6–7, 160–163
    early acting factor, 160–161
    IgE regulation, 226–230
    IgG sub-class regulation, 8
    IL-6 interaction, 127
    isotype switching, 161
  in B cell activation, 50–54, 73–78
    as competence factor, 73–74
    IFN antagonism, 75
    with IL-5, 78–79
    in phenotypic alterations, 74–75,
      76
    signal transduction, 51–54
    species differences, 7
    synthesis, 76–78
  in B cell differentiation, 119–122
    IFN-γ inhibition, 124
    IFN interaction, 119–120, 121, 122
    IL-5 synergism, 123, 125, 127
    IL-6 interaction, 121
  in B cell proliferation, 4, 5, 79–84
    activation stimulus, 79–81
    autocrine B cell stimulatory
      factors, 81–82
    and IFN-γ , 82–83
    and IL-1, 82
    and IL-2, 83–84, 86–87
    and IL-5, 84
    leukaemic B cells, 81
  CD23 induction on B cells, 101
  in isotype regulation, 177–179, 184–
    185
  in lymphopoiesis, 68–69
  physico-chemical properties, 19–21
  signal transduction, 254–255
Interleukin-5
  in B cell activation, 78–79
  in B cell differentiation, 122–125
    IFN interaction, 124
    IL-2 interaction, 124
    IL-4 synergism, 123, 125, 127
  in B cell hyperactivation in lupus,
    222

  in B cell proliferation, 88–90
    characterization of IL-5, 88
    for human cells, 89
    IL-2, 87
    and IL-4, 84
    and B cell subpopulations, 89–90
  in isotype regulation, 181–182
  in lymphopoiesis, 69
  physico-chemical properties, 20–21
  in specific antibody responses, 163–
    164
  species differences, 7
Interleukin-6, 215
  in antibody response, 6
  in B cell differentiation, 116, 126–
    127, 184
  in B cell proliferation, 95–96, 97
  in cardiac myxoma, 223
  in diabetes mellitus, insulin
    dependent, 224
  in EBV-transformed cell growth,
    204–205
  in HIV infection, 220–221
  identification, 116
  and IL-4 induction of IgE, 162
  and Ig secretion, IL-4 interaction,
    121
  in isotype regulation, 184–185
  multiple myeloma cell production,
    205
  physico-chemical properties, 21–22
  in rheumatoid arthritis, 223
  in specific antibody responses, 166
Interleukin-7
  in lymphopoiesis, 67–68
  physico-chemical properties, 23
Interleukin-8, 99
Isotype regulation, 173–174, 176–193
  germline transcripts in, and
    cytokines, 186
  IFN-γ in, 179–181, 187
  IL-1 in, 182–183
  IL-2 in, 183–184
  IL-4 in, 177–179, 184–185, 187
  IL-5 in, 181–182
  IL-6 in, 184–185
  mechanisms, 186–188
  T helper cells in, 173
    subsets, 176
  TGF β in, 185–186

Isotype switching, IL-4 in, 161
  mechanism, 162–163

Leishmaniasis
  resistance, 134
  susceptibility, and lymphokines
    production, 176
Leucocyte function adhesion antigens
    (LFA)
  expression on B cells, IL-4 in, 75
  in T/B cell contact, 156–158
Leukaemia
  chronic lymphocytic, B cell autocrine
    growth in, 204–205
  hairy cell
    interferons for, 92
    TGF growth inhibition, 98
Leukaemic B cells, 58
  IgE secretion, corticosteroids in, 102
  proliferation
    IL-1 from, 204
    and IL-2, 86
    and IL-4, 81
    IFNs and, 91
    TGF β growth inhibition, 98
Leukotriene B4, B cell stimulation, 102
Lipopolysaccharide (LPS)
  B cell activation, 72
  IgG1 secretion, 119
  and IL-4 in B cell proliferation, 80
Low molecular weight B cell growth
    factor (LMW BCGF) in B cell
    proliferation, 92–94
  IL-2 synergism, 87
  and IL-4, 84
  receptor, 94
Lupus erythematosus, systemic, 221–
    222
Lymphomas
  Burkitt's, CD23 expression, 201
  Hodgkin's, cytokine disregulation in,
    236–237
  immunoblastic B cell, autocrine
    growth potential, 205
  non-Hodgkin's B cell
    interferons for, 92
    TGF growth inhibition, 98
Lymphopoiesis, cytokines in, 66–71
  IL-1, 69, 71

IL-3, 66–67
IL-4, 68–69
IL-5, 69
IL-7, 67–68
in vitro models, 66
TGF β, 71

Major histocompatibility complex
    (MHC)
  and B cell activation, 5, 77
  expression on B cells, IL-4 in, 74
  in T/B cell contact, 145–146, 153–156
Mast cells, cytokine release in IgE
    regulation, 235
Myeolomas, multiple
  IL-6 and, 95, 205
  interferons for, 92
Myxoma, cardiac, 223

Neoplasia, B cell, autocrine growth in,
    204–205
  see also Leukaemia; Lymphomas
Nerve growth factor (NGF), 101
  physico-chemical properties, 31–33
Non-Hodgkin's B cell
  interferons for, 92
  TGF growth inhibition, 98
Ontogeny of B cells, *see*
    Lymphopoiesis, cytokines in

Parasitic infestations, cytokine
    disregulation in, 240–241
Phorbol esters
  B cell activator, 73
  and IL-4 in B cell proliferation, 79–
    80
Phosphoinositide (PI) pathway, 40–41,
    42, 48
  G-proteins in, 41, 43
  IL-4 activation, 51, 52
  surface Ig in, 44–45
Polyclonal B cell activators (PBA), 72–
    73
Proliferation of B cells
  assays, 255–257
  complement factors in, 98–99
  feedback mechanisms, 102

Proliferation of B cells, *cont.*
 IFN in, 4, 5, 90–92
  early stage action, 92
  IL-2 synergism in, 87
  IL-4, 82–83
  leukaemic B cells, 91
  normal B cells, 91
  in vivo effect, 92
 IL-1 in, 94–95, 96, 97, 182
 IL-2 in, 84–88, 183
  activation requirements, 84–85
  interactions, 86–87
  leukaemic B cells, 86
  in vivo lack of effect, 87–88
  in vivo/in vitro responses, 85–86
 IL-4 in, 79–84
  activation stimulus, 79–81
  autocrine B cell stimulatory
   factors, 81–82
  and IFN-γ, 82–83
  and IL-1, 82
  and IL-2, 83–84
  leukaemic B cells, 81
  and other cytokines, 84
 IL-5 in, 88–90, 181
  B cell subpopulation, 89–90
  for human cells, 89
  late acting, 88–89
 IL-6 in, 95–96, 96, 97
 LMW BCGF, 84, 92–94
 TGF β in, 97–98
 TNFs in, 96, 97
 in vivo, 102–103
Protein kinase C (PKC)
 activation, 45
  and EBV activation of B cells, 197
  by IL-1, 56
 B cell activator agonists, 73
 translocation, 155
Proto-oncogene expression, 57

Receptor signalling in B cells, 40–63
 gene expression control, 56–58
 lymphokine receptors in, 49–56
  IL-1, 56
  IL-2, 54–55
  IL-4, 50–54
 second messenger systems, 40–41,
  42, 43

 G-proteins in, 41, 43
 surface Ig in, 44–49
  alternative pathways, 46–47
  biochemical signalling, 44–47
  Fc receptors in, 47–49
  phosphoinositide pathway, 44–45
Receptors, cytokine
 epidermal growth factor, 33
 family, 20
 IFN-α and β, 26
 IFN-γ, 27–28
 IL-1, 14–16
 IL-2, 17
 IL-3, 18–19
 IL-4, 19–21
 IL-5, 20–21
 IL-6, 21–22
 IL-7, 23
 nerve growth factor, 32–33
 TGF β, 31
 TNF α and β, 27–29
Reed-Sternberg cells, EBV in, and
  Hodgkin's disease, 237
Retinoic acid, and B cell differentiation
  block, 217
Rheumatoid arthritis, 222–223
mRNA transcription, 57

Somatostatin, 101
Substance P, 101
Surface immunoglobulin (sIg)
 in B cell receptor signalling, 44–49
  alternative pathways, 46–47
  biochemical signalling, 44–47
  Fc receptors in, 47–49
  phosphoinositide pathway, 44–45
 sIgM expession, IL-4 in, 53–54, 75,
  77
Systemic lupus erythematosus (SLE),
  221–222

T cell replacing factor (TRF)
 actions on B cells, 115–116
 IL-2 as, 5–6
T helper cells
 see also Cellular collaboration in
  antibody response
 in contact-dependent antibody
  response, 159–160

in isotype regulation, 173
  and IL-1, 182
subsets, 174–176
  and isotype regulation, 176
  lymphokine patterns, 175–176
T–B cell interactions, *see* Cellular
  collaboration in antibody
  response
Thymus-dependent (TD) antigens
  binding in B cell activation, 72
  and IL-4 in B cell proliferation, 80
Thyrotropin (TSH), 99, 101
Toxocariasis, cytokine disregulation in,
  240
Transforming growth factor (TGF)
  in B cell differentiation, 131
  in B cell proliferation, 97–98
  B cell stimulation inhibition, 207
  in isotype regulation, 185–186
  in lymphopoiesis, 71

physico-chemical properties, 29–
  31
Tumour necrosis factor (TNF)
  in B cell differentiation, 130
  in B cell proliferation, 96–97
    IL-2 synergism, 87
    and IL-4, 84
  B-CLL cell response, 204–205
  in HIV infection, 220–221
  physico-chemical properties, 27–29

Vasoactive intestinal peptide, 101
Vernal conjunctivitis, cytokine
  disregulation in, 238–240
Virus infections, IFN-γ in antibody
  response, 180
  see also Epstein-Barr virus (EBV);
    Human immunodeficiency virus
    (HIV)